RETURN TO NATURE!

The True Natural Method of Healing and Living
and
The True Salvation of the Soul.

Paradise Regained

By ADOLF JUST.

THE CARE OF THE BODY—WATER, HUMAN CURATIVE POWER, LIGHT, AIR, EARTH, FOOD, FRUIT CULTURE.

AUTHORIZED TRANSLATION
FROM THE FOURTH ENLARGED GERMAN EDITION
BY BENEDICT LUST, NATUROPATH.
EDITOR OF "THE NATUROPATH AND HERALD OF HEALTH," DIRECTOR
AND PROPRIETOR OF THE AMERICAN JUNGBORN,
BELLEVUE, BUTLER, N. J.

VOLUME I.

PUBLISHED BY
THE TRANSLATOR, B. LUST, 124 EAST 59TH STREET,
NEW YORK, U. S. A.

COPYRIGHTED 1903
BY
BENEDICT LUST, NEW YORK,
AND
REGISTERED AT STATIONERS' HALL,
LONDON, ENGLAND.

ALL RIGHTS RESERVED.

NEW YORK
THE VOLUNTEER PRESS
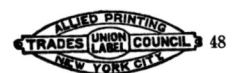
38 COOPER SQUARE

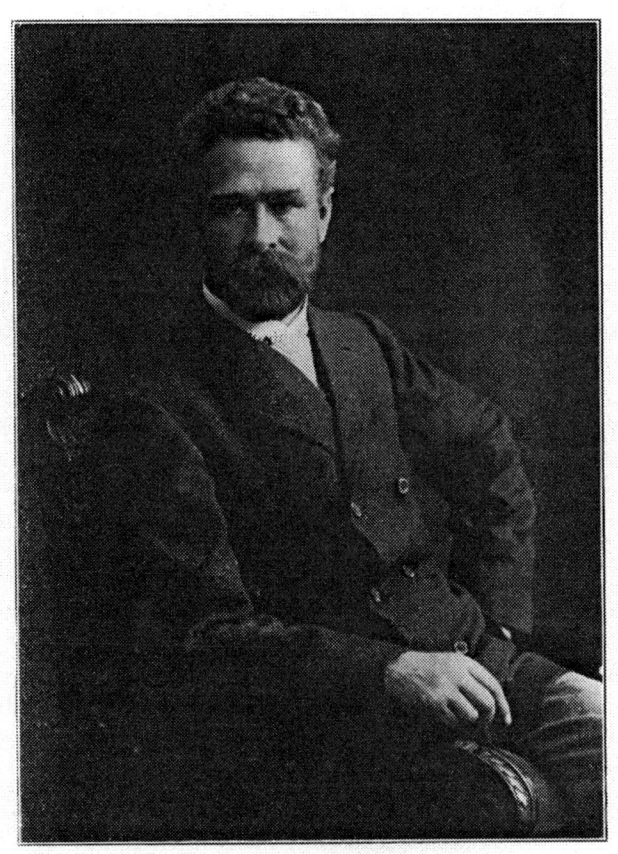

"Return to Nature!"—Adolf Just.

DEDICATION.

IN translating the present work I had in mind that large number of the English speaking people of the world who are to-day suffering under the lash of medical superstition, quackery and charlatanism; men and women and children who for want of proper education and understanding are groping about in darkness, and are constantly being imposed upon by human vipers who live and thrive upon the suffering and ignorance of their less fortunate fellowmen. *"Return to Nature"* was written by a man humanely inclined, and with a heart for the lowly as well as for all men who work towards the betterment of Humanity. May this volume be the means of spreading and propagating, health, peace and happiness, hope, faith and enlightenment in the thousand homes. It was in this spirit I undertook its translation and with this wish I respectfully dedicate it to the English-speaking people of America, and throughout the world.

THE TRANSLATOR..

Naturopathic Sanitarium "Jungborn."

BENEDICT LUST, Director & Proprietor

POST OFFICE: **BUTLER, N. J.**   RAILROAD STATION: **BUTLER, N. J.**

Teleg. Address:
LUST,
BUTLER, N. J.

Tel. Connection

For country messengers an additional fee of 25 cents is to be prepaid at the Telegraph Office.

Butler is a station on the New York, Susquehanna and Western Railroad.

THE JUNGBORN was founded in 1896.

AMERICAN
Mother Institute
OF THE NEW AND TRUE
Nature Cure.

AN IDEAL PLACE

Near Echo, Greenwood and Pompton Lakes, in the most beautiful parts of the Ramapo Mountains, the Highlands of New Jersey.

Greater and Quicker Successes

Than by any of the preceding Nature Cure Methods.

NEW PICTURESQUE PARKS, SPLENDID SPRINGS, GRAND CASCADES.

Large Reconstructions

Property more than fifty acres in circumference, enlarged and improved. At the entrance of the lovely and well protected Grace Valley.

Greatly enlarged in 1898 and 1904.

Most romantically situated on the top of a hill, about 15 minutes walk from the depot, "Jungborn" comprises a large area of woodland, laid out with shady walks along two picturesque brooks of clear water, known as Grace Valley Brook, and Regeneration Brook, and with its beauty-spots in the shape of quiet nooks, sheltered from the sun, its numerous springs along the hillside, its grand view into the Ramapo Mountains, is an ideal resort for lovers of nature.

TRANSLATOR'S PREFACE TO THE ENGLISH EDITION.

MOTTO: *Nature ever shows the true and perfect way,*
Therefore learn betimes ne'er from her paths to stray.

The Simpler Life is the demand of the hour. The confusions of a complex civilization, the disintegration of the old-fashioned home, the distractions of international discord, the perplexity of the individual mind wavering between the evolution of Science and the revolution of Theology—all these disturbing elements have settled moodily into a sense of universal unrest, that pervades the mingled atmosphere of nations.

Poets, preachers, philosophers, even diplomatists and politicians have propounded causes and proposed cures innumerable. But the dream of Individual Peace and Universal Harmony is as yet but a beautiful vision of prophetic revelation. And realization seems too remote to reckon with.

Simply because we humans have persistently sought *Peace from external conditions.*

One single attainment would bring the concept from the clouds into the concrete—*Be at peace with yourself.*

This is not moralizing.

Nor philosophizing.

Nor rhapsodizing.

It is the energizing impulse that constrained Adolph Just to renounce the grimy smoke, mental fog and moral miasma of artificial civilization and seek from the clear pure horizon-vantage of Nature the secret of Health, Happiness and Universal Oneness.

This book reveals the secret.

It is so simple, easy and unpretentious that the world's greatest scientists, doctors and savants have quite overlooked it.

Would you be whole, in body, mind and spirit? Would you live to be twice threescore-and-ten, each year growing younger, happier, better?

Would you feel consciously superior to cooks, doctors, druggists and undertakers, and everlastingly immune to all forms of

Dis-ease? Would you, incidentally, halve the cost of living, and lift housewifery from the drudging routine of three-meals-a-day-and-a-lunch to the imperial freedom of meal-time abolished?

Would you evolve from a wretched, dyspeptic, fearful pessimist into a cheery, strong, courageous optimist?

Would you thrill in tune with every bird and flower and rill in "God's great out-of-doors," finding your own divinity reflected in every living thing?

Would you become the supreme embodiment of Health, Beauty, Grace, Power, Truth, Wisdom, Love?

Then return to Nature—that's all. For Nature is the true interpreter of the Infinite: no other voice whispers truths so potent to awaken, arouse and inspire Humanity.

But one word more as regards my functions as Editor of the English Edition. Animated by a deep spirit of veneration and respect for the humanitarian author, Adolf Just, I have made but very few alterations and corrections. I have ventured to amend the translation in so far only as it appeared to me to be indispensable for the better understanding of the English and American public.

In conclusion I give expression to the sincere wish that every reader of this book may be as much benefited by "Returning to Nature" as I have been.

BENEDICT LUST,
Naturopathic Physician,

American "Jungborn," Butler, N. J., U. S. A.,
July 4th, 1903.

PREFACE TO THE FIRST EDITION.

I publish my book in celebration of the opening of the Jungborn.

The vernal sun is again shining in the sky, the gloomy Winter is gone. Snow and ice have yielded to the warm, bright sun, new life is sprouting in field and meadow, in wood and glen, the Easter bells are tolling, the festival of the resurrection has come.

I wish at the same time to add a friendly Easter greeting to all those who have already emerged from darkness to light, to all those whom my book may happily lead out of gloomy, dark, desolate, frosty paths into bright, sunny cheerfulness, to all my friends far and near.

AD. JUST.

Jungborn, Stapelburg in the Harz,
    Easter, 1896.

PREFACE TO THE FOURTH EDITION.

When I had finished the first edition of this book, and sent it as a message of glad tidings into a world full of disease and suffering, full of worry and restlessness, full of misery and unhappiness, the earth was putting forth its first green, and resurrection songs filled the air.

Three years have passed since then, men have not despised the glad tidings, but received them with joy and enthusiasm. The Jungborn, which is the heart and main artery of the enterprise, already blooms and prospers.

But in the meantime it has become necessary to expand and perfect my book in important respects.

While I am engaged on this fourth and enlarged edition, nature appears in her brightest colors. Solemnly and joyously the bells are announcing the festival of Pentecost. The spirit of Pentecost is about to descend.

During the past three years my cause has become widely known all over the world. But the cause is nothing without the spirit. In many places the true spirit is still wanting; sometimes, indeed, even an unclean spirit threatens to beset the cause.

May this new edition, with its many improvements, foster and spread the true spirit!

Filled by this sincere wish I send these old and many new teachings once more into the world, to all men and women who are seeking and longing, who are weeping and lamenting, who are groaning and sighing.

ADOLF JUST.

Jungborn, Stapelburg in the Harz,
  Pentecost, 1899.

TABLE OF CONTENTS.

Dedication	v
Translator's Preface to English Edition	ix
Preface to the First Edition	xi
Preface to the Fourth Edition	xi
The Voices of Nature	1
The Primitive and the Present Condition of Mankind	2
How I was led to a true Natural Method of Healing	3
Reason and Science, and the Voices of Nature	6
The Jungborn, its Purposes	8
The Natural Bath	10
The old Natural Method of Healing and the true Natural Method of Healing	11
Vincent Priessnitz	14
Mistakes of past Water Applications and the incorrectness of Full-Baths	14
The Bath of the Animals in the natural state	16
The Natural Bath of Man, its Description	18
Details of the Natural Bath	20
The Origin of Acute and Chronic Diseases	24
The Effect of the Natural Bath	23
Goethe's "Faust"	26
The Application of the Natural Bath and its Significance	23
Wounds	46
Operations	46
Rubbing and Stroking of the Body	48
Cures by Stroking of women and men (shepherds, etc.) in the country	49
Masseurs and Masseuses	50
The Application of Human Healing Power after the Natural Bath	51
The Explanation of the Curative Effects of Rubbing and Stroking	52
Who is gifted with Human Healing Power?	53
What more is to be considered in the application of human Healing Power	53
Light and Air	54
Light and Air, the true vitalizing Agents	55
The great mistakes and omissions of the past, with regard to Light and Air, and their Consequences	58
The true and perfect application of Light and Air (the Light-and-Air Bath)	60
Light-and-Air bathing Details	61
The Sunbath	65
Light-and-Air Huts and Cottages	66
Injurious Gaslight	67
Our Clothing	71
The way clothes should be made	71

Health Shirts, Shoes, Sandals, Stockings, Gloves, Suspenders	72
Trousers for Men and Women	74
The Corset	75
Swathing clothes for Children	76
Going Bareheaded	77
The Purpose of Clothes	79
Jesus and Clothes	80
Furniture	82
Curtains	83
Beds	84
Earth Power	85
Man and his relation to the Earth	85
The Myth of Antaeus	86
The significance of Ancient Myths	86
The Bible	86
Sleeping on the Ground	88
False use of Reason, Science	89
The great significance of Going Barefooted	93
Additional directions for Sleeping on the Bare Ground	98
The present need of sleep, a consequence of unnatural living	96
Details with regard to Sleeping on the Bare Ground	102
How can one daily exploit the Earth-power?	102
The Fear of Catching Cold	103
Further Remarks on the Origin of Acute and Chronic Diseases, and the significance of Air with regard to them	106
The injuriousness and danger of the Fear of Catching Cold	110
Earth Bandages and Earth Compresses	119
The Rationale of Earth Bandages and Earth Compresses	119
The great significance of Earth Bandages	119
Directions for Earth Bandages	121
No Blood Poisoning through Earth Bandages	121
Earth Compresses	122
Significance and Application of Earth Compresses	123
Directions for Earth Compresses	124
Earth and Sand Baths	126
Earth and Clay as Skin Purifiers	127
How Shall we Bury Our Dead?	129
Nutrition According to Nature	132
Science and the Question of Nutrition	132
Fruits, Man's Natural Food	134
The greater and lesser Disadvantages of the Foods hitherto used	136
Fruit Diet	137
Fruits alone contain healing juices	139
The Nut our Chief Food	139
Milk, Bread, Vegetables, and other transitional Foods	140
The great mistakes of Contemporary Vegetarians	142
Dr. Densmore and his Teachings	144
Unripe Fruits	145
Vegetables and leguminous foods	146
Tropical fruits	147
Sugar very injurious	147
Details with regard to nutrition according to Nature	148
Ought man to Drink?	149

What ought we to Drink?.	150
Effect of a Natural Diet upon the Soul.	154
The myth of the Danaids and the Hydra.	155
Sexual sensuality, Modesty, Prudery, and True Morality.	156
Jesus and Nutrition According to Nature.	156
Natural Mode of Life the foundation of the Scheme of Jesus	157
John the Baptist and his Food.	159
The Bible and the Natural Food.	161
Meat and Alcohol.	163
Man is not a Beast of Prey.	163
Climate	165
The use of Alcohol occasioned by the use of Meat.	166
The danger of Alcohol.	167
The Bible, Jesus, and the Meat Diet.	167
The Tree of the "Knowledge of Good and Evil".	168
Did Jesus partake of the Easter Lamb?.	171
What is the Serpent in Paradise?.	173
Jesus and Alcohol.	174
Fire	174
Fire the origin of Civilization and Anti-naturalism.	174
The myth of Prometheus.	175
Cooked Food, Warm Baths, etc.	176
The significance of Living on Raw Fruit.	177
Cinderella	178
When Ought we to Eat?.	180
The directions of Nature with regard to the Time of Eating	180
The significance of the Holy Communion.	181
The Natural Food, Care, and Education of Children.	182
The Duties of a pregnant Woman.	183
Immorality within Marriage.	184
The care of new-born Children.	184
Milk as food for Children.	186
The fear of Bacilli.	186
Fruit as food for Children.	187
Jesus and the Children.	189
Vaccination	190
Prevention of the great Dangers of Vaccination.	191
Serum and Diphtheria.	191
Children's Diseases.	192
Specific present-day Dangers and Sufferings of Children.	192
The Dress of Children.	193
The only true Education of Children.	195
School Education.	195
The Calling which Children are to Choose.	196
Cases and Cures.	197
What value attaches in general to testimonials of Cures?.	197
Inflammatory Rheumatism.	198
Serious Nervous Diseases.	198
Serious Trouble in the Head and Deafness.	199
Serious Stomach Trouble and Tuberculosis of the Spinal Cord	201
Retention of the Urine, incipient Dropsy.	201
A high degree of Nervousness.	203
Pneumonia	203
Disturbance of the Digestive Function.	203
Dropsy	204

Throat Trouble	204
Scab on the Head	204
Tuberculosis of the Spinal Cord	205
Toothache	205
Tuberculosis of the Bones	206
Typhoid Fever	206
General Debility	207
Convulsions	207
Fistula of the Rectum	208
Blindness	208
Cholera Nostras, or Diarrhoea	209
Sexual Disease	210
The Dangers of Sexual Aberrations and the present false treatment of Sexual Diseases	211
Diabetes	212
Boils	213
Chronic Headache	215
Tetter	215
Snake-bite Poisoning	215
Disease of the Spinal Cord and Obesity	216
Chronic Inflammatory Rheumatism	217
Miscellaneous; rejuvenation, intellectual vigor the result of true Natural Healing	218
Large wound from the Bite of a dog	218
War, a Curse to Mankind	219
The significance of Earth Bandages in War	220
Influenza	221
General Remarks on Cases and Reports of Cures	222
General Directions with regard to the application of the Natural Method of Healing in every case of Sickness	223
The Fear of Infectious Diseases	227
The Freedom of Man	228
Sea and Mineral Baths, High Altitude Sanitaria	228
When Ought we to Submit to a Natural Cure?	229
The ancient Germans, once the strongest Men in the World	231
My Relation to the Old Method of Natural Healing	231
All innovation and progress in the Natural Method of Healing are in the beginning always opposed by the adherents of Natural Healing	232
The Mistakes of the prevailing Natural Methods of Healing	233
Everyone his own Doctor	237
The Errors and Dangers of all Medical Examinations	238
The great Importance of Everybody being his own Doctor and enjoying perfect Liberty	240
Truth and Honesty in the Natural Method of Healing	241
Trust in God and Charity	243
Agriculture, Fruit Culture, Veterinary Science and Vivisection	246
Agriculture and its latest Mistakes	247
The Poverty of Agriculture	248
Fruit Culture instead of Agriculture	250
The Cultivation of Nuts	251
The original Food of the ancient Germans	252
True Natural Veterinary Science	253
Mistakes and Crimes in the Breeding of Animals	254
The terrible Cruelties and Horrors of Vivisection	256

Mental and Physical Work, Fruit Culture, and Sport............	257
Rest and Work..	257
Mental work detrimental.................................	258
Sport (gymnastics, bicycling, etc.) contrary to Nature......	261
Physical Work..	262
The Great Significance of Fruit Culture...................	263
Happy Homes...	263
Goethe's Mistake (in "Faust") with regard to a Natural Life	265
Civilization, Science, Art, and true human Happiness........	268
The Family, the Home, and the Country.......................	269
The Family and Marriage of Civilized Man.................	270
Love and conjugal happiness in a true Natural Life.........	271
At Home and Abroad......................................	272
The Love of one's Country................................	272
The Emperor...	273
Ideals and Poetry...	274
Contemporary mankind without Ideals.....................	274
Science and Poetry.......................................	274
The Poetry of the Bible...................................	275
Conclusion	277
The Soul's Life...	277
Supplement	281
The Arrangements, Aims and Purposes of the Jungborn. The Contents and the Significance of the following volumes (Vols. I and II) of my Work.........................	283

THE VOICES OF NATURE

In communicating my ideas concerning health, the cure of disease, and human happiness I am merely obeying a serious, powerful, inner command.

Man originally came from the hand of the Creator absolutely healthy and good, without any blemish in body and soul. The handiwork of the almighty, all-good, and all-wise Creator could not indeed have been from the start an imperfect and defective, a diseased and sinful, a miserable and unhappy being.

In paradise man lived originally free from sin and disease, in perpetual joy and unclouded happiness. But man lost paradise—was driven from it. The ancient myths, especially the myths concerning paradise, which we find among all civilized peoples, embody the profoundest truths regarding the original state of man and the primitive history of mankind.

True health is no longer met with among mankind. Everywhere on earth disease and decadence stare at us in infinite variety. From the cradle to the grave men are beset by pain and suffering in all their forms. Not nobility of soul and brotherly love, but hate, envy, jealousy, brutality, vice, and crime rule in the world. It may truly be said that we behold contemporary man only in care and sorrow, in misery and suffering, in unhappiness and despair.

I, too, have had to drain the cup of suffering to the dregs. A serious nervous trouble, the disease of the century, and which was caused chiefly through inheritance, began early to undermine my health.

During this period I passed through all the phases of misery and unhappiness, and, as already remarked, was obliged to drain the cup of suffering to the dregs.

My ailment was a very serious one, all remedies, including

those of the nature cure, proved unavailing, or at best gave only slight relief.

The greatest distress compelled me to pursue my studies farther and farther, in search of truth and help, and in this way I discovered the only sure path to health and happiness, and the only effective remedies. By passing through this severe school of suffering I am perhaps the better fitted to preach the truth to my fellowmen and to point out to them the *true cure* and help. Since I, too, have passed through all the mistaken paths along which mankind is journeying to-day, I am perhaps the better fitted to raise a cry of warning and lead my fellowmen away from them.

I intend to show in the following pages in what way alone we may escape all illness and suffering, and thoroughly cure all pain and disease. But we shall then see that in this way we can also free ourselves of all sinful impulses, of vice and despair, find rest and peace of mind, and return to true religion and to God.

I do not intend to write a book of precepts on health and happiness according to some artistically conceived plan, but I shall communicate my views simply and precisely in the same order in which, after much wandering, I came upon the path that led me to nature, and consequently to health.

In my sufferings I naturally consulted, first, the old-school physicians. I called on celebrated doctors and university professors, but they could not help me.

In the direst distress and despair I finally lost the high opinion of science which I had acquired through education and schooling. What did I care for science; in my despair I wanted help and nothing but help.

I now heard of the good results of the nature cure method, and turned to it. I began to go barefoot, to apply Kneipp douches, Kuhne baths, packs, steam baths, massage, vegetarian diet, etc. This for the first time gave me real relief and improved my condition. But I wished to go still further along this line, to achieve still greater success, to reach indeed the highest aim.

I placed my greatest hope in the nature cure method. By following it with the greatest perseverance I wished to regain my health, the highest happiness.

But finally my confidence was undermined and shaken. The realization of my high hopes, my complete recovery, was still delayed. Besides, I saw so much quarreling and controversy among the individual champions of the nature cure method. One or another process was represented as false, or even injurious.

Were the opponents right or wrong? Could it be that the nature cure method was even harming me? Or were all my sacrifices again in vain? If I got no help from the nature cure, where then was I to place my faith? Was I simply to resign myself to my fate? The dissensions among the nature cure people were at least suspicious.

These trying doubts cost me much distress, and I know that many patients have suffered greatly from similar depressing and tormenting doubts.

At that time, in my wandering and despair, there suddenly appeared a bright star which I have steadily followed ever since, and which has brought the greatest and most significant change into my life. I greatly desire that before long it may become the guiding star also of all mankind, who would then no longer languish under the heavy burden of disease and invalidism.

Who tells the children of nature in distant countries, the animals of the woods how they are to bathe, what they are to eat, and how to avoid danger? The voices of nature alone: *instinct and the organs of sense (the sense of hearing, smelling, tasting, etc.)* are their guides.

> "Man while he striveth is prone to err.
> —Goethe, "Faust."

We can therefore never expect to get any correct information from the men of to-day (not even from their writings) concerning our welfare and happiness.

Neither can we allow men to teach us the care of our health and the curing of our diseases.

But nature does not err; she is still the only one to teach us what is right.

Men who no longer listen to the voice of nature become the victims of a thousand different diseases and miseries. But the creatures of pure nature, on the other hand, the animals of our forests, are free from sickness and from everything else as well that corresponds to the sins and vices of mankind.

> ". . . Every prospect pleases,
> And only man is vile."
>
> —Heber.

To-day, indeed, there is not a spot left where man has not interfered with nature* for the worse. Therefore we may find even in free nature, in the forest among plants and animals, single instances of taint and disease, but these are still so rare, compared with the infinite sufferings and the great misery of mankind that the words of the poet quoted above still hold good.

The creatures of nature are, indeed, free from disease. But they also fall easy victims to it as soon as they are withdrawn from unmolested nature, and no longer stand in the relation to light

---

*Man in his misguidance has powerfully interfered with nature. He has devastated the forests, and thereby even changed the atmospheric conditions and the climate. Some species of plants and animals have become entirely extinct through man, although they were essential in the economy of nature. Everywhere the purity of the air is affected by smoke and the like, and the rivers are defiled. These and other things are serious encroachments upon nature, which men nowadays entirely overlook, but which are of the greatest importance, and at once show their evil effect not only upon plants but upon animals as well, the latter not having the endurance and power of resistance of man.

To him who cannot see the defects caused by man himself, and who doubts the absolute perfection of nature, one is tempted to say:

> "Thy sense is shut, thy heart is dead:
> Disciple, up! untiring, hasten
> To bathe thy breast in morning-red!"
>
> **—Goethe, "Faust."**

and air, earth and water, and no longer receive the nourishment appointed for them by nature. Therefore our domestic animals are much more subject to sickness than the animals of the forest.

When we look at nature with an open, unprejudiced mind, and are not blinded by the teachings of science, we must arrive at the clear conclusion that man has become sick and miserable only because he no longer heeds the VOICES OF NATURE, and has thus everywhere transgressed the laws of nature, and lost his way.

Nature is forever unassailable in her justice; she punishes every transgression of her laws, but likewise rewards every return to obedience.

In all cases, and in all diseases, therefore, man can recover and again become happy only by a *true return to nature*: man must to-day strenuously endeavor, in his mode of living, to heed again the voice of nature, and thus choose the food that nature has laid before him from the beginning, and to bring himself again into the relation with water, light and air, earth, etc., that nature originally designed for him.

Nature speaks intelligibly and gives her precepts plainly to all creatures; to the animals as well as to man.

Nature does not intend man to remain in such great ignorance and confusion concerning the true course of life and the true methods of cure that he will fall out with his fellowmen in discussing these subjects and become a victim of tormenting care and doubt. We must only no longer listen to men, but go for information to nature.

But nature speaks in a different manner than man. She offers her lessons not in books, not in dusty tomes; she expresses her will to her creatures plainly and clearly through *instinct, the organs of sense,* etc.

In addition to these, rational man is also gifted with *conscience*.

Primitive peoples in distant parts of the earth still preserve these only safe and sure guides on the road of life. It is well known that these children of nature are gifted with such keen organs of sense (seeing, tasting, hearing, etc.) and such sure instinct as to readily recognize all danger and all things harmful to them.

These primitive people recognize, for instance, quite plainly every poisonous plant without ever having studied botany or indeed anything else.

Civilized mankind, consisting of the more highly developed human race, originally also followed the only safe guiding stars on the sea of life, and escaped all suffering and disease as long as they persisted in this course. But there lurked a danger for them in their higher *intelligence.*

Man is gifted with intelligence that he may recognize, in contradistinction to the animals, his connection with God, God's goodness and love, and enter into filial relation with God and lead a higher life. His intelligence constitutes his highest excellence.

But man used his intelligence for the purpose of separating himself from nature; he early refused to listen to the voices of nature, and followed the inspirations of his reason. He wished to be teacher and law-giver on his own part, and made of himself "the little God of the earth." With the aid of his reason, his intellectual "faculties," he engaged in special, arduous studies and researches, on which he reared a system of laws according to which he arranged his life, his food, his clothing, his labor, education, etc. *Civilization* began.

Out of this false use of his reason grew *science.* In this way science rests on error and is followed by disaster.

We shall here especially consider the *science of medicine,* with its teachings and demonstrations in chemistry, anatomy, physiology, etc.

The voices of nature have always been true to man, but science is the cunning serpent in paradise which deceived man from the start, led him astray, and gave him false instruction.

The more man listened to the teachings of science, especially of medicine, the more he became a victim of disease and misfortune, although science was extolled from the beginning as the dispenser of happiness and blessings.*

The only way, therefore, how man can be cured of his diseases with certainty and can again secure entire happiness is to abjure science and all things scientific.

It is very difficult, to be sure, to protect one's self altogether from this cunning serpent at present; for men have been obliged to listen to science from early childhood, and have imbibed its poison from innumerable books; many have sacrificed their entire fortune and their health to science,—in short, men everywhere have worshipped at the feet of this celebrated goddess.

When man is just beginning to allow himself to be guided once more by nature, in a simple manner, without any doubts and subtleties, the cries and exclamations of science are heard to interfere from all sides. In hygiene and pathology then the talk is of bacilli, albuminous matter, nutritive salts, colds, etc., etc. Man is then easily led astray again.

Let man therefore be guided solely by the voices of nature (instinct, conscience, organs of sense, etc.).

It may be objected that it is easy to see how the animals are safely guided by their instinct, but it is hard to understand how for the present man can be led by nature in the same manner.

To be sure, man has not listened to the voices of nature for a long time. Instinct and conscience have consequently grown silent, and the organs of sense have become weakened. But nevertheless we can still be led by them easily and safely. Well does the great Goethe say:

> "Quite softly speaks a God in our breast,
> Quite softly yet perceptibly He shows us
> Which we must seize, and which to flee."

---

*It is still a risky thing to attack science, notwithstanding the fact that precisely her most faithful and honest devotees are the most afflicted with disease and suffering. I need refer only to the many nervous and broken-down savants. Our opponents here remind us of the great and beneficent researches, discoveries, inventions, etc. But I trust that those who read my book will no longer be dazzled by the great "achievements" of science or the great blessings of civilization, that are said to have grown out of it for man.

When I began to heed the voices of nature once more, everything was soon clear to me. On the important points I soon knew everything that was necessary for me to know, and which I have recorded here in my book. There was no need of a long period of laborious research and investigation.

Everything that I have written in the following pages I learned from nature alone; her voices alone have guided me.

Let the reader judge for himself whether these teachings of pure and simple nature appear to him plausible and true. At all events I know that they have so far met with the most enthusiastic approval and acceptance on all sides, and that the good they have already done is greater by far than is generally believed. I have often had the opportunity to convince myself how much lost happiness my book has again restored, how many a blessing it has wrought.

The more man sets his face again toward nature, the more his conscience and instinct will reawaken within him, and the more acute will his organs of sense become. He is still surrounded by many happy creatures, children and especially animals, who have preserved these higher guides of life, and from whom he can learn the true course in all emergencies.

If man, therefore, has gained sufficient power of resistance to the seductions of science, he may still easily be led by the hand of nature, and will then surely soon recover health and true happiness. He will no longer be tossed about upon the ocean of life, like a ship without a rudder, destined to be dashed to pieces against rocks and reefs.

THE JUNGBORN.

When after a long, long search I came from error to truth, from night to light, from disease to health, I was seized by a great desire to impart my experiences to my fellowmen and to let them profit by them.

I determined to place the strength and vigor which I had but just regained, entirely at the disposal of the great cause. I resolved to become the champion of nature, to work for her, and to point out the right way which will lead men from dreaded night to joyous light, to true health and complete happiness,— those purblind and deluded men who no longer understand nature and who abuse her marvelous goodness to their own destruction. The mere thought of devoting my life entirely to nature and her great truths was indeed blessedness.

I soon began to write this book.

But I also founded "Jungborn," in the Hartz, between Isenburg and Hartzburg. This is, first of all a model institution for the true natural life, where those who wish to make arrangements for such a life at home in their own gardens can find the pattern. It was also meant to show, from the start, how the most intimate communion with nature can be re-established, and at the same time to demonstrate in practice how easy and what a blessing such communion is.

In the meantime the Jungborn has fulfilled its purpose completely. After its pattern many have already made the requisite arrangements in their own homes or gardens.

Other similar institutions are coming into life.

The Jungborn has now also practically demonstrated the correctness of the return to nature methods and its significance for the welfare and salvation of man.

For the rest it has always been my aim to show how we can lead a natural life at home, under ordinary circumstances, and establish a relationship with nature, for in this way alone can my book be of service to the masses.

It was necessary to mention the Jungborn here, as I shall have occasion to refer to it.

A detailed description of the Jungborn and its arrangements will be found at the end of this volume.

THE NATURAL BATH.

Within the last century great and gifted men have taken up the nature-cure method. Their genius led them to the ways of nature. Priessnitz, Schroth, Graham, Rausse, Rikli, Kneipp,

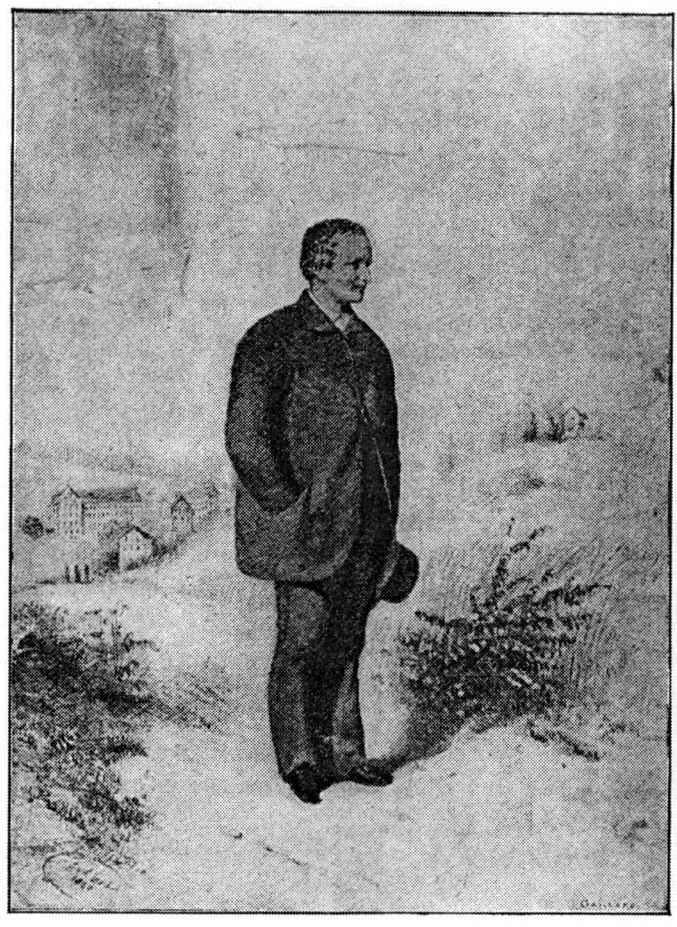

VINCENTZ PRIESSNITZ,
Father of the Natural Healing Method.

Kuhne, Densmore, Trall and others have already achieved great things, and have won for themselves immortal honor, for from darkness they penetrated into light.

But these men have by no means been fully and clearly conscious that they must allow instinct alone to lead them, and they have not strictly and carefully followed the other voices of nature, which I have often mentioned. They have not sufficiently studied the ways of children and animals, those beings who still possess the true guides of life in a higher degree than the adults of modern civilization. They have not considered with sufficient care many of the contrivances and intentions of nature. Therefore their systems and teachings have not been perfect; they have contained mistakes and errors. These systems have now partly been forgotten, and in the course of time will be entirely swallowed up in the sea of oblivion.

After mankind has deviated from nature for thousands and thousands of years, it is very evident that they can only gradually regain a true insight as to which are their duties toward nature and her laws.

All the men who have hitherto built up the nature cure methods are deserving of our highest praise. We must by no means heap reproaches upon them and accuse them, because their systems are faulty and because they did not yet reach a complete natural method.

The nature cure method has evidently inspired the most serious and largest movement that civilized mankind has yet seen. It concerns itself with the health of the individual, that greatest of worldly possessions upon which such an infinite amount of well-being and happiness depends, and which is the only possible safety and redemption from all misery and evils—from final ruin. Therefore we may not remain silent or conceal anything concerning any person, but must above all things always keep our eye upon the great cause, and subjugate everything—every other interest and even every person—to this cause.

From this point of view I shall not hesitate to uncover the

mistakes of former nature cure methods, of the old vegetarianism, etc. But in doing so I do not wish to hurt any one.

I shall now advance a mode of life and a curative system which has nothing whatever to do with science, and in which we allow ourselves to be guided, as I have frequently stated before, by the great teacher, "Nature," alone. Thus at last a beautiful, bright morning sun will rise from dark chaos, which mankind shall greet with joy.

We now have a *simple* nature-cure system; as simple as the great teacher, nature, herself. This nature-cure system is the same for *all* diseases and *all* cases, even as the origin of all diseases has but *one* cause, an unnatural mode of life; and there exists a *unity* in all the laws of nature and in all her manifestations. All the former nature-cure methods will gradually dissolve in this one true nature system.

In this method there is nothing to be learned in the usual sense of the word; every one who has but freed himself from the spell of modern wisdom and science can apply it. Through it men become free from all dependency on and slavery to the entire fraternity of physicians, doctors of medicine as well as nature doctors.

Nature does not err, therefore in her the errors and contradictions which are now keeping so many away from the nature-cure method, do not exist.

The invalid who allows himself to be guided entirely by the hand of nature is led gently, without severity and distressing deprivations, much more gently, and more pleasantly, quickly, and more surely than by the former nature-cure methods, back to health, strength, and vital energy unto a fresh, green meadow full of flowers and sunshine. And above all, the severest and most desperate diseases, in the presence of which the ordinary nature doctor is helpless, loosen their grip and drop off before Nature.

The true nature-cure system penetrates with its healing power into the innermost recesses of the mind and soul. Dark veils are lifted from the mind; even the soul participates in the

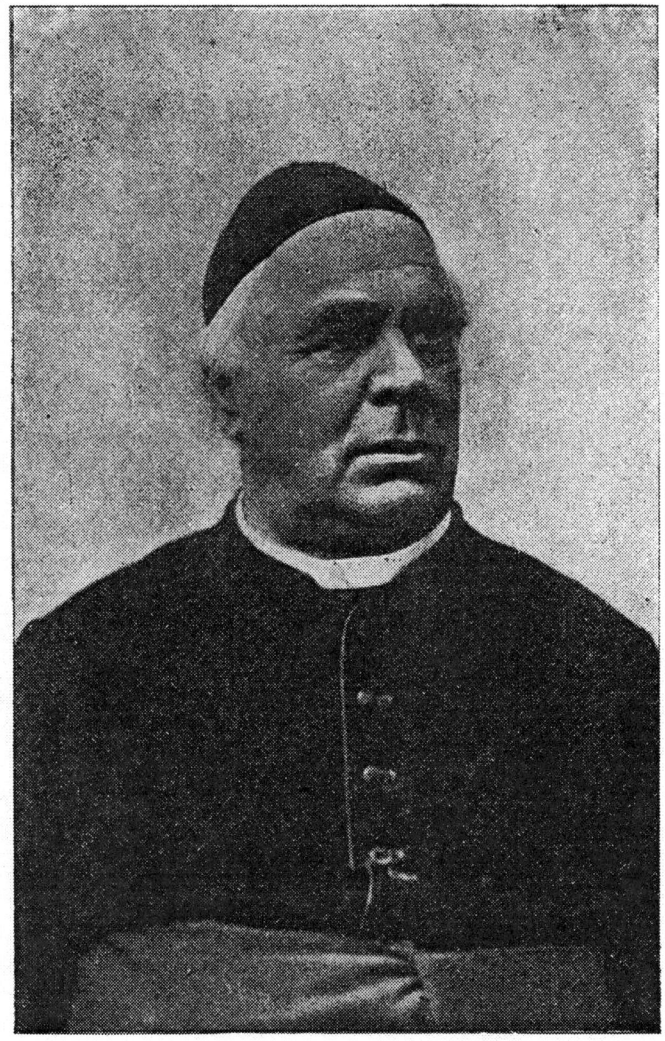

VERY REV. MGR. SEB. KNEIPP,
Founder of the Kneipp Water and Herb Cure in Woerishofen, Bavaria.

healing balm. Man is released from vice and crime, hatred, envy, and malevolence. Peace, joy, brotherly love, happiness once more take up their abode in the breasts of the unhappy human beings of to-day.

Now at last the morning of a new Spring dawns for humanity; paradise is regained.

As I have said before, I once fled from the error and confusion, the strife and dissensions of men to nature. Here alone I found rest, peace and truth.

When in the present century mankind instinctively turned their faces once more toward nature, it became evident to them that all diseases had their origin in impure matter in the blood, in the body—in disease germs or foreign matter. On the basis of this correct discernment people, in treating the sick, soon refrained from exorcising the devil with Beelzebub by introducing more foreign matter and poison into the body, as medical science does by drugs, medicines, etc. They sought rather to cleanse the sick body of its foreign matter, and that, indeed, with but one natural remedy—with *water*.

In this respect the peasant Vincentz Priessnitz was the pioneer. He is therefore to be considered as the real founder of the present nature-cure method.

The nature-cure method was in the beginning only a *water-cure method,* and only *water-cure* institutions were at first established.

Therefore it was my first endeavor to obtain from nature herself directions for the right use of water applications.

In my endeavors I did not observe that an inner voice directed me to a special use of water,—namely, the instinct.

But I learned from foresters that the animals of free nature which follow only their instinct, take a bath according to definite rules.

I began to observe them, and reached the following conclusions:

The natural bath does not consist in jumping into the river and taking a full bath. *The full bath taken in the river or in the bath-tub is contrary to nature.*

Land animals not only take no full baths, they are actually afraid of them. One need only to throw an animal (especially a monkey) into the water and see how eagerly it makes for the

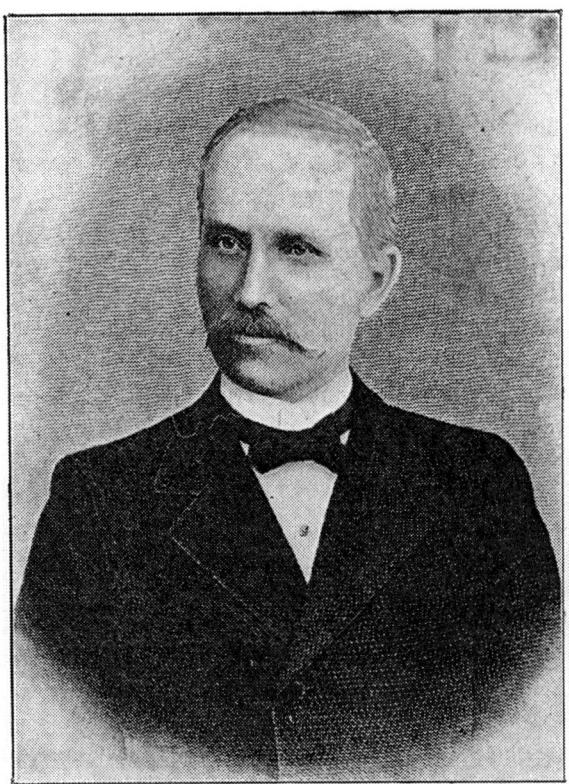

LOUIS KUHNE, OF LEIPZIC,
Founder of the Kuhne System of Natural Healing, Exemplifying the Oneness of All Disease.

shore. To other water applications also animals submit only under compulsion and most unwillingly.

Individual exceptions which occur among domestic animals that already lead unnatural lives prove nothing to the contrary.

On the other hand the higher land animals (mammalia), especially wild boars and deer, *in free nature* (in the forest) are in the habit of lying down in small muddy swamps or pools, at first only with the *abdomen,* and *rubbing* it to and fro in the mud.

Hereupon the animals rise and generally sit for awhile with their posterior, their anus, in the mud. After awhile they roll in the mud for a moment with their whole body, and then rub themselves against the earth, trees, and other objects. Hunters call this bathing of the animals "wallowing."

The birds, on the other hand, go to brooks or springs, and by immersing their necks throw water over their bodies by means of the hollow that is formed between the neck and the trunk, and by splashing themselves with their wings. Then they *rub or scrub* their body with their head and bill and their wing-elbows, if I may so call the wing joint which corresponds to the human elbow.

It has always been vainly asked why it is, for instance, that the stag, the king of our forests, this beautiful, otherwise so cleanly animal, that carefully avoids soiling his lair, and in many other respects shows himself most cleanly, can lie down in such muddy water to bathe, while birds will bathe only in clean water.

I am of the opinion that mammals bathe in the mud only *because they can thus rub and scrub the abdomen and the sexual organs,* which they could not do in clean running water with a hard bottom.

Birds, on the other hand, because they are built differently and can rub themselves with several limbs, do not require the mud for the purpose of rubbing and scrubbing.

The explanation that the mud is required because it enables the mammals to *rub* themselves, is considered a most plausible one by all foresters, too.

We see then that the more highly developed animals bathe.

The roe, the chamois, etc., do not bathe, probably because these species have been placed by nature upon high mountains and rocky regions where water is not always to be had. Neither do beasts of prey bathe. It is likewise quite evident why they do not bathe.* The bath has a quieting influence, but beasts of prey cannot allow themselves to be quieted; they must be bloodthirsty and wild; their place in nature requires it, otherwise they would lack the incentive and the capacity to win their prey. It is the meat diet that develops these bloodthirsty cravings. ||

There is no reason, however, why man, the highest creature, should not bathe. It must rather be assumed that nature prescribes a bath for the preservation and strengthening of his highest physical and spiritual powers.

Men have, indeed, always had an instinctive longing for baths, and even if the inner voice no longer plainly indicates the right kind of bath, every one still feels a need to cool the abdomen, the anus, and the sexual organs by means of water.

Thus we see that animals bathe in different ways according to the construction of their bodies. Mammals take their bath in a different way than birds.

Now whoever has carefully watched animals at their bath and has observed the pains they take to rub or cool the sexual organs in the mud (or water), easily takes the hint of nature and comes to see what the natural bath for man ought to be, especially when he attempts to take a bath in the open air where no artificial apparatus or other aids are to be found.

---

*It cannot be called a bath if our domestic dog goes into the water on a hot day.

|| It is easy to see how beasts of prey become bloodthirsty through a meat diet.

The hunter's setter only brings the game to bay, but does not attack it so long as he is fed on vegetable food alone, but as soon as he is given meat he begins to bite and kill.

I knew an ape in a zoological garden that was very gentle and good-natured. But when he was fed on meat he became vicious and snapped even at his keeper for whom he had had the most friendly feelings.

Beasts of prey must, indeed, be savage and bloodthirsty in order to win their prey.

I shall now proceed to describe the *natural bath*. Since most people must, for the present, take their bath in a room, and have not always an opportunity to bathe in the open air, they must naturally have a basin or tub. It may be any sort of basin or tub in which a person can comfortably sit with his knees drawn up.

The following cuts show tubs that can now be procured in the market.

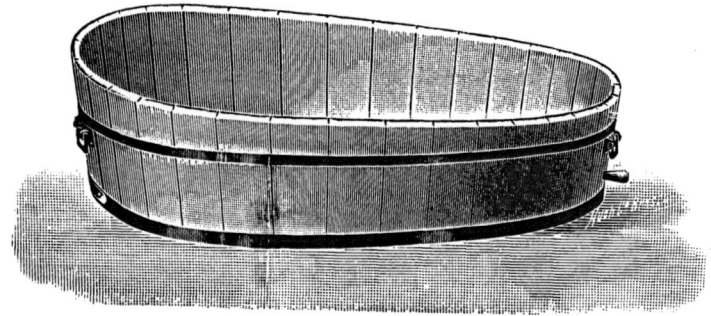

Tub for the Natural Bath No. 1.

The bather sits down in the tub, which contains *naturally cold* water, about three and a half inches (8 cm.) deep, so that the seat, the feet, and the sexual organs are for the most part in the water. Only the seat and the feet touch the bottom of the tub, while the knees are quite aways above the water.

The knees are now spread apart, and the water is vigorously dashed over the abdomen with the hollow of the hand. The throwing of the water is followed by a brisk *rubbing* of the abdomen in the middle, on both sides, and all over with one or both hands. After this alternating process has been carried on awhile, the woman rubs the region of the groins and the *external* part of the sexual organs with the open hand *under water* (the sexual organs are supposed to be submerged). The man also rubs the region of the groins, the testicles, and the dam (the region between the sexual organs and the anus) with the open hand, *under water*. Hereupon the entire body is rapidly washed with the bare hands. A second person can assist in rapidly washing the body. Then the body is rubbed with the bare open hands (*not with a towel or flesh brush*) until it is completely dry.

The body ought never to be dried with a towel after a bath.

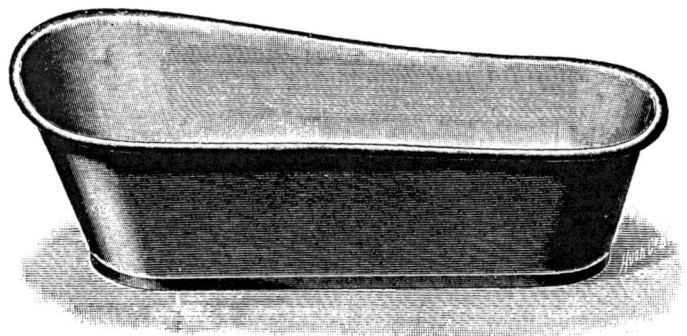

Tub for the Natural Bath No. 2.

The rubbing with the hands can be done by the bather himself. This is at the same time a beneficial bodily exercise. But the rubbing can also be done profitably by a second person. I shall return to this further on.*

After the bath it is advisable to go about naked for a time in a cold room with open windows, or, still better, in the open air. But care must be taken to restore warmth; rapid, vigorous walking or physical work are the best means of bringing this about, or, where neither is possible, wrapping in woollen blankets or bedding must be resorted to. Restoring warmth through the sun, the best warming and invigorating agent we have, is highly to be recommended.

---

*The bath of the sexual organs, after the manner indicated, is very important, especially for women; it is especially effective and healing in cases of sexual excitement and irritation.

Bath tubs Nos. 1 and 2 are made of zinc; No. 3 is made of wood, and is therefore more appropriate and desirable. The bath in the wooden tub is the most beneficial.

For the open air bath tubs of stone or cement are the most appropriate. They must not be too narrow.

The duration of the bath must be regulated entirely by the temperature and condition of the bather. Here again everybody must observe his own inclinations somewhat, and heed the inner voice. On cool days from two to five minutes are sufficient. If it is warmer, or very hot in Summer, the bath may last as long

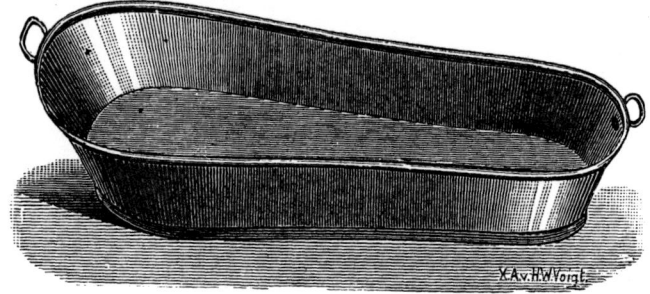

Tub for the Natural Bath No. 3.

as ten minutes and over. One-half of the time of duration of the bath is to be devoted to the abdominal rubbing, the other half to the rubbing of the sexual organs.

The time thus indicated for the duration of the bath does not include the time for the washing of the entire body and the rubbing of it till dry. With respect to the number of baths every one must again consult himself.

A daily bath may be taken in the warm season, or we may bathe twice a day if it can be done in the sun, in a room, or still better in the open air. In colder seasons it may be sufficient to bathe only once in two or three days. Sometimes it is even advisable to suspend bathing entirely for a time.

As a matter of course hot fever patients and strong, vigorous persons can bathe longer and more frequently than chilly patients and weak anæmic persons.

I have often observed that many people prefer to take a short bath and repeat it at frequent intervals; others prefer it a longer time and less frequently. This is also the case among animals in the free state of nature.

It is advisable never to warm the water for the natural bath. It is also best to take the bath, if at all possible, in an unheated room, in which even the windows are open.

At the end of the bath the feet and the anus should always be scrupulously washed. This insures their cleanliness, which is very important.

It is clearly the most natural and the very best way to take the bath in the open air.

The opportunity to take the natural bath in the open air can be found almost everywhere, for a little water is always to be had where there are people.

The full bath, however, cannot always be had in free nature. It is possible only in a few places: only where there happen to be large brooks, rivers, ponds, or lakes. The opportunity for the natural bath in the open air is, therefore, much more commonly and easily found than for the full bath.

The position of the person in the natural bath is comfortable and desirable.

The natural bath differs from all other water applications especially in that the bather does not sit or lie in the water quietly, but is continually *rubbing* special parts of the body, and finally the entire body, with the *bare hands;* not with a towel or the like.

All water applications hitherto have differed from this natural bath, therefore they were not according to the prescriptions of nature and could not produce the proper results and were often even harmful. Nature insists in every respect on having her dictates obeyed.

The natural bath is in every way simpler and more beneficial than any water application that has heretofore been used. It requires but little water (no warm water), and can be taken alone, without the help of a second person. The bath-tub required for it is simple and more easily handled than other bath-tubs. Every one can easily have one standing under his bed, ready for use in the morning after rising.

Therefore this bath will surely come more and more into

favor in families and with the public than other more complicated modes of bathing.

If one does not happen to have an appropriate basin or tub at hand, for instance, while traveling, one can take the bath nevertheless, in a simpler form. Any wash basin will answer.

One sits down over a wash basin containing cold water, washes the anus and cools the sexual organs by pouring water over them with the hollow hand for a few minutes. Then the abdomen is speedily washed with the hand, and finally the whole body, whereupon the work of drying by rubbing is begun.

In this manner a bath can be taken anywhere and at all times, and it is the easiest, simplest bath possible.

Even taken in this way it is well to go about naked for a while after the bath.

This always enhances the efficacy of the bath.

The natural bath, taken in any form whatever, far surpasses in its effect all water applications hitherto employed.

As I continued to think about this new kind of bath, it became more and more clear to me that a bath of this sort must be necessarily superior to all others. The primitive man, evidently, was often obliged to walk about for weeks, perhaps months, in the wet; perhaps even in the snow. He was most likely also obliged to stand still in it for a length of time, and also to sit down with his seat in the wet. The feet and the posterior, therefore, must have been designed by nature to endure wet and cold. But whatever nature has made a necessity for her creatures, she has at the same time made their greatest blessing. When, therefore, present-day man keeps his feet and the anus *artificially* warm, parts where congestions (piles, etc.) so often occur, being caused by internal inflammation, then he deprives the body of its greatest blessings and does it much harm. Therefore many nature doctors order their patients to walk barefooted in the wet for hours, and even days, to stand in it for a short time, forbid the sitting on polsters, in order not to heat the anus artificially, and recommend injections that are to be retained. It is well known that accumulation of the fœces at the extreme end of the rectum, piles, etc., on the anus, which are productive of heat there, affect the head very injuriously. A thorough cooling with water of those parts must therefore have the effect of relieving the head. By immersing the seat and the feet in water the circulation is at all events regulated. An intense cooling of the abdomen, which being the source and *actual* hotbed of disease, where, as is well known, great heat is generated in sickness, must be of the greatest importance.

In the natural bath nearly all the means are united by which the chief representatives of the nature-cure method of to-day attempt to heal disease: going bare-footed, standing in the water, avoiding the heating of the anus, the enema, the light-and-air bath, the abdominal compress, the abdominal bath, the water bath, the cooling of the sexual organs, Kneipp douches, massage of the abdomen and of the whole body. Just this simultaneous co-operation of all these means is the design of nature and the natural bath is therefore of the highest efficacy and benefit to mankind.

These natural and effective means are of course always accompanied by severe *healing crises*, which may manifest themselves in distressing sensations and pains, since the powerful reactions which are produced at once begin to dislodge and expel the foreign matter.

The more natural a remedy is, the severer the crises may often be.

But these healing crises are not at all of a nature to be dreaded; they are rather always to be welcomed.

The crises occur only in the beginning, and we must above all things not allow anything to prevent us from bathing.

Man fell out of harmony with nature, he no longer subsisted on fruit which the earth offered him freely, he no longer went naked, and he transgressed the laws which nature gave him concerning air, earth, water, etc. Consequently he became ill. Only by returning to the harmony in which nature had originally placed him, can he regain health. Man must once more be led by nature; for this he needs no skill and need not learn or know anything. He must rather, in order to find the right way to health, unlearn all the unnecessary and false things that one is obliged to learn to-day; he must first of all discard all the wise ballast that burdens and oppresses the mind and the soul, and that in reality only blinds and stupifies mankind. When man once more listens to the voices of nature, he must not want to KNOW anything; he must not even aspire to know why his diseases are healed or his health is strengthened by arranging his life according to the dictates of nature, or how the processes in his body, the phenomena in his mind and soul are to be explained. The present-day KNOWLEDGE of men is unreliable and only too easily leads one astray.

Man must once more yield himself to nature in childlike faith.

All our anti-natural habits cannot, however, be eradicated at once. Neither do I here wish to pour out the child with the bath, but will make concessions to the present tendency of man always to demand an explanation for everything.

Therefore I shall occasionally state my views concerning the origin of disease, and offer an explanation of the great effect of the natural bath and the other nature remedies to be specified later.

Disease is caused by the introduction into the human body of unnatural food, that is, such food as nature has not intended for man and for the assimilation of which his digestive organs are not adapted. The unnatural food is then either not sufficiently, or not at all, digested. Unassimilated remnants remain behind, constituting foreign matter within the body, which interpenetrates it in all directions, enters into fermentation,* and becomes the cause of all disease, all pain and suffering in man.

Like the want of water, light, etc., powerful emotional influ-

---

*In these days it is usually **chronic disease** with which we have to do. If the fermentation is powerful, it produces a revolution in the body, during which the latter tends to eliminate the foreign matter suddenly and violently. We then have **acute disease** (colds, typhoid fever, pneumonia, etc.). When the body is no longer strong enough for an attack of acute disease, chronic disease **appears.**

ences also foster and cause disease by paralyzing and disturbing the nervous and digestive function of the body, and by aiding or favoring the formation of foreign matter.

The fermentation of the foreign matter produces heat, wherein chiefly lies the injurious and dangerous element of disease.

In order to cure disease we must above all aim to lower the internal heat of the body. But it is also necessary to stimulate the vitality of the body, that force, by means of which the body firstly, draws the true benefit (repair) from food, but, secondly, also expels the foreign matter (disease-matter) through the skin (transpiration), urine, fœces, etc.,—the force which constitutes the real life of man.

It is readily to be seen that both of these ends must be achieved by means of the natural bath.

By the application of cold water to the abdomen (the seat of all disease) and to the sexual organs (the centre of the nervous system), we secure the most immediate and effective lowering of the internal heat of the body. The nerves are stimulated to action by rubbing during the bath, and the cooling of the interior of the body, as well as the stimulation of the vital force, is thus best accomplished by way of the sexual organs.

It is of great importance that by means of the bath the anus becomes thoroughly cooled and cleansed.

All remedies that have not been taken from nature, and are not in accordance with her, prove futile; no matter how often, apparently, they may have operated beneficially and effectively. There are too many deceptions here. The injury that inevitably accompanies all unnatural remedies, sooner or later, always comes to the surface and causes them to disappear again, unfortunately only after much harm has been done. Such unnatural, or not strictly natural, remedies come and go, therefore, and will never find an abiding place of refuge.

We see accordingly new remedies rising to the surface daily in medicine, only to disappear again as quickly as they came. To-day carbolic acid, to-morrow salicylic acid, now antifebrin, again Koch's lymph is the elixir upon which the safety and happiness of mankind is said to depend, until it has become clear that they work only harm and disaster. At present we calmly allow ourselves to be most seriously injured by remedies whose dangerous character can reveal itself only in the future.

Dr. Faust, who in company with his deceased father had so often dispensed medicines and magic draughts, and to whom the populace does homage and offers thanks on Easter Day, is made to break out into this reproachful lament by Goethe:

"Couldst thou but read within mine inmost spirit,
　How little now I deem
That sire or son such praises merit!

This was the medicine—the patient's woes soon ended,
　And none demanded: Who got well?
Thus we, our hellish boluses compounding,
Among these vales and hills surrounding,
　Worse than the pestilence, have passed.
Thousands were done to death by poison of my giving,
And I must hear, by all the living,
　The shameless murderers praised at last."*

Since I look only to nature when I want to know the right thing to do for my health and my wellbeing, I always find that everything that I have recognized as strictly natural, that is, as thoroughly in the spirit of nature, has on trial always proved itself to be the *right* thing entirely. Where nature is accurately observed, experiments to prove the correctness of a procedure are superfluous. When nature's intentions are perfectly understood,

---

*At the end of the last century the sickly tree of humanity sprouted once more and grew a twig of rare vigor. The great Goethe saw the light of day. This lofty genius could not attain to the full truth in his time, and his last words upon earth were, "More light!" But still he came near to a recognition of our cause, the truths of nature. In Goethe's "Faust," at least, we find the absurdities of civilized mankind exposed in the most masterly manner and described in magnificent poetry.

we can at once confidently rely upon them as correct, just as primitive man and the animals in the free state have always eaten and bathed without first convincing themselves of the right way by experiment. This has likewise been shown by the natural bath.

After the first bath of this kind I at once felt benefited and refreshed in a way that I had never experienced from any other water application. Almost all who besides myself have tried this new bath have been surprised by its agreeable and positively good effects.* All experienced a very strong but pleasant sensation of coolness, and after the bath a much better and more agreeable bodily warmth. The points that were especially commented on were the exceedingly stimulated digestion, warm feet for the entire day, increased action of the skin as shown by a slight perspiration, unusual vivacity and cheerfulness, remarkable vigor, and other favorable manifestations.

I could here mention innumerable reports that I have received concerning the efficacy of the bath, both by letter and by word of mouth, the latter always with a happy, beaming face. But I send it into the world simply on its own merits and without flourish of trumpets.

Whoever understands nature, and knows that everything which is in the spirit of nature and according to her dictates must result in the greatest blessing for mankind, will welcome this bath, and to him it will bring blessing and happiness in abundance. Let those who care nothing for all-wise nature and everything for the "science" of men, of sick men, and who flounder from one error to another, scorn and deride it!

---

*Only a few were frightened by the healing crises brought on by the baths. In one person, for instance, who suffered from chronic lung trouble, a lung trouble put in its appearance after a few days: the chronic ailment had become acute, a most favorable sign. The same person also declared that sun baths did not agree with him, that they gave him pains in the body, while these pains only showed that the foreign matter (disease germs) in his body were being loosened by the sun, preliminary to being thrown off. Patients who show such little appreciation of nature and her healing forces, will probably never regain their health.

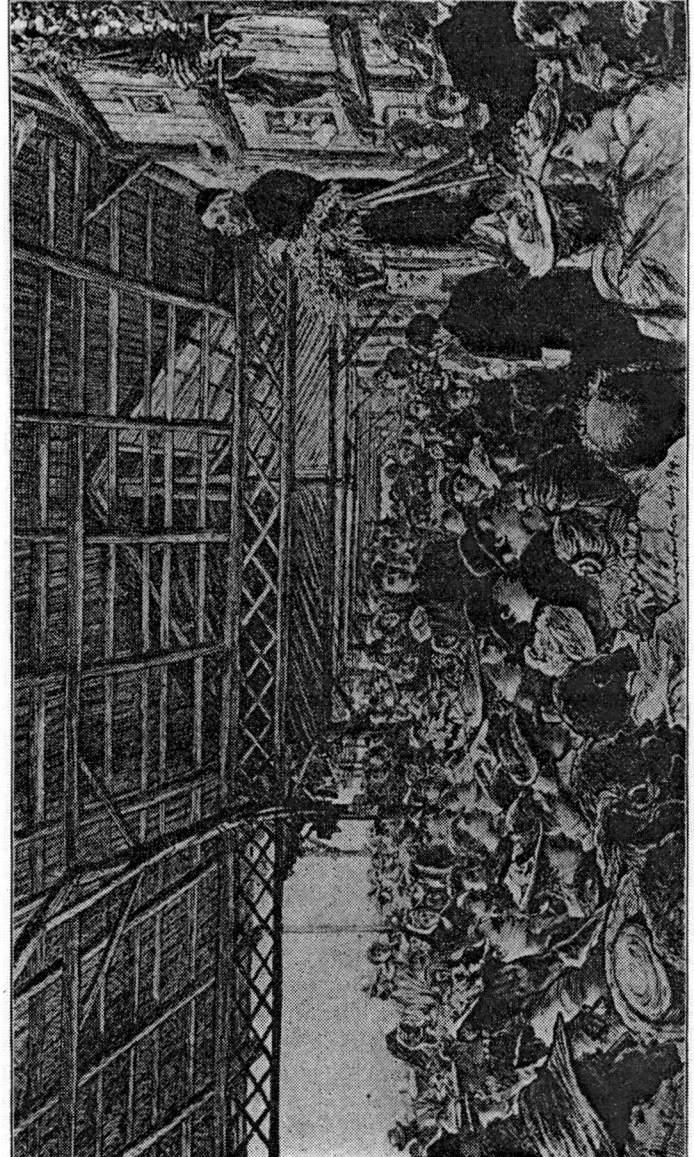

Father Kneipp Lecturing to his Patients on the Natural Method of Living and Healing.

In sending my bath into the world, I wish to give it only a few directions on the way. I disapprove, on the whole, of the warming of the water; it is against nature.* It is not so difficult to sit with only the posterior and the feet in entirely cold water, once the abdomen and the sexual organs have been washed and rubbed and the interior especially of the abdomen has been cooled off and the blood is once more driven towards the extremities. But if for all that one cannot stand it very long in Winter, which does not easily happen, one can take a very short bath, or even dispense with it altogether. In this case we have still another resource, namely, going naked, or the earth compress on the abdomen, of which I shall speak more in detail later.

The water ought not to be too deep—about as deep as the width of the bather's hand; for adults at most three inches. The rubbing and the exercise after the bath must not be executed according to any definite rules, or any system of massage or gymnastics, but entirely according to one's own feeling and inclination.

Whoever has the opportunity (and the opportunity can always be found if it is only sought) can take his bath in the *open.* Man originally had to take his bath in the open, and in the open he must again take it regularly, if he is to derive the full benefit of it, just as food partaken in fresh air always tastes better, and does more good than when it is eaten in the room and in impure air.

Women can discontinue their bath during their monthly periods.

The other remedies of nature, however: walking barefooted, the air-and-light baths, earth compresses, etc., women need not avoid during this period. They are especially beneficial at that time.

The bath can always be taken in rivers (near the shore when they are deep), in brooks and small ponds.

In the room, if it is heated, the windows can always remain

---

*In order not to discourage beginners, they may be allowed to warm the water a little or to take the bath in a warm room.

open to some extent. The early morning, or at least the forenoon, when one has not yet broken one's fast, or has eaten very little, is the best time for the bath.

All fishes (water animals) try to avoid the air, while all air creatures take great pains not to get their bodies into the water and, while taking their bath, as little as their bodily structures will allow. Man is the highest light-and-air creature. If the air should suddenly be entirely withheld, he could live only for a *very short time*. But even if only a very small part of the air due him is withheld, he at once loses vitality and is weakened, just as the fish begins to die when he is taken out of his element, the water. But now the body is almost entirely immersed in water during a *full bath*, and the skin, through which the body ordinarily absorbs quite a considerable quantity of air, can neither absorb nor throw off the bad, used-up air. The body is therefore weakened and injured by a full bath. If the full bath lasts only a very short time, perhaps only several seconds, the benefit which the body derives from the cooling, for which a few seconds suffice, may be somewhat greater than the harm done by depriving it of air. But if the full bath lasts five, ten, fifteen minutes and longer, as is customary in our bathing institutions, it is always very injurious. But if we deprive only a part of the body, or separate organs, of air,—for instance, the hands by means of leather gloves—these are always injured and lamed. In our sitz-baths, hitherto, the abdominal organs were always surrounded by water from all sides. These were therefore shut off from the air and rendered more or less inactive, so that they could not work in the right way during the bath. Thus the effect of these baths was essentially weakened. Neither was the water thrown over the entire abdominal surface in the sitz-bath, and there was no *rubbing*. In the natural bath everything that interferes with the full effect of former water-applications is done away with, and this is the explanation of the great results that are only now being achieved by water.

It is to be hoped that the natural bath will now be welcomed by the public at large, by rich and poor, by high and low, and carry to old and young the blessing and wellbeing which the kind mother, nature, has always intended to shed upon mankind with lavish hands. Let no one say that he does not need the natural bath because he is well. For it is plainly not the first intention of nature to cure diseases by the bath, but rather to keep her creatures well, bright and happy.

As Winter succeeds Autumn, and night the day, according to stern natural law, so man, leading an unnatural mode of life, breathing impure air, using tobacco, alcohol, coffee, etc., must fall a victim to disease. This does not always manifest itself in the form of what is called disease nowadays, but disease is nevertheless present, and will make itself felt plainly enough.

The child at school is inattentive and indolent and learns his lessons with difficulty; often he is ill-bred, and becomes a prey to sin and vice. He is punished, often severely enough. But the poor fellow is in fact only ill, and suffers his punishment innocently. The husband and father is unkind, harsh, often even brutal toward his wife and children—toward those whom he loves. Later he is filled with remorse, not knowing that only his nerves have been overheated by the use of alcohol, tobacco, and other modern poisons, and that he, too, is ill.

Others are directly driven on to the path of vice and crime. They are put into houses of correction and penitentiaries, instead of being cured and made whole.

The young wife becomes whimsical, irritable, hysterical.

>"With the cestus loosed—away
>Flies illusion from the heart."

Conjugal happiness is not realized, as had been expected, and the heaven dreamed of in reality turns into hell. The young girl who entered wedlock with the fairest qualities and a good heart, an angel, becomes a vixen. But do not reproach her, poor thing, for the unnatural life which married people almost always lead bears fruit and demands as its first victim the wife.

The plants and animals of the forest, in the state of nature (not the plants of the fields), retain their health, beauty, youthfulness, and goodness up to a certain period, fixed for the individuals of the same species, when they die suddenly, with only a few exceptions which here again have been caused by man's interference with nature.

Among men, in modern times, one becomes shortsighted in childhood, another hard of hearing, one loses his teeth, another his hair, many suffer from nervous troubles, and even are enveloped by mental darkness. The young girl who is a celebrated beauty to-day, suddenly falls away, grows thin and pale, or becomes bloated and ruddy soon after her marriage, and appears offensively homely to the man whom she had so recently charmed.

Many people are favorably situated, but nevertheless give themselves no end of care and trouble. Even millionaires are sometimes troubled by the care for food.

> Care at the bottom of the heart is lurking:
> Her secret pangs in silence working,
> She, restless, rocks herself, disturbing joy and rest.
> * * * * * * *
> We dread the blows we never feel,
> And what we never lose is yet by us lamented!
> —Goethe, "Faust."

All these evil spirits that disturb the peace in hovel and palace and destroy the happiness of peasant and king will largely be dispensed with and put to flight by the natural bath.

This new, or rather old bath will give to man in the present fierce struggle of existence youthful freshness and vigor, and a serene calm in the hurry and scurry of life. I have seen animals chased by dogs until they became faint and desperate, seeking the bath to sooth their nerves and recuperate themselves. Would that the unhappy men who are to-day hounding each other until they are incessantly gasping from exhaustion, and their nerves are ever vibrating,—would that they might seek peace and strength in the bath!

The immediate effect of the bath is to so cool the abdomen, and to stimulate the vitality (digestion) to such a degree that it will reject the foreign matter, remnants of insufficiently or not at all digested unnatural food, and thereby prevent a real attack of sickness in most cases where a sensible mode of life is otherwise observed.

With the regular use of the natural bath many a stroke of paralysis, also melancholia, typhoid fever, cholera, cancer, consumption, etc., will never develop.

The effect one experiences from it, is such as to allow one to expect these results.

The body's power of reaction is also considerably strengthened by the bath. It is this power which originally was instantly aroused to activity to ward off and eliminate any injurious matter that was introduced into the body (just as the first cigar causes sickness and vomiting.)

As an effect of the natural bath some find that their cigar no longer agrees with them, others experience an antipathy against the use of beer, as well as against all alcoholic and spirituous liquors, and against meat. Most people feel themselves again drawn towards nature, and many certainly will yield to this attraction, and adapt themselves more and more to nature in their mode of living. Thus the bath will cure those who to-day call themselves well.

But I would have the natural bath enter also the sick chamber and carry its message of joy to the weak and fever stricken, to the gouty and lame, to the blind and deaf, to the nervous sufferers and consumptives who groan and lament there.

Here every gleam of hope that penetrates the night is still looked for, and every word of comfort is listened to, but many are sighing: "The message well I hear, but faith, alas, is wanting." Yes, the faith in a helper and saviour is often put to a hard test here. The sick have been deceived so often and have buried all hope.

But whose advice has always been asked, so far, and whose help has been implored? Many an idol who has been worshipped, ought to have been examined, his high titles and false modern glitter ought to have been torn from him, and it would have been found that he was of stone and clay.

They had confidence in a physician who prescribed medicines, and if one objected that he had heard much good said about the nature cure method, the answer was that the prescribed remedies were also taken from nature and were therefore good. Yes, everything is taken from nature, even the tobacco and the alcohol which cause so much distress to-day, and every poison that kills immediately if taken even in the smallest quantity. These remedies are mostly prepared from poisonous plants and minerals. Primitive men, who have never had any instruction in botany, and animals know poisonous plants at once, without tasting of them, and flee them as their enemies. But even to us, in spite of our spoiled taste, poisonous plants and "curative" minerals and metals in their natural state, taste exceeding bad, which plainly proves that, made still worse by artificial preparation through chemical processes, they are in *every* case bad for us. When we are sick they are of course more injurious than when we are well.

However God still speaks to us often and plainly enough in many different ways, "Thou shalt not eat of the tree," but even to-day we so often disregard the command of the All-wise and All-powerful One, that man is again and again driven from paradise for his disobedience.

Others have so often heard of the great successes of the nature cure method, that they blindly trust themselves to the "nature doctors," and think that now they are absolutely in the best hands. But even here many a hope is not realized.

We can still easily and with certainty discover what is necessary for the preservation or restoration of our health if we only go to the right source—NATURE. A nature doctor advises us not to eat fresh but only stewed fruit. But we see that nature produces only fresh and not stewed fruit, therefore fresh fruit must in all cases and conditions be better, for what nature produces is always the best. The changes which man brings about in her products always deteriorate them. Another recommends eating freely of Graham bread. We see, however, that sparrows as well as the horses, like to eat the kernels of rye and wheat, but man does not seem to find them agreeable in their natural state. Animals also like wheat best in its *unripe* or *half-ripe* state, and generally with the accompanying straw, while Graham or groats-bread is always made of entirely ripe kernels and without the straw. Furthermore, we observe that horses and other animals, when they are fed much on oats and wheat, especially when they are not at the same time doing very arduous physical work, grow stiff in the legs and become vicious. What a sensitive creature our horse is, and how easily it sickens, especially the pleasure horse, that is chiefly fed on kernels! How much more beautiful, fleeter, more enduring and hardy are the wild horse and the zebra, which subsist on grasses alone! In the Graham bread, moreover, the grain is considerably changed from its natural state by the grinding and baking. It is well, therefore, not to follow the above counsel, and eat only very little of the groats-bread if one cannot do without altogether. Our present leavened bread, to be sure, is still less to be recommended.

Steam baths are also frequently prescribed, but nature has never equipped any of her creatures at birth with a steam apparatus, and there is no contrivance in nature that in the least approaches a steam bath, so that it could be considered even as a weak substitute for one. Therefore steam baths are in every case harmful, even if all nature doctors should be of a different opinion. The future will judge of the steam bath; single voices are even now raised against it.

We see, then, that nature everywhere still speaks very plainly to us, and if we will only begin and try, we can learn to understand her language more and more, even if it is not taught in our schools.

Some people, indeed, have become almost entirely deaf to it in the course of time, especially those who have received their knowledge of health from universities and those places where receipts and laws of health are concocted systematically against the voice of nature. Here food-stuffs and the like are tested in retorts, to ascertain their ingredients, and their action upon each other; and *corpses* are supposed to shed light upon the processes that transpire in the living body.

> Alas! in living Nature's stead,
> Where God His human creature set,
> In smoke and mould the fleshless dead
> And bones of beasts surround me yet!
> —Goethe, "Faust."

But primitive men had never seen chemical tables, and the horses and deer in the forest never examine the corpses of their sisters and brothers, the construction of their stomachs, the length of their intestines, etc., etc., in order to ascertain what is the right food for them, and what they ought to know to insure their well-being. It is *not* the intention of nature, then, that we should acquire the knowledge of our welfare in this way, it is rather directly opposed to it, and must, therefore, always lead to great errors. In the retort nothing but dead matter is manipulated, while in the human stomach, parts and supplements of the living body, are produced. The effects of chemical elements upon each other cannot be compared with the effects upon the nervous system of the *living* man. In the processes of the human body, in nutrition, and in life in general mysterious forces are at work, into which we have never penetrated and which we shall probably never understand. To be sure, the men of to-day are incessantly and without rest making researches, for here again a curse of the Deity is being fulfilled. "A fugitive and a vagabond shalt thou be on earth," but,—

> Mysterious even in open day,
> Nature retains her veil, despite our clamors:
> That which she does not willingly display
> Cannot be wrenched from her with levers, screws, and hammers.
> —Goethe, "Faust."

Elements and matter and processes which are of importance in the retort, may be of no benefit to the human stomach and to the nerves of man, they may even work the greatest injury. This sort of science has consequently always been fraught with harmful absurdities*. But errors impress especially young people with their stamp which cannot easily be effaced and always leaves a trace behind,—young people who are susceptible to external influences and who by virtue of the prevailing false education surrender themselves unconditionally to the "authorities," the sources of all wisdom. Physicians who intend to throw overboard the ballast received at the university and put aside the errors taught them there, must therefore always remember that a special effort on their part is necessary to this end, and that they must especially rid themselves of all pride which seeks to give to shallow things an external value.

All nature doctors must regard it as their ideal aim to develop the people to the point where each will be his own physician.

It is of course always easier and pleasanter to let others think for us, or perhaps not think for us. But if people wish to pursue a course that will certainly lead them to true health, to the springs of life, each must be his own doctor.

But if to-day I recommend to a patient the natural bath, may he trust me? Certainly! Without hesitation! I myself have nothing to do with it, or at most only in so far as I have had the good fortune, as it seems, to have been the first to receive from the hands of nature the bath in this form. For the rest, I merely show that the creatures of the field and meadow, of the forest and glen, which still clearly understand the precepts of nature, know this bath and apply it to their advantage. Although largely suppressed, our feelings, instinct, and conscience are still suffi-

---

*Let it not be objected that the venerable science of medicine cannot thus be steeped in error. It began with man's fall from nature, grew step by step with his unnatural mode of life, is explicable or inexplicable like this, and will finally disappear with this mode of life. Besides, we learn from history that also other errors were current among men for centuries and longer and were countenanced by science, for instance, witchcraft.

ciently active to recognize the true course that we ought to pursue. We can still learn by means of the sense of taste that of the foods in the natural, unchanged condition it is not the cabbage, nor the potato, nor meat, but the fruits, berries, and *nuts* which have been set apart as food for us. So, too, those who have tried all of the various baths soon experience from the use of the nature bath such a sense of comfort and well-being that they can no longer doubt its supreme excellence.

Let us confidently resort to the bath, therefore, in such disturbances of the health as are nowadays called disease, even in desperate cases where many a remedy, which certainly must have been more or less anti-natural, has already failed. But when a patient nowadays turns away from those dangerous and injurious medicines, and takes up the safe remedies of nature, the disease has generally reached such an advanced stage, largely owing to the medicines and otherwise false treatment, that the still more important remedies of light, air, diet, earth, etc., are now also necessary. But everybody stands aghast at the thought that he should go naked even for a little while only, especially at low temperature, be it even only inside the room with open windows; and his dismay becomes still greater when a life without meat is suggested to him, from which he thinks all his strength is derived. He can more easily make up his mind, however, to take the bath, especially in the form of the natural bath, which does not necessitate the immersion of the whole body, or even half the body, in cold water. Well, then, let us make a beginning with the bath.

Water is indeed nature's own remedy, with which she has intended to attain great ends for her creatures. Especially if employed in the form desired by nature, one can understand the words of the Bible: "And the earth was without form and void— *and the Spirit of God moved upon the face of the waters."* and it becomes clear why it was in baptism that the Holy Ghost descended upon Jesus, and that the water bath became a holy sacrament of the Christian church, a symbol of physical and spiritual health.

But to-day one is deaf, another nearsighted, one suffers from swollen feet, another is humpbacked, with some the liver is out of order, with others the kidneys, here we see one writhing in epileptic fits, there another is in the clutches of insanity and mental darkness. Many totter to the grave as consumptives, others are shunned by society because they are the victims of syphilis. Now you will certainly ask me, "And is this one bath to cure all these diseases, and is this the only water application to be used in all cases? It seems altogether to be too simple a thing." My answer is: "Yes, in ALL cases always only this ONE bath." In this manner the curing of diseases is of course most *simple, but everything that is truly natural is necessarily also most simple.* All disturbances and abnormal manifestations in the body as well as in the mind and soul are only the consequences of disobedience to or transgression of the laws of nature. There is therefore also but *one* way to health: the return to nature and the employment of her remedies, and she prescribes no other form of water bath than the one under consideration.

The fact is that in nature undefiled and pure everything is good and beautiful, that is, sound, and that in man, too, in the degree in which he again returns to nature and avails himself of her remedies all disturbances and deviations from his original ideal state of body, mind, and soul can be overcome and repaired faster or slower in proportion to his defects and his remaining vitality...If we therefore scrupulously and in every respect endeavor to learn anew the precepts of nature, and in so far as our bodily and mental energy and other circumstances permit, strive to obey them zealously, we shall be doing our duty, which of itself will result in our greatest good and welfare.

The perfectly beautiful and good human being, that is, the perfectly healthy man, is perhaps best represented by the Apollo of Belvidere and the Venus (Aphrodite), the two most important works of Greek art. Since we have no examples for comparison, we cannot form a true idea of the intellectual and spiritual state of man such as it would have been among the most highly developed Caucasian race if he had never fallen away from nature,

—of his wonderful energy, of the keenness and clearness of his intellect, of his gentleness, of his kindness and love, in short, of his God-likeness.

As man truly returns to nature, he approaches this ideal state more and more in every respect, physically* as well as intellectually and spiritually.

How closely he will approach it, depends on his hereditary taint, on his age, on his remaining vitality, and on the degree in which he lives in conformity with nature.

Children, of course, have the best chances here. They should therefore, above all, be again led on the road to paradise and especially be made to take the bath. We shall often be surprised then to note how much better behaved they become, and how much more easily they learn at school, for dulness and stupidity are diseases, just as the higher degrees of these forms, mental night and insanity, have been recognized as diseases.

Barrenness and painful labor are also great abnormities. Through the use of the bath, this partial return to nature, the curse of civilized woman will disappear for the greater part. The act of child-bearing will pass off without pain and without entailing special exhaustion, as is the case among all creatures in the state of nature. The mother will be greeted by a much more lovable and a healthier child which she will be able to nurse herself, and thus fulfil her sweetest duty. In this regard my experience has already furnished me with the most favorable results.

Disease, especially *chronic disease,* begins, as we have already seen, with man's transgression of the laws of nature. Unnatural food, as I have said before, can be digested only with difficulty, if at all. Our nervous energy or vitality is weakened by various harmful influences. In this manner more and more undigested matter, "foreign matter," accumulates in the body. This is the

---

*Only the means of nature, such as the bath, lead to true beauty of the body; these alone will smooth away many a wrinkle and roughness of feature. All other means are of no avail, and do more harm than good. Would that our young girls and women gave heed to this!

cause of chronic diseases. From the abdomen this matter passes through the entire body in gaseous, liquid, and solid form.* It changes the shape of the body, and causes disturbances in mind and spirit. Body, mind, and soul are in the closest and most intimate connection, of which everyone can become convinced by his own observation. The body endeavors from the start to get rid of food-remnants and foreign matter through the excretory organs by the natural way of the fæces, urine, exhalation, perspiration, etc. But if the foreign matter continues to accumulate it cannot all be removed in that way. Thereupon the body attempts to eject it by force, stimulated thereto by a variety of causes, which as fresh air, drafts, dampness, etc. These revolutions in the body are called *acute diseases;* the lighter forms, such as catarrhs, etc., are generally known as colds. The more serious forms, such as measles, scarlet fever, diphtheria, typhoid fever, cholera, etc., are always accompanied by fevers, which are a violent fermentation of the foreign matter.

The acute diseases, therefore, dreaded as they are to-day, are to be regarded in the light of most favorable healing crises and should be greeted with joy. They become dangerous only under wrong treatment, under treatment with medicines, for instance, and by shutting the patient off from fresh air, which weakens the body and paralyzes its functions, so that the foreign matter which is in a state of agitation cannot be ejected and may cause great distress, even death.

A cold in the head, for instance, is always very useful and really a good thing if the phlegm (the foreign matter) is thrown off in great quantities. And a child dies of measles only in case they do not develop, that is, when the rash, which contains the foreign matter, does not come out thoroughly.

While disease is in process, heat develops within the body, from the motion of the foreign matter, the friction of the particles against each other, which constitutes the fermentation. This heat

---

*How a foreign substance can traverse the body is illustrated in the case of a soldier who received a bullet in the shoulder which after the lapse of a year came to the surface in the leg.

is formed especially in the abdomen, the real seat of the disease. When the body in acute diseases, that is, in acute fevers, agitates the foreign matter powerfully, the heat rises to a dangerous degree. This can then be brought down considerably by the natural bath. As soon as the water, especially if it is very cold, touches the abdomen of the patient, he is wonderfully relieved and refreshed. But the bath at the same time increases the vitality of the body, which is thus essentially aided in the work of throwing off the disease germs in order to completely attain its end. This is soon shown (sometimes, however, not until a few days have passed) in copious sweating and a more abundant discharge of urine and fœces.

In an acute disease, therefore, whether it be a simple cold or something more serious, like diphtheria, typhoid fever, cholera, etc., one ought to take the bath and then try to sweat, either in the sun or by wrapping one's self up in woollen blankets in bed. A light-and-air bath in these cases is especially beneficial. Care ought to be taken above all to have a constant supply of *fresh air* night and day by keeping the windows open, even in winter at a low temperature. The diet also ought to be carefully chosen and as near to nature as possible. The favorable results will then be surprising, and our subsequent good health will convince us that in bringing the illness about, nature had the best of intentions. It goes without saying, of course, that the sooner one begins with this method of cure in the case of acute diseases, the surer and the more permanent will be the result. If we resort to it only at the last moment when the patient is often far gone, the hope of recovery is but slight.

Medicines paralyze the body and bring its eliminatory functions to a standstill. This nowadays is called healing acute diseases. Such cures are of course followed by the greatest injury to the body, and entail chronic troubles, such as nervous prostration, cancer, epilepsy, consumption, etc.,—troubles very prevalent in these days and are largely a consequence of medicine and vaccination.

In the advanced stage of *chronic diseases* the vitality of the body (the digestion) is at a low ebb, the eliminatory organs (the kidneys, stomach, and intestines) are completely paralyzed, the activity of the skin is always wholly inadequate. The body is no longer capable of the violent elimination of foreign matter,— is no longer capable of acute disease. The foreign matter begins to ferment in the body (internal fever),—in the case of one, chiefly in the lungs, in the case of another, in the legs, of one in the eyes, of another in the brain,—or it paralyzes the entire nervous system, when we reach the worst form of chronic disease, nervous prostration. We now have the diseases which are commonly first described as chronic diseases: consumption, cancer, syphilis, diabetes, epilepsy, gout, open sores, insanity, etc. In these diseases the foreign matter in the body plays havoc with and undermines it more and more. The body is no longer strong enough to eliminate it gradually or eject it suddenly by force. Persons suffering from nervous prostration, the insane, consumptives, etc., therefore rarely, if ever, catch cold, and rarely, if ever, are seized by acute diseases, like typhoid fever, etc. This is not a good sign, it is rather a very bad sign for the patients. In *individual* cases, however, the natural bath and the other natural remedies increase the vitality of the body so rapidly and to such a degree as occasionally to bring about acute troubles like catarrh, coughs, fevers, and other distempers, although these appear only rarely and in an extremely mild form, so that one can feel their harmlessness and liberating influence. Boils, carbuncles, etc., are also formed, constituting as they do only the outlet for the foreign matter.

These affections are under all circumstances to be regarded only as favorable symptoms.

It is precisely at these times that the body must be assisted in its eliminatory functions by the natural remedies (bathing, fresh air and light, and a natural diet), so that the acute disease may be exploited to the greatest possible advantage of the body. Above all, let us not be too timid in such cases.

Other accompaniments of a natural mode of life, of bathing, of natural diet, and going naked, such as temporary emaciation, weakness and debility, bad looks, pains in the limbs, etc., indicate only favorable crises and need not disquiet any one. We must remember that the application of really natural remedies can never result injuriously, and that whatever happens must therefore be favorable to health, however dangerous it may appear from the modern point of view.*

For severe chronic diseases, of course, the new bath proves itself to be wonderfully effective. Here, too, in the course of time, enormous heat has developed, especially in the abdomen of the patient, who gradually has become almost parched. The mucous membrane of the rectum has dried up, so that the fæces can no longer move on, and a dangerous constipation prevails. If the surface of the abdomen is now cooled with very *cold water,* and is thoroughly rubbed during the process, the digestive organs are at once stimulated, and the poor patients again experience for the first time a delight to which they have long

---

*One disagreeable feature connected with the nature cure lies in the circumstance that especially in periods of crises so many busybodies incessantly annoy the patient with warnings, sage counsel, etc. Healthy and more sensible persons have no time for that sort of thing, and are aware, moreover, that they know too little about the matter to express any opinion concerning it. But those poor unfortunates who have become mentally crippled by illness, who do not understand things, who are dissatisfied because of their superficiality, and consequently always become bores, soon prove a veritable nuisance to those attempting the new mode of life. Everyone must study for himself how he can best keep at a distance these unhappy creatures, but in all cases in such a way as not to hurt their feelings. We must be gentle and considerate to those also who scorn and ridicule us for adopting the natural mode of life. They are mostly persons who are instinctively aware of their false mode of life and the troubles engendered by it, but who either lack the necessary energy, or who have not yet met a favorable opportunity to depart from their false course. They are especially in need of our sympathy and consideration. We must forgive them if in their diseased condition they occasionally give way to ill-temper. It is, however, only in the beginning of the cure that one is disagreeably and painfully affected by what has just been said. We soon experience a calm and contentment which nothing can henceforth disturb.

been strangers, and a joyful hope and the certainty of recovery is born.

Let no one be surprised if in order to cure chronic diseases, for instance, swollen feet, eye and ear troubles, cancer of the nose, or open sores on the legs, the abdomen is treated with water.

The foreign matter has originated in the abdomen, from there it passed to the affected parts, and it must now go back to the abdomen, to be discharged from there.

Even in the very severest chronic diseases, nervous troubles, insanity, cancer, consumption, etc., which are nowadays generally considered as more or less incurable, the greatest improvements, even complete cures, sometimes take place in a most incredibly short time, in several weeks or several months, with this natural treatment.

As a general thing, however, chronic diseases, from which the patients have usually suffered for many long years, require even by this method patience and perseverance, for the vitality of the sufferer can only slowly and very gradually be restored, so that a cure can be achieved. But much, very much, can still be gained here—much more than is considered possible, according to the results of the curative methods at present prevailing. Of course, in very special and severe cases of exceedingly long standing, often only an improvement, sometimes no result at all, can be reached. Help is indeed sought sometimes from this cure by veritable death candidates.

When *wounded*, animals put the injured part into the water to cool it, and lick it incessantly between times. The nature-cure method of to-day also first cools thrust, cut, burn, and ulcer wounds with water, and then applies linen cloths dipped in cold water to them, varying the thickness of the cloth with the size of the wound, whereupon they are wrapped with woollen bandages. Much better, indeed, would be a compress of moist earth. I shall speak of this again further on.

The licking of wounds, so far as that is possible, is also very good. I have recently experienced a striking result in the case of a skin trouble in a new-born child, by the mother's licking the part. Of course, one must not lick a wound in the center, but the skin round about it, which is free from pus and other impurities.

In the case of larger wounds, however, the natural bath must be used in addition, and if possible the other remedies of nature, which will be spoken of further on. These remedies are necessary likewise for the cooling down of the internal heat, and to increase the vitality so that it can repair the injuries of the body. In this manner one can soon become convinced of the brilliant cures that are achieved.

We note also that among animals in the natural state the greatest injuries and wounds are effectively healed in an astonishingly short time precisely through a perfectly natural mode of life. An animal in the forest sometimes has a leg shot off or torn away by a trap; the wound heals completely in a very short time, and the animal continues to live on as if nothing had happened.

I know of a deer that was shot through the body in the region of the ribs so that on the side where the bullet came out the ground was covered with blood. After a few days the deer was driven in a corner that was fenced in. In spite of its large wound it then jumped with the greatest ease over the high fence. In this case the bullet had not, of course, touched any of the vital parts, such as the lungs, heart, etc.

Formation of pus and similar phenomena that accompany wounds in man are merely eliminatory processes of the body. Like acute diseases, they are favorable symptoms, and become harmful and dangerous only in consequence of false treatment. Never treat boils by means of steam baths, nor apply partial steam baths to the affected parts.

But above all, and in ALL *cases, let us abjure the use of the knife and the scalpel on the human body. Cutting and operating is in the crassest contradiction with the processes of nature, and is always followed by the most serious consequences, although they may not always manifest themselves at once.*

Whoever thinks that it is not always possible to get along without the knife and the scalpel, ought in serious cases first try *all* the means which nature offers, and *these in the right proportion and form.*

Nature disdains all bandages, even in the case of rupture (rupture of the legs, ribs, etc.), and broken limbs never heal wrongly, as happens so often to the doctors in spite of bandages and splints.*

Thus we have seen that the water bath, taken in the right form, is of the greatest significance and effect.

In the JUNGBORN, where the bath is mostly taken in the open, it has from the start given much enjoyment and delight, and has always been splendidly successful. I have often seen the most timid and discouraged spirits soon become lively and bright, courageous and daring through the bath.

It is also the most appropriate means for leading mankind once more back to nature.

---

*In asserting that operations are unnecessary in the nature-cure method, we must not go too far. For instance, bad teeth are among the infirmities caused by an unnatural mode of life. Now if we want to avoid operations altogether, we must not have teeth extracted or filled. To be sure, with a more natural mode of life, and especially by the use of earth compresses, these things may in great part be avoided, and the suffering from toothache also.

But the cutting of the hair and nails may also be considered as unavoidable operations. The animals in the state of nature, however, need nothing of the sort. And yet they do not become unsightly. Everything regulates itself in free nature.

In still other cases (also in natal deformities) pain can be avoided by an operation, the use of limbs can be made possible, or other advantages can be gained. But these exceptional cases are of an entirely different nature from the many cases in which apparent advantages are gained nowadays, while on close inspection we find that the health is seriously injured and more and more undermined, until sometimes even death ensues from surgical interference with nature.

In all diseases, acute as well as chronic, and also in wounds, physical and mental rest is a great desideratum; for the body needs all its energy to recuperate.

It enables us to avail ourselves of ever more important remedies of nature, and to rise to ever finer health and higher earthly happiness.

RUBBING AND STROKING OF THE BODY.

I have already called attention to the importance of rubbing during the bath.

When a child has had a fall and runs crying to its mother, the latter does not long consider what physicians and books say as to the first thing to be done in emergencies, etc., but in her overflowing love and sympathy she involuntarily rubs and strokes the painful spot.

Who has not heard of the "wise" women and men (shepherds and the like) who formerly used to work wonderful cures in the country by means of rubbing and stroking?

These simple, sound, and also pious country people did not devote themselves to healing as a business. They even thought their service would do no good if they took money for it. They acted in the spirit of the words:

"Freely ye have received, freely give."—Matt. 10:8.

The help which they gave their fellowmen had to be an act of brotherly love. Within the last decades science and civilization, education and enlightenment, have spread wonderfully. We are proud of this achievement. But we are nevertheless often sorely tempted to exclaim: "There are more things in heaven and earth than are dreamt of in your philosophy."

We have long shrugged our shoulders contemptuously and derisively when speaking of the women and men who performed those cures by stroking. In their place to-day we have masseurs and masseuses. These masseurs have received special training. They have studied the anatomy of the body, the position of the various muscles and nerve fibres. The present-day masseurs, however, do not accomplish in weeks or months what those illiterate and untaught men and women of the country formerly accomplished at a sitting or in a few days. There was a charm about them that forthwith caused the disease to disappear.

Our masseurs treat sick people day after day. We soon observe them to grow pale and get sick themselves. But it also happens that one or another of these pale and sick masseurs suddenly regains his health.

By the stroking and rubbing of the body vitality and health are always transferred from one person to another. The diseased parts of the body are thereby invigorated, and this constitutes the principal effect and advantage of rubbing and stroking. The training of the masseurs is useless; it is even disadvantageous.

Liquid and gaseous substances intermingle the moment they come in contact with one another.

The soul of man is also a substance, the very finest ether-substance. But the substance which constitutes the soul of man is concentrated about a center. This center is the will-power. The mutual interchange and mingling of men's souls does not, therefore, take place like the mixture of gases; mutual likes and dislikes, love, indifference and hate, play a great part here.

The interflow of two human souls, their mutual attraction or repulsion, is moreover even visible to the eye. It has already been photographed, and there are pictures which plainly show it.

Furthermore, the souls of two people can pass into each other so completely that it may indeed be remarked of them:

> "Two souls with but a single thought,
> Two hearts that beat as one."

Now these country people possessed an abundance of vitality and health, and they still had a heart full of love for their suffering fellowmen and a firm trust in God. That is why a magic healing power emanated from them.

When a masseur has for some time continuously treated sick people, he loses much vitality and health and becomes sick himself. If it now happens that for a time he shall treat persons who are in better health than he is, he becomes well again. It is plain, therefore, that as a rule one cannot derive much good from a masseur; one may even lose what health remains. To the present-day masseur massage is a business, and not a pleasant business at that. He must make a living and do his work for the money there is in it. He cannot consult his affections or his inclinations.

Here, again, one must exclaim:

RETURN TO NATURE!

The mother who rubs and strokes her child in the fulness of her love, can effect the speediest and best cure provided she is not herself weak and sick. But even so the mother will give the last glimmer of her life to her child.

I said that in rubbing and stroking vitality and health are transferred. It may also be said that animal heat is transferred.

The more animal heat one has, the healthier one is. Animal heat, therefore, is the same thing as vitality and health. Therefore only those persons who have warm hands are fitted for stroking and rubbing. Sick people always have cold hands and cold feet.

Persons whose heart is with us, parents or loving friends, are therefore the most appropriate persons for rubbing and stroking if they are at the same time healthy.

Of course, I here mean healthy people only in the present, customary sense. Strictly speaking there are no entirely healthy people among civilized men to-day.

Strong, healthy persons from the laboring and serving classes, who have not become enervated, bloodless, and weak from mental work and a refined mode of life, and who are mostly engaged in physical work in the open-air, are very well adapted for rubbing and stroking. But the transmission of vitality is not the same between all persons. This depends on the mutual affections (sympathies) existing between the respective persons. There must above all be no feelings of repulsion on either side, otherwise there will be no result.

One must therefore select vigorous, healthy, and sympathetic persons. They must not only be physically agreeably, they must also be well-meaning and lovable. Selfish, thieving and lying people cannot help us. They rather anxiously strive to keep their vitality and warmth for themselves, and in no way desire to impart them to others.

We must beware not to consider ourselves better than others on account of our education, social position, wealth, and suchlike illusions, and thereby hinder the mutual, purely human affections. It is always to be remembered that whoever sows love will reap love.

The freer a man is from all present-day science, the more childlike and innocent he is, the happier is he, and the more can he be of service to his fellowmen.

It is desirable that a person should not know about, or at least not think about, the transference of vitality and warmth through rubbing and stroking. His only concern should be to help his fellowman, and to free him from his suffering, and he must accordingly have the good will, earnestness and perseverance necessary for it.

If this is the case, the person will not require any special instruction regarding rubbing and stroking.

Every sick part of the body can now be rubbed and stroked in the case of pain, swelling, gout, etc. In headaches, for instance, the stroking and rubbing of the neck is very beneficial. Stroking the calves and the abdomen is of great benefit and increases the general wellbeing.

The parts which are to be rubbed or stroked must always first be moistened with water (not with some kind of oil or fat).

The rubbing and stroking must be done quietly and firmly, but sometimes also with a light touch. The right way is easily found.

The best time for the transference of vitality and animal heat for the general invigoration and strengthening of the whole body is at the end of the natural bath.

When the entire body is wet from the bath, it draws in with

actual greediness the vitality and warmth of the person who is rubbing it dry with the bare hands.

Whoever, therefore, can avail himself of a suitable personality to rub him dry after the natural bath, may under certain circumstances derive great benefit from it, and greatly facilitate the healing of his trouble.

In nature everything depends on action and reaction; the whole universe is held together by mutual attraction and repulsion and consequent exchange.

It is a well-known fact that plants thrive better in company with others than if they stand alone. It has also frequently been observed, among domestic animals, that an individual fares better when stalled and fed in the company of another.

But more than plants and animals are human beings dependent one upon another. Man's whole and perfect happiness lies in social life, in mutual love and support, and much of his health depends upon it. The sick are especially dependent on the love of their healthy fellow-creatures.

It is known that men have often been rejuvenated and wonderfully cured by the influence of other persons. Sick persons, having accidentally come into friendly intercourse with young, healthy persons, soon became well, without knowing the cause of their sudden convalescence. Many have experienced rare benefits with regard to their health on becoming engaged or getting married on the basis of a pure and noble love, which brought about a perfect spiritual harmony between the contracting parties. Much vitality can be communicated by the sleeping together of two persons. By this means old men have often been rejuvenated by young men.* But these instances of rejuvenation

---

*In a book entitled "The Transference of Nerve Force" (infection by health), by C. Buttenstedt, we read of a large number of cases in which wonderful rejuvenation, healing, and even revivification has been effected by the transference of vitality in all periods of life. Buttenstedt deduces from these facts the possibility of regaining health at any time, of rejuvenating our life, and prolonging it at will. He expects very greatly to extend the duration of human life. Butten-

and healing have always been the result of happy accidents and were connected with a great many circumstances.

The way for a general application of this force has not yet been found. But let us only grasp the hand of nature again, she will lead us on to the fountain-head of health and happiness.

As soon as we have found our way to the natural bath, the magic means of the transference of health is always open to us. Almost everybody has a friend or a servant, or knows of some other suitable person with the requisite qualities as above described, who can rub him dry after the bath, or at least assist him in it. But one must always be grateful for this help; it must not be rewarded with hard cash, but with sincere gratitude. Otherwise the result would grow continually less.

Never force a dependent to rub you dry; the person charged with this task must do it willingly and joyfully. We must treat our dependent fellowmen in such a manner that they will lend a helping hand out of love for us.

I need not lay down any special rules for the rubbing after the bath. It is done with the bare hands, and as quietly as possible.

The transference can easily take place from male to female, and *vice-versa*.

But sensuality must hereby in no wise play a part. The persons engaged in the process must remain strictly noble and pure, otherwise the harm will be greater than the gain.

Married people who desire to rub each other dry after the bath must also observe this rule. And it must likewise be borne in mind if vitality is to be transferred through opposite sexes in other ways than after the bath.

When men have been accidentally killed, by lightning and the like, they have frequently been recalled to life by being thoroughly and perseveringly rubbed down by strong healthy persons.

---

stedt furnishes a great deal of important information regarding these matters, even if he aims too high at times.

Besides, Buttenstedt writes very entertainingly and fascinatingly, and his book is well worthy of perusal,

If such rubbing can bring even the dead back to life, it is easily to be seen of what advantage rubbing and stroking must be in strengthening us and in curing our troubles and diseases. Wonderful results may indeed be achieved in many cases.

Let us, therefore, return to nature! A realm of health will then open unto us, a realm of sunshine and earthly happiness. Our weak pulses will soon begin to beat more vigorously, our sick breast will heave with new hope.

LIGHT AND AIR.

Man was created naked by nature, and in the beginning lived naked for a long time. "And they were both naked, the man and his wife."—Gen. 2:25; and according to the intentions of nature he was always to go naked. This is the design of nature which nothing can change.

Going naked is in accordance with nature, and consequently right.

Everybody knows that light-and-air creatures, plants as well as animals, pine away in dark places and become more and more lifeless. But if they are brought to light, they instantly wake up and become full of life. It is as if one could see this, even in plants, which soon regain their healthy color. In the case of animals we can plainly see how they brighten up, jump, and run about.

To-day man lives, clothed as he is, with the greater part of his body in the dark. Let him, for once, throw off his clothes, especially in the open air, in the woods, and he will directly feel how new vigor and life reanimates the body. Immediately all the organs begin to work more vigorously, the digestion, the vitality is increased, and a rapturous sensation of wellbeing passes through the almost lifeless sick organism.

When animals are confined in dark places, the process of transpiration still goes on, *and the internal heat which is developed in sickness is still thrown off,* while the wearing of clothes prevents this in man. *Going naked temporarily,** even in the room with as many open windows as possible, but better still in the open, in the woods, proves of wonderful beneficency and efficacy, and *is more strengthening than any other means.*

The light at once reanimates the vitality of the body, which, moreover, being now entirely free from clothes, need not partly reabsorb through the skin, the bad used-up air which it had thrown off, and can take in more pure air.

This explains the immediate remarkable invigoration of the organism, and the wonderful effect of the light-and-air bath. The importance of the light-and-air bath in the preservation of health, the curing of diseases, acute as well as chronic, and also in the healing of wounds must become evident to even the dullest understanding.

And yet it is hardly ever used even by nature doctors, although it is the simplest and cheapest remedy, and one that is always available.

In acute diseases the greatest danger lies in the *acute fever.* It is therefore always necessary to reduce this.

To-day recourse is first had to water, which is applied in the well-known manner, as cold washes, packs, and the like.

But the fever returns again and again, and increases more and more. In diphtheria the danger of suffocation becomes greater and greater.

The nature doctor himself now grows uneasy and loses his composure.

· Without the wind is howling as if he would call out that he, too, is there; that he, too, has a great and important place to fill in the economy of nature; but the nature doctor does not hear. He leans against the window, the cool air blows in and cools his heated brow, he feels it to be a comfort, but still does not understand what message the breath of air is bringing him.

---

*Going naked temporarily is called in the nature-cure method taking a "light-and-air bath." But I do not see why we cannot speak plain so that everybody can at once understand us.

The patient who during a high fever has lost his reason and understanding (divine gifts often falsely employed), and disregards them, follows once again exclusively his instinct, a sure guide.

The child, stricken with diphtheria, tosses to and fro on his bed. He would throw the covering from him if he could.

The delirious typhoid patient strives with all his energy, which nature seems to have increased in the violent fever, to escape outdoors, but past the water basin in which he had just been immersed in cold water, screaming and chattering—he wants to fly out of the window into the icy air.

Everybody near the patient becomes excited and alarmed. Nature speaks here almost as through earthquake and thunderclaps. But the doctor remains deaf. He did once indeed attentively listen to the croaking voice of the professor who delivered a scientific lecture on the cure of lung troubles and who died a few years later of consumption; but the mighty voice of nature he heeds not. Nor does he understand it.

Full of love, and trembling with anxiety for her suffering darling, the mother sits beside the bed of the child stricken with diphtheria. Again and again she covers him carefully. *Sancta simplicitas! O, saintly simplicity!*

The grown-up typhoid patient is attended during the night by a guard of three or four strong men, so that he may in no case follow the voice of nature.

But although man wilfully rejects her offers, nature is nevertheless intent on showering on him in every possible way and by all means her blessings and benefits.

There is a story of how nature lulled to sleep the watchers, these hirelings of human unreason, so that the patient, without clothes, might escape through the window into the frosty Winter night.

In a neighboring house, it is related, nature resorted to still more drastic measures to save a fever patient: the clear night of Winter was suddenly rent by tremendous thunderclaps, as if God were in wrath.

Suddenly, with a crash, lightning struck the house of the patient. Everything was ablaze. People awoke from their sleep and ran and fled in wild confusion, the patient with the rest, naked as he was.

The bells were tolling, men and women with diseased and excited nerves ran aimlessly hither and thither; one was trying to save his nightcap, another the washbasin with the water.

When they had somewhat regained their senses, they thought of the patients, and started, as they believed, in search of their dead bodies.

However, they found them doing finely, the fever had entirely left them, and to the surprise of everybody they began to improve and grow well from that time.

Nature annihilates with lightning only what is rotten and decayed, only what is *diseased,* and thus sternly punishes disloyalty to her laws.

Lightning does not kill the healthy animals of the forest, but the sick domestic animals and still more sick man.

If all the ignorance and stupidity in the world could be embodied in One Being, and if God should strike it with His lightning, millions upon millions of His children would again become happy creatures and be a pleasure to look upon.

Such and similar stories are related everywhere and of almost every sick chamber.

I am firmly convinced of the actual occurrence of cases in which delirious fever patients have passed some time outdoors, in the severest cold, almost naked, with the happiest results.

I have been positively assured of the actual occurrence of a number of such cases.

On the other hand I am myself aware that many, if not most of such tales, have been exaggerated by popular fancy, if they have not been invented altogether.

But where do we find deeper truths than in popular myths and folklore?

Nor do I doubt that many a patient who in the agony of death rushed into the open, nevertheless died.

As I have already shown, the natural bath is accompanied by the most wonderful effects in the healing of acute diseases, in which it promptly allays the dangerous fever. But obviously the natural bath cannot be employed for as long a time and as frequently as the light-and-air bath, which consists in temporarily walking about in a state of nudity.

Domestic animals which are compelled by man to live very unnatural lives, and which pass their time almost continually in dark, narrow stalls, in the foul atmosphere of their own dung, often feeding on unnatural food, like decayed turnip leaves, etc., frequently fall seriously ill. But we never find among them high, dangerous fevers; we never find that sick animals grow delirious like a typhoid patient.

Every veterinary physician will confirm this; that is if he is not told beforehand that his testimony is to be used in favor of the natural cure.

The diseases of domestic animals would pass off still more mildly if on the appearance of the first symptoms they were driven into the open, in all sorts of weather and temperature, instead of being anxiously shut off from all light and air in narrow, dingy stables.

In men the fever reaches dangerous degrees and often becomes fatal only because the internal heat cannot continually stream out and cannot be kept down by *very cold air*, as is the case among animals which are *naked*.

The heat of the body is reduced by the cold of the air in the same way as a hot liquid is cooled by placing the vessel containing it into cold water.

It ought, therefore, to be the nature doctor's first concern, when he is called to a sick person, to take the clothes or the bedding from his body, and if he cannot take him into the open-air, at least to let him go about or lie naked in the room, with as many windows open as possible, even in the coldest winter day, from fifteen to twenty minutes according to the temperature, or in summer from one to three hours.

In Summer the cool of the morning can be used for this purpose. The colder it is the surer will be the effect.

Egypt was once beset with darkness for three days. It seems as if mankind were to be visited with such an evil for over three thousand years.

Colds! is what every aunt and cousin, every Philistine exclaims, and even the nature doctors cannot entirely free themselves from the fear of them, although they well know that colds, like acute diseases, are nothing but curative crises, and are therefore *under all circumstances* most favorable symptoms, and not only entirely harmless under correct treatment, but always of the greatest benefit to the body.

The weed that has grown rank in their brains at the university, has so entirely overrun them that it can never again be quite eradicated.

Oh! that God would once again send a great man, possessed of all wisdom and the eloquence of angels, to put to flight the fear of colds and of *light and air,* the greatest benefactors of mankind, which could make many a one well and happy again and save many a precious life!

Especially for man, who is the highest of the light-and-air creatures, *light and air* are the true life-elements. According to nature's design he ought to move in them naked, day and night, Winter and Summer.

But since in this respect man has sinned against nature for such a long time, the return to nature here becomes an all the more pressing and immediate necessity. It is greatly to be regretted that man cannot yet manage to go naked for a sufficiently long time to secure the full benefits of light and air. How can he ever do too much in this respect? Can he go naked longer than day and night Summer and Winter?

It is a mistake to assume that man was originally covered with hair and that now, having lost his hairy fur, he cannot be without clothes. Only very few human beings (individual, rare exceptions) are hairy; the rest, including men who have hitherto lived entirely, or almost entirely, naked, are not hairy. The hands, the forehead, the neck, and other parts of the body which have so far remained free from clothes, are without hair. Nature has surely fitted out man, the highest of her creatures, with a naked skin for the reason that he should come into most direct contact with light and air, the preservers of all higher life. He must, therefore, now suffer all the more from the wearing of clothes, and has so much more to gain from going naked.

The very circumstance that light and air cause colds proves how very much they stimulate the vitality, and as draughts and cold air are the most fruitful source of colds we see that they are the most favorable and best means for curing diseases.

The reason for the provision of cold, of Winter, in nature is to interrupt the fermentations of the earth, of plant and animal life, to kill all bacilli, bacteriæ, microbes, tubercles, and such like organisms. But such an effect is to be desired above all in the sick body of man.

Many a person could soon kill the organisms producing the itch if he would only go naked in the open air on cold Winter days, just as many consumptives could by such a light-and-air bath most surely kill the bacilli in their lungs after awhile, which are the product of the foreign matter fermenting there.

The weak and the sick, more than the healthy and strong, are the very persons who are in need of such a cooling down of the inner heat and a strengthening of their vitality. They ought to be persuaded, therefore, to take the light-and-air bath above all things else and in every kind of weather and at all temperatures.

When I once asked a nature doctor why the light-and-air bath was in such little use, especially in fevers, he replied: "There really have not been enough experiments made with it as yet."

The course in our high schools and colleges lasts many years, a course of medicine requires five years, and in this long time, which for the sake of greater proficiency is even extended by most students, not enough "formal education" has been acquired to enable a "thinking" nature doctor to conclude from his own observation of the processes in nature and from the important part which light and air, warmth and cold play there, and without the aid of previous experiments, that the light-and-air bath is the most *harmless* (! ! !), the most effective, and indeed the very best means for the preservation of health and the cure of diseases, both acute and chronic!

However, I can assure such timid men that the many trials which I have made with the light-and-air bath, in the most varied cases of sickness, have yielded splendid results, as I well knew beforehand.

For the most part, after I had explained matters to them, the patients submitted willingly and gladly to the light-and-air bath from the start.

Young people as well as old, who had become exceedingly delicate from the wearing of much woollen underclothing and by shutting themselves off from light and air in other ways, went at once and without passing through intermediate stages naked into the open air, *in wind and weather, in rain and snow storms, even at low temperatures.*

Some were so weak that they could hardly walk to the place where the light-and-air bath was to be taken. Directly they were naked they began to feel stronger, and could always walk home more easily and quickly than they had come. There were among these light-and-air bathers not only some very weak, but also some very old and venerable people, over seventy and eighty years of age.

In acute diseases, especially in high fevers, the patients always experienced such a refreshing, strengthening effect that they would not leave the open window even on the most urgent pleading of frightened relatives. In one case even cold air of fifteen degrees Reaumur was streaming in at the window upon the completely naked body.

The improvement and convalescence, especially in acute cases, was so rapid and striking that the people about the patient were full of astonishment.

At Jungborn it was in the cool season especially that the light-and-air baths created the greatest enthusiasm,

In speaking about cold light-and-air baths, moreover, the thing sounds much worse than it is, just as a storm appears much more uncanny to us when we are sitting in a warm room than when we are sitting right in the midst of it.

One does, indeed, gain a good deal of bodily warmth and energy through the light-and-air bath, so that it becomes more and more easy to take, and seems less extraordinary as we go along. Of course, the light and air bath on beautiful Summer mornings is the most pleasurable; first the delightful coolness of the fresh morning, then the warm sunshine, and again the agreeable change of a cool shade. But we must take our light-and-air bath as we can have it, and in Winter there is the advantage that the cooling off is much more powerful and does not require so much time as in Summer.

After what I have said of the light-and-air bath there is, I suppose, no longer any need of assuring a reasonable person that in *no* case has there been any bad effect from it. In a few cases of very serious chronic disease, I could indeed have wished that a bad cold or some other acute disease had been contracted. I should surely have taken advantage of that for the good of the patient, but I have not yet had the good fortune to experience such a favorable case. If a cold does set in, it becomes still more important to continue diligently to take the light-and-air baths. The vitality is in this manner raised more and more, increasing the body's ability to throw off foreign matter, while at the same time the heat that is thus produced is cooled, so that the patient experiences no distress, but soon feels relieved.

It is absolutely necessary that the nature doctor should be perfectly clear in his own mind with regard to the light-and-air bath, and should remain perfectly calm. If a cold should frighten him, and he should now shut the patient off from the air in a warm room, and perhaps even have recourse to medicines, the body would be weakened, the foreign matter that has been set in motion is obstructed, and the cold can so become very disagreeable, even dangerous.

But certainty and quiet wins, as I always convince myself, the layman first. Therefore let every one try first for himself the light-and-air bath and then for his family, trusting to wise nature and her beneficent means more than to the advice of erring men.

I have often marveled how men, and women as well, in consequence of the wonderful effect experienced from the light-and-air bath, continued it with true enthusiasm, not only in Summer, but even in Winter before an open window.

It is not the fault of the public if the light-and-air bath is not generally introduced, but of the Naturopaths alone. For the people are not educated to think for themselves in caring for their health, but always to hear without judging what is preached to them.

It is most natural and best to go naked day and night, Summer and Winter, taking the light-air bath without interruption The old Teutons in our part of the country went almost entirely naked, with a loose hide at most thrown around the shoulders.

This was even more true, in proportion as they clung to nature in their diet, subsisting on the fruits of the forest, in addition to only on milk, and, to be sure, on meat, but on the meat of healthy animals, and not on the *increasingly artificial preparations* of agricultural products, nor on alcohol and other stimulants.

But what man among the present effeminate, and enervated generation could still continuously go naked, even if there were no other difficulties in the matter? Therefore each must decide for himself how long and how often, according to the temperature and opportunity and time at his disposal, he can take the light-and-air bath. The dictum here is: *the more and the longer the better.*

Much more effective than in the room, of course, is the light-and-air bath in the open, in the woods. In our forests there are countless places where one can take it undisturbed early in the morning, which in summer is the most appropriate time. Where there is a will, there will also be found an opportunity and a way for the light-and-air bath.*

Public bathing places offer a very favorable opportunity for light-and-air bathing in the open. There one can at any time go naked unmolested, as long as he likes, of course, with bathing trunks. It would be the simplest thing to enlarge our public water-bathing institutions and make arrangements for light-and-air bathing.

But those who have no opportunity for light-and-air bathing in the open, especially women, can take it daily in the room by open windows, in summer as well as in winter. One can, of course, begin with it on the very coldest days. Especially children ought to have a light-and-air bath from the day of their birth,—if in the room, preferably in the morning on rising. They will soon delight and revel in it. In this way a hale and hearty generation may yet perhaps arise. It is advisable not to wear any clothing whatever during the light-and-air bath, no shoes and stockings, no bathing trunks, etc.

In cold weather, especially, one ought to take a great deal of exercise during the light-and-air bath by walking and running.

It is of course peremptory to become thoroughly warm again after the light-and-air bath. This is best accomplished by brisk walking or by physical work, also by housework, or by wrapping in woollen blankets or bedding.

It is a mistake to think that the light-and-air bath is taken for the purpose of feeling colder. We take it in order to feel warmer at all other times, for it is well known that he suffers most from cold who is always sitting about a warm stove.

The effect of going naked in the room is most excellent.

If the natural bath, including a wash of the entire body and a thorough rubbing, is taken before the light-and-air bath, the blood is forced to the extremities and to the surface of the

---

*At night also the body takes in purer air and is cooled during the light-and-air bath. Therefore it may also be taken at night.

skin, and the light-and-air bath can be endured more easily and for a longer time. One trial will confirm me in this.

It is also very beneficial, besides taking the light-and-air bath, to go bareheaded in the rain.

Besides taking the light-and-air bath, one ought to go *barefooted* whenever there is time and opportunity for it.

Drying with towels after a water-application, also after bathing the head and going barefooted, is contrary to nature and ought to be dispensed with.

One ought to take as much exercise as possible in the open air.

The windows in the bed-room must always be open at night, Winter and Summer.

One kind of light-and-air bathing is the sunbath. You lie on the ground, preferably in the woods, without clothing. But if the sun is very warm, novices must protect themselves against burning by a covering of porous cloth, or still better, fresh leaves and branches.

Farther on I shall explain how one can protect himself best against getting burned, by rubbing the body with moist earth. Getting sunburned is not really harmful and dangerous, but it may become very painful and unpleasant. It is therefore advisable to avoid as far as one may the scorching of the body by the sun. But if it should nevertheless occur, the remedy to be applied is cold water and wet compresses (also compresses of moist earth). The customary oils and salves should be avoided.

In the hot sun the sunbath must not last too long. One can take the light-and-air bath by alternating between sun and shade.

It is of great importance that the sunbath should be taken lying on the earth, not on mattresses or even roofs, as has been sometimes done. Man belongs to the earth.

I shall speak more in detail also of the great influence which the mere earth exerts on man in all cases where he comes into direct contact with it.

A2

If there is no opportunity to take the light-and-air bath naked, the next best thing is to take it only lightly dressed in the open or in one's room, as the case may be. The face should always be protected against the sun.

After the sunbath one must always see to the cooling of the body by means of the natural bath.

LIGHT-AND-AIR HUTS AND COTTAGES.

One great benefit to health comes from sleeping in huts and cottages situated entirely in the open, and which at all

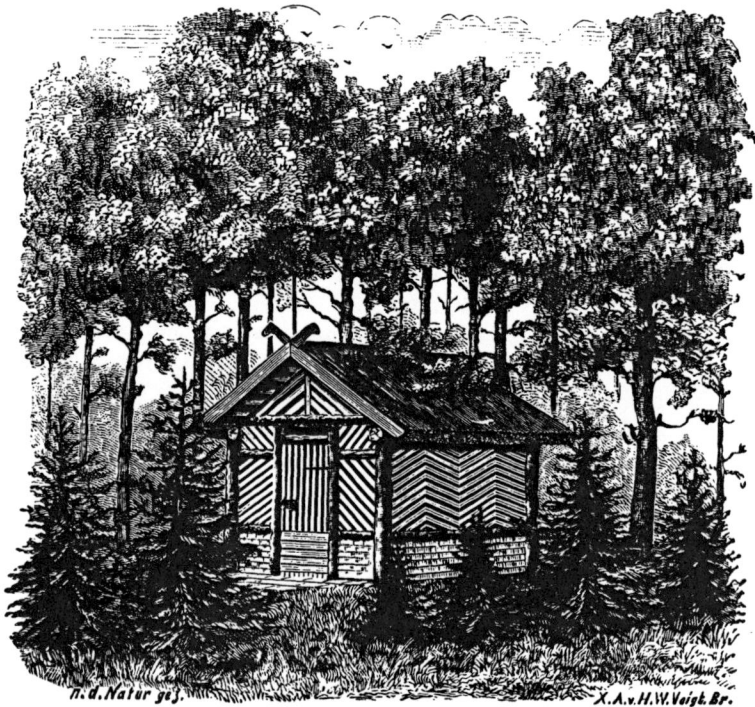

Light and Air Hut in a Woodpark, Near Brunswick, Germany.

times offer free access to light and air.

We call them *light-and-air huts* and *light-and-air cottages*, but there is nothing about them in the way of appointments that would make of them special hygienic apparatuses and institutions.

They are huts with a roof to keep the rain from coming through, but without walls, or only lattice walls. For protection against stormy weather they are provided with curtains. For winter (for they may be used also at this season) they can be kept warm and made to keep out the snow by means of straw and partition walls penetrable by the air.

It is still better to erect more perfect cottages, with thicker walls, adapted to real dwelling purposes. But they must be sufficiently provided with windows, blinds, ventilators, etc., to permit the ingress, when open, of plenty of fresh air. "The ceiling must be provided with ventilators which may be opened when windows and doors are closed." I refer to the illustrations of the light-and-air huts of Jungborn.

Pure, fresh air is required by the body especially in the night, when it is chiefly engaged in the work of digestion. Therefore sleeping in such a hut is very important. More than is at present the case, owners of gardens, parks, and woods ought to build such light-and-air huts and cottages for dwelling purposes.

The rooms of houses, even if they are in the woods, are apt to be penetrated with the odors from the cellar, the kitchen, closets, garbage heaps, etc. The air is vitiated, moreover, by the circumstance that several, often many persons live in a house side by side, and below and above one another, and that stone walls retain foul odors a long time. They are therefore never filled with entirely pure, unvitiated air. But this is the case in light-and-air huts.

Absolutely pure air is of the greatest importance in the healing of all diseases, whether catarrh or typhoid fever, cholera, rheumatism, cancer or scurvy, a fresh wound or a running, open sore.*

---

*While speaking of the great importance of pure, unvitiated air I want to call attention to another very dangerous enemy in our pres-

Health is the foundation of all happiness, man can enjoy earthly pleasures only in the measure of his health. Only when this shall have come to be more widely recognized, will people begin to appreciate and build light-and-air cottages.

Living or sleeping in one of these beautiful cottages, surrounded by nature, will then no longer be a matter for surprise, but will be regarded as infinitely preferable to occupying dark and dingy apartments in cities, poisoned by foul odors, the breeding places of all diseases which not alone weaken and undermine the body, but are also the cause of all the defects of the mind and soul, of idiocy and insanity, of lust and self-abuse, of vice, and crime, of hate and envy, of contention and strife, in short, of all the ills of the earth.

One need not be afraid of freezing in one of these open light-and-air cottages during low temperature. In the open, in the woods one can sleep very comfortably in a light-and-air cottage during the coldest winter, if one has only a few feather beds or quilts, because the body develops more heat when breathing pure, fresh air than it does when breathing the foul and stuffy air in houses.

The light-and-air cottage protects the sleeper and his clothing during the night against rain. During fair weather it is advisable to place the bed outside the cottage and sleep entirely

---

ent mode of living—I mean **gas light**. In apartments with gas fixtures, even if gas is not used, flowers never thrive; they soon begin to wilt and finally die. Shrubs and trees along promenades and in parks in the neighborhood of gas mains likewise often die. The smallest quantities of gas escaping from the stops and fixtures affect the organism most injuriously. The bad, poisonous air of the cities originates largely from the gas works. The pallor and poor health of office workers are chiefly caused by gas. In sanitaria and hospitals gas is a thing unknown. Any other kind of light (petroleum, etc.), is less injurious than gas light. The electric light is, of course, superior to all the others. It is to be regretted only that where there is no water power for the production of electric light, recourse must be had to steam, whereby the nuisance of smoke-stacks belching forth enormous masses of dense, suffocating smoke is still more increased.

in the open. To this end take a strawtick or a quilt (woollen or cotton) covered with coarse linen or thick burlap for mattress, and a quilt for covering, so that the whole outfit can be easily transported, and place the mattress on the ground.

We shall thus soon become aware that nature rewards every step that is taken toward her, for it is still more beneficial and healthful to sleep entirely in the open than in a light-and-air hut.

In the open where we can soar unhindered to the stars, and where soft zephyrs waft about us, beautiful nights are truly enchanting, and all the infirmities of the body and soul heal quickly.

> Dann gehet leise
> Nach seiner weise,
> Der liebe Herrgott durch den Wald.

> With footsteps holy
> Then walketh slowly
> Our beloved Lord through the woods.

Seriously considered there is nothing ostentatious or ridiculous when a man once more puts up his bed outside of a house, entirely in the open, where hare and deer, stag and boar, and so many others of God's creatures retain and preserve their clear, bright eyes, their physical activity and strength, their perfect health, that precious talent which the Lord has entrusted to them. These do not do as the men who to-day neglect their health, yes, even trample it under foot, so that their entire earthly existence is embittered by misery and disease and it will be difficult for them in the time to come to account for the talent entrusted to them. We shall soon see farther on how sleeping on the bare ground is a most natural and healthy practice.

I must observe also that light frame dwelling houses are more healthful than those built more massively.

More small houses ought to be built again, surrounded by

gardens and trees, if possible. Our present large, barrack-like houses with thick stone walls in narrow, stuffy streets are obviously not conducive to health.

In cities, therefore, people ought to try to live on the outskirts.

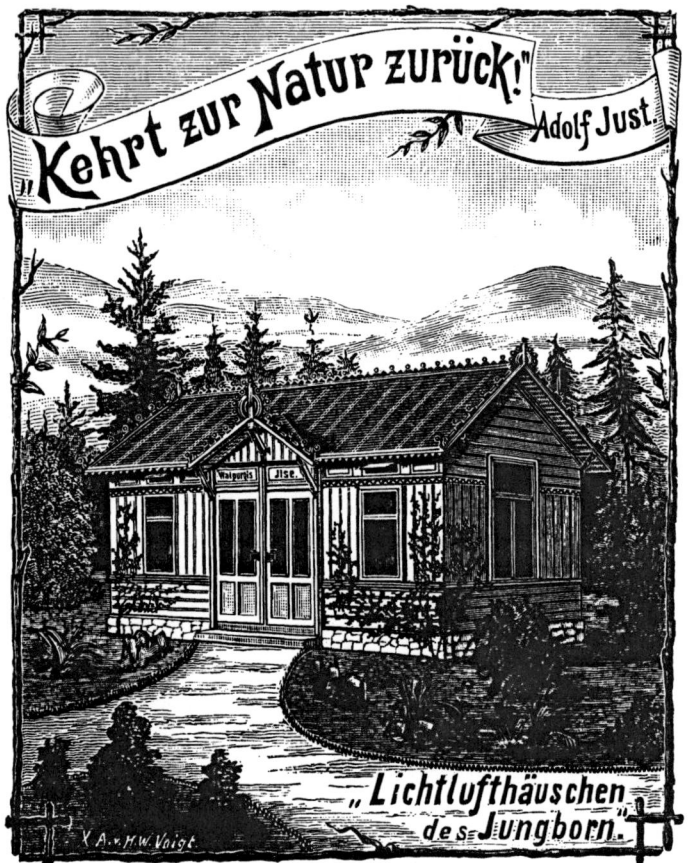

Light-Air Cottage in Jungborn, Germany.

Dwelling houses ought always to be so built and the rooms so arranged that very much light and air can at all times stream in.

So-called architectural beauty need not, therefore, be neglected. But here, too, it were well to aspire towards greater naturalness and simplicity.

OUR CLOTHING.

According to the intentions of nature man should go naked; his body is constructed for this mode of life. If this were not so, he would have perished before the time came when he had invented the requisite tools and machinery for the making of clothes. Therefore, strictly speaking, man ought not to wear any clothes whatever.

All dress with which we drape the nude body only for a moment is contrary to nature, and always injures health. We no longer have any idea of man's original state of health, of his physical and spiritual powers, the duration of his life, and his higher capacity for happiness; and for this reason we do not recognize what inconceivable harm the wearing of clothes and the consequent deprivation of the body of light and air have brought to mankind.

There are to-day still a number of nations within the temperate zone who go naked the year round, Summer and Winter (for instance, the Fire Islanders and others). But a few years ago the newspapers published accounts of a European—a certain Captain Schmidt—who went naked during his voyages in all zones.

I suppose I need not here enter into the reasons why we cannot at present expect that all men should suddenly go naked again.

But it is of great importance that in the choice and construction of our clothing we should strive to allow as much light and air as possible to have access to the body, and to offer as few obstacles as possible to the transpiration of the skin.

Of late a sufficient variety of porous material for men and women's clothing has been put on the market, but the garments must not only be very porous and airy, they must also fit the body very loosely.

No one need to-day dress so peculiarly and in such poor taste as to attract attention, but neither need he be the slave of an absurd fashion or place any value on beautiful clothes.

It has indeed been observed that "fine clothes make fine men." This is very discouraging. But let us hope that a better opinion may yet prevail later, and that we may yet learn to appreciate higher things.

Many different kinds of *health shirts* have made their appearance. They are still very faulty. I cannot recommend woollen shirts, for wool worn next to the body makes the skin too tender. No one would ever think of covering or bandaging a wound or ulcer with wool. But what is bad for the injured or sick skin cannot be very good for the sound skin.

Many cotton shirts are still not porous enough; often they shrink upon washing and become like felt.

Linen shirts, also, besides being too heavy, are often not porous enough.

Some shirts are too fine and thin, and consequently adhere too closely to the skin.

And in many health shirts the quality of durability leaves still much to be desired.

All these faults must be considered when buying shirts— this important article of clothing of the present.

At Jungborn *Mahr's* shirts are worn, in the manufacture of which many of my wishes have been considered by the manufacturer.

These JUNGBORN SHIRTS are in great favor and have so far

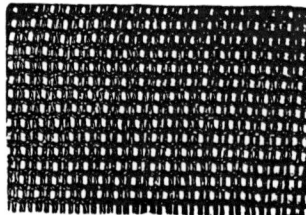

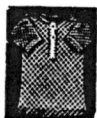

Net or Air Cell Shirt.

answered their purpose in every way. The accompanying figure shows the material of which they are made. It is VERY POROUS AND NOT TOO FINE, so that the shirt does not cling too closely to the body. It is cream colored, but might as well be white, of course. In illustrating the material, I wished merely to give a sample of a design.

Above all, people sin against their feet to-day. The feet excrete more morbid matter than any other part of the body, as is shown by their perspiration. Therefore the feet ought to be uncovered at frequent intervals. Unfortunately the very reverse is the case at present. The feet are squeezed into tight leather shoes, to the greatest agony and injury of the people's health.

LEATHER SHOES ought not to be made tight fitting. Cloth —that is, canvas—shoes are much more healthful than leather shoes. Canvas shoes can be had everywhere nowadays. Rubber and leather are especially bad for the skin. Therefore leather shoes, leather gloves, rubber suspenders and the like ought to be avoided. Thin cotton STOCKINGS are better than woollen ones.

GLOVES ought to be dispensed with entirely, but if they must be worn preference should be given to thread and worsted gloves. SUSPENDERS, also, are to be had of strong, elastic cotton material. This is the kind worn at the Jungborn.

Above all, people should go BAREFOOTED again.

There are, of course, still many prejudices to be overcome before we can go barefooted again without attracting attention. But we should not be too timid in this respect, but take courage and boldly set a good example, for we are thereby advancing a great and important cause. Such a cause deserves sacrifice, and we shall soon find followers.

If we lack the courage to go barefooted in the streets of our cities, we ought at least to do it in the country, on walking tours, etc.

But every one can certainly go with bare feet in *open* SANDALS in his own house, his own room, and in this manner one may enjoy splendid comfort.

I for my part cannot see why the wearing of sandals should

not be beautiful. The ancient Greeks, and the kings of antiquity whom we see pictured with sandals looked stately indeed. Present-day sandals still have many faults. They sometimes rub and press the foot. The Jungborn sandals, which have been made according to my directions, and are shown on the accompanying cut, are free from these defects. They leave the foot free, as far as that is possible, and are comfortable. This cut, too, may serve as a pattern.

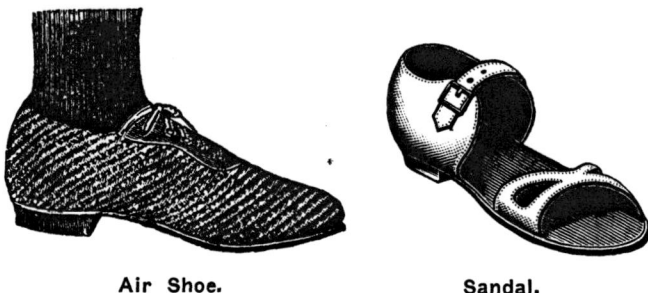

Air Shoe. **Sandal.**

TROUSERS were held in great contempt among the ancients. Whoever wore trousers was considered a barbarian. The toga, a loose garment with rich folds, was looked upon as the genteel dress.

Nevertheless the men of to-day will probably not soon exchange their trousers for a toga or any other simple cloak. It is not easy to attempt anything against this preference. But men might at least discard their drawers and other underwear.

It is, however, quite incomprehensible why women and girls, even very little girls, should wear drawers. I don't want to inveigh against the custom here too strongly, but I am firmly convinced that many female troubles, womb troubles, difficult labor, hysterics, etc., would not occur if women did not wear drawers, and if the air could circulate around the abdomen.

Let who will act accordingly.

A terrible monster has found refuge in the wardrobe of our girls and women—the CORSET.

The old instruments of torture which are exhibited as the relics of past times, and which are intended to prove the cruelty which men were once capable of, do not impress me as more terrible than the corset of the present day. The aforesaid instruments of torture, moreover, were employed for the punishment of great criminals, who suffered torture under compulsion; our girls and women, however, compress their body by means of

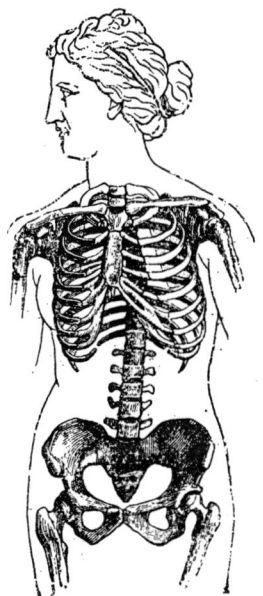
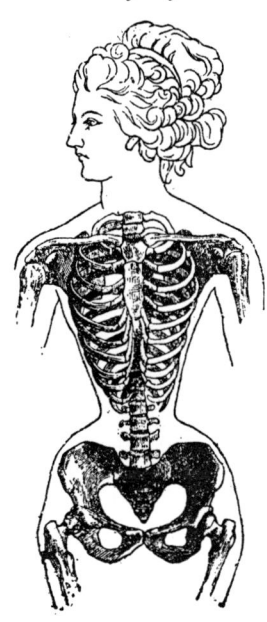

Natural size of waist.   Reduced size, caused by tight lacing.

the corset until they can hardly breathe, and so commit this cruelty against themselves voluntarily. This is a strange riddle.

Women have gradually become accustomed to their sufferings; therefore they can hardly realize them any more. But in reality no less suffering is occasioned by the corset than was once caused by the old instruments of torture.

Much has been said and written against the corset, but mostly in vain. I shall not waste any more words on the subject. As long as fainting fits, hysterics, and all sorts of weakness and misery are taken for joy and happiness, and pale, pitiable figures are looked upon as models of beauty, the corset will continue to hold sway.

When men shall have been sufficiently punished for their follies in this regard, God will surely let them come to an understanding of themselves.

There are nowadays plenty of suspenders and similar expedients, of which women can avail themselves if they wish to wear loose garments which shall in no way compress the body and in the least impede the free circulation of the blood.

The so-called LUISEN-COSTUMES (named after Queen Luise of Prussia) would most nearly meet hygienic requirements.

It is time the swaddling-cloth, in which new-born babies are placed and whereby they are from the start seriously injured in their development, were discarded.

Children have much more vitality and animal heat than adults. They can stand being naked a great deal better than older people.

They instinctively seek to throw off their clothes entirely at frequent intervals. They are in a state of exultation whenever their swaddling-bands and clothes are removed. Let us, therefore, heed the voice of nature and allow the children frequently to lie and go about naked. But always have them lightly dressed.

If you will cease to be too solicitous with regard to their clothing, good mother, your children will one day be very grateful to you. Their gratitude will be greater than you can imagine.

Going BAREFOOTED is the greatest joy of children. Let us allow them this joy, and not be unreasonable by restraining them from following the paths that lead away from the modern diseases and sufferings and an early grave. If we are reasonable in this regard, they will no longer in the future cause us so much anxiety, sorrow, and bitter suffering.

But why do mothers, without knowing it, turn their tender love into hard cruelty, and deny to their children—their greatest treasure on earth—the purest joys which nature holds out to them, causing them thereby suffering and bitter woe their whole life long? Who can solve this riddle?

Let us only look at the fresh and hearty street urchins in the country and at the gipsy children who go barefooted and wear scant clothing, ragged and more than porous, allowing the wind to whistle through. After that no one need any longer be in doubt as to what to do to keep children healthy.

Going BAREHEADED is likewise a good practice, alike for children and for adults. Why do we take off our hat on saluting a person, or on serious, solemn occasions, for instance, at church, at funerals, or at prayer? A still, small voice yet reminds us that covering the head, the seat of intelligence in man, is contrary to the intentions of nature, to God's command, and consequently sinful. On solemn occasions we involuntarily refrain from committing this sin.

Nature originally adorned the head of man with long, wavy, curly hair, which especially in woman ought to envelop the beautiful body in long, golden tresses. But man abuses this wonderful, natural adornment when he covers his head. He destroys it, moreover, and that is very foolish and sinful. The head of the Saviour never wore a covering; it was adorned only by a crown of thorns.

The more thoroughly the head is covered, the more does the hair suffer, until it entirely disappears.

Here it is plainly seen that instead of becoming more handsome we grow more homely when we destroy the ornament of nature, for a *bald pate* is certainly homely.*

Hats and caps should be light and porous, with no leather inside of them. They may be provided on the inside with strips

---

*All who desire to regain better hair must live according to nature (water, light, air, diet), and leave the head uncovered whenever possible. Temporary earth compresses (see farther on), by which foreign matter is withdrawn from the skin of the head, will prove serviceable. The natural treatment will provide the hair with more favorable conditions for its development.

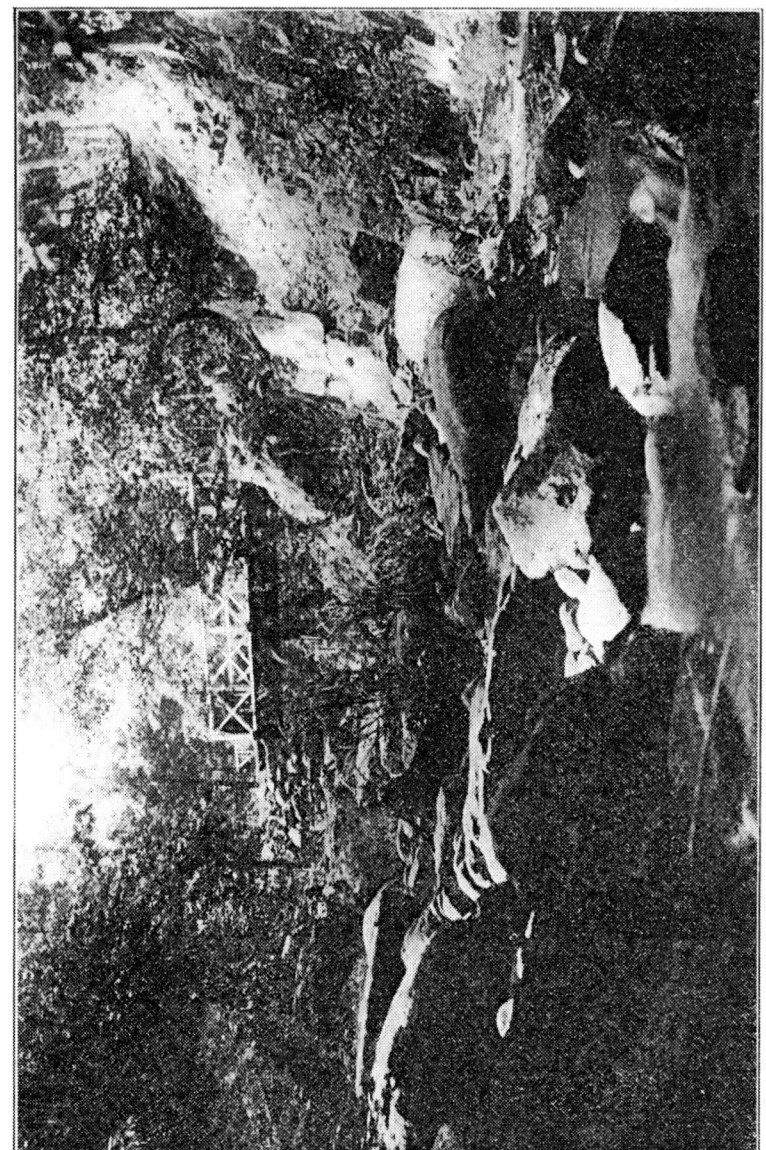

Brook in the American "Jungborn" Park, Bellevue, Butler, N. J.

of cloth (woollen). But it is advisable to avail one's self of every opportunity for going bareheaded.

In our houses and rooms the head ought to remain uncovered. And we should always go bareheaded on getting outside the city limits.

If men could only be prevailed upon to once more go barefooted, bareheaded, and if possible with a bare breast, like sailors, an incalculable gain would be theirs. They would thereby take an immense step toward nature, and a great breach would be made in the endless ranks of chronic diseases.

Nevertheless we need never go so scantily clothed as to be always cold and to make one's life miserable.

If we will only in every way begin to live a more natural life, we shall gradually acquire so much animal heat, that we shall gladly, and of our own accord, discard one warm piece of clothing after another. We shall not only be able to easily do without them then, they will even become oppressive.

Many a person, on merely hearing of a natural life, will anxiously think of the many clothes, furniture, and the like, which have hitherto brought him comfort and enjoyment, and which in future he will have to discard. But this is an entirely false fear.

Let everyone for the present keep his clothes and enjoy his other comforts. But in returning to nature many of these attributes of civilization will gradually become not only superfluous, but more and more an uncomfortable burden. They will then be cheerfully discarded, and the greater simplicity and freedom from wants will be sure to create increased joy and happiness.

Therefore let us return to nature! We shall thus enter upon the way that leads to gladness and joy, to happy simplicity and freedom from wants.

Clothes are required to-day only because of our effeminacy and because without them we cannot live and move in society without giving offence and causing embarrassment. This is the purpose that clothes serve for, as far as necessary, otherwise they are of not the least use to us.

We should not wish to shine and charm by our clothes, or to gain through them any factitious value.

Thus we shall no longer feel the same concern about our clothes, and they will become indifferent to us. They will no longer worry us so much, or take up so much of our time and thought, and this will, indeed, be a great relief.

We shall especially no longer care to stick and hang rings, bracelets, chains, and other gewgaws on our limbs and about our body.

. Jesus, the world's Saviour, exhorts His followers not to wear two coats, and He says further:

"He that hath two coats, let him impart to him that hath none."

Jesus would have pursued a false course, as did all mortals who came before Him and after Him and strove to make men happy once more and pleasing to God, if He had not above all led them back to nature. The Saviour and His teachings would in that case long ago have been engulfed in the sea of oblivion, just as those philosophers and sages have been forgotten who did not recognize the claims of nature.

In Jesus' time there was a small sect, called the Essenes by their contemporaries, of whom the Roman historians Josephus and Philo give us an account. These Essenes lived strictly natural lives, partly as hermits in the desert and on the mountains. In this manner they hoped to live a joyous, happy life on earth, free from sickness and want, and thus to prepare themselves for heaven.

The teachings of these Essenes, as the historians report them, have so much in common with the teachings of Jesus, as they are handed down to us through the New Testament, that an unbiased and unprejudiced mind cannot resist the conclusion that Jesus was an Essene. Even theologians do not deny it.

I shall return to this later. Now the historians inform us that the Essenes avoided every superfluity and always possessed only one white cloak, their sole bodily attire. This cloak evidently served the purpose of supplying the most indispensable covering for the body. The Essenes did not wish to give themselves a handsome appearance, or to charm and shine by means of their dress. Therefore they wore their one cloak until it was entirely used up, and could no longer supply the most necessary covering for the body. Not until then did they provide themselves with a new cloak.

The frequent teachings of Jesus in regard to a natural mode of living have in the course of time almost been obliterated, or are entirely overlooked, or receive at least only a very superficial symbolic interpretation.

In truth, however, the injunction, "He that hath two coats let him impart to him that hath none," was meant by Jesus to be understood in the same sense in which it was understood by the Essenes, and was meant to be taken literally. Strictly speaking, therefore, every Christian ought to give away all his many clothes to the poor, and keep absolutely only one garment for himself.

Everyone must decide for himself, of course, how far under existing conditions and opinions he can go in the way of wearing a dress according to the requirements of nature and the teachings of the Saviour that is least injurious to health, and to what degree he can attain to simplicity and freedom from wants in the matter of clothing.

But in getting new clothes we ought at least to begin more and more to consider the demands of hygiene, and to have more regard for simplicity, especially in the dress of women. When all is said and done, plain and simple clothes appeal more to the sense of beauty than all our present insane fashions.

The women who dress in a plain and simple manner, and do not make of themselves thoughtless slaves of fashion, but rather defy fashion, can only be the gainers. They will in this way everywhere be sure of sympathy and respect.

But let us no longer do homage to sinful vanity.

All who strive to make themselves attractive by means of costly clothes ought to heed the words of the Saviour:

"Consider the lilies of the field! And yet I say unto you, that even Solomon in all his glory was not arrayed like one of these."—Matt. 6:28.

Only nature is beautiful, whatever is unnatural is ugly.

The flowers of the field, the squirrel in the woods that sprightly and joyously flits from tree to tree, the graceful deer that gayly skips over brush and stone, the bird in bright plumage that merrily sings its song—all are beautiful. Beautiful, too, was the Grecian woman, adorned by her flowing hair and the magnificent symmetry of her limbs, and robed in a light, flowing garment. The beauty of the Samoan women is greatly celebrated to-day,—these children of nature who but scantily clad roam the forests of their island in perfect innocence and guilelessness and with most charming grace, subsisting almost entirely on the fruits which nature still offers profusely and freely.

But dudes and fops, those prematurely old youths with bald pates, pointed shoes, monocles, and other foppery, are ugly and disgusting.

Ugly and repulsive, too, are those anæmic girls and women, resembling ghosts and scarecrows, who with laced bodies, riggings on their heads, with dangling and clinking chains, rings and spangles, walk the streets and boulevards of our cities. There is nothing winning about them, they rather offend every true and natural feeling.

Jesus went into the minutest detail in laying down His precepts. He forbade His disciples even the use of a cane:

"Provide neither two coats, neither shoes, nor yet staves."—Matt. 10:10.

It is more natural and, therefore, more healthful to walk without a cane. Nature is very strict, indeed. Whoever will give proper heed to it will himself feel that it is more beneficial for the body to walk without a cane.

But not only in our clothes, also in the way of furnishing

our houses there prevails to-day much luxury that is unnatural and injurious to health.

In this respect we have also departed very far from that original state of nature when men dwelled under God's dome, under the starry heavens, under the shady canopy of trees, and sat and reclined on the bare earth. Nature herself then undertook the furnishing of the home, she used flowers, shrubs, and trees.

In the first place upholstered furniture ought to be shunned and discarded. In sitting and lying on soft bolsters certain parts of the body become overheated. Blood will accumulate in these parts, and cause disturbances of the circulation, weariness and languor, effeminacy and enervation generally. I for my part could never understand how people could really feel comfortable in a room stuffed with the most luxuriant upholstered furniture, which is at the same time the best of dust traps. Upholstered furniture might be replaced by rattan furniture with cane seats. Simple wooden chairs, benches and tables, such as one formerly found exclusively in the country, are better than upholstered furniture.

Much absurd usage prevails also in the decoration of windows. In the country people formerly never put up any sort of curtain or shade before a window. The light could stream in unhindered and continuously, and this was right. In refined families it seems to be considered a pity that houses have windows through which the light can enter, and they seem to deem it necessary to drape them.

They, consequently, not only provide the windows with shades which may be drawn together in case we wish to shut off the view of the interior from passersby, they also drape them with thick, impenetrable material which darkens the room permanently. But in this way the rooms are not only made unwholesome, but also uncomfortable.

If the windows must be decorated, why not use some transparent material, arranged in a way, moreover, to bar out as little light and sun from the room as possible.

I want to devote a few words in this place to our BEDS. Man passes nearly half his time in bed. In bed he expects to recuperate, to gather strength, and to further his health. A great deal more attention ought therefore to be paid to beds, so that they may be made to conform to the requirements of nature.

In the first place the bed, also, ought to allow the air to circulate freely. The outside air must mingle freely with the air under the bed-covers, which has become vitiated by the transpiration of the body. The feather-beds of to-day make this mingling of the air exceedingly difficult. Feather-beds ought to be discarded, therefore. Woollen quilts make the best covering. The cover that is next to the body ought to be rather thin, so as to more easily fold itself around the body. The quilts ought to be covered with very porous material. Under such woollen covers the body develops a more agreeable warmth.

For a mattress the old-fashioned strawtick is most appropriate. Straw enables the air to circulate freely, is very warming, without heating unnaturally. But it would not do to let a straw fall on the carpet of our present-day elegant bed-chambers. Therefore the old-fashioned strawtick will not, presumably, be admitted again.

But mattresses may also be made of other vegetable material, such as soft seagrass, oat chaff, and the like. Mattresses are best made entirely of wool like the quilts. Horse-hair and wool may be used. Horse-hair will prevent the wool from becoming so matted together from pressure in the course of time as to keep the air from passing through.

The head should not be raised during sleep by means of pillows, or only very little.

It is greatly to be recommended to lie entirely *naked* under the covers (*without a shirt*). One is much warmer in bed without a shirt than with one.

Airy mattresses are already in the market. Everyone is in a position to gradually replace individual parts of his old bedding by more hygienic pieces.

THE EARTH-POWER.

The fish belongs to the water, here alone can it live and thrive. The bird is destined for the air,—that is its realm. "Wie im Reich der Luefte, Koenig ist der Weih" (as the hawk is king in the realm of the air). If the bird wants to rest, it alights on a tree; it rarely touches the earth. (Of course, I do not here speak of the land fowl.)

But man walks on the earth.

As long as man wore no shoes or clothes, he was always in direct touch with the earth, both when he moved and when he rested.

This direct connection with the earth was originally in no wise disturbed.

Such a close connection of man with the earth is therefore the intention of nature. It corresponds, moreover, to a holy, inviolable law of nature, the transgression of which will always sternly be avenged.

In my earnest and untiring efforts to return more and more to nature, to penetrate more and more to a knowledge of her laws, in order to place it in the service of my fellow-men, I have made this discovery, which will certainly prove of the utmost significance.

I observed plainly that going barefooted in the room and on boards was in no wise so effective, so refreshing, and so invigorating as going barefooted on the bare earth, even if the sand or the turf was completely dry. Foresters and forest laborers have assured me that it agrees much better with them, and that they derived much more strength from their rest if they lay directly on the earth in the woods instead of on a bench or other contrivance.

We still possess a splendid treasure of myths from the time of the old Greeks. Among them is the story of Antæus.

When the giant Hercules was in the service of Eurystheus, he was ordered to fetch the golden apples of the Hesperides. But the golden apples of the Hesperides were guarded by the giant Antæus, the son of Geea, the earth goddess. Hercules closed with Antæus, and during the struggle Hercules observed that Antæus always was refreshed and strong when he stood upon the earth, but became weak and powerless as soon as he was separated from the earth and lifted into the air. Therefore Hercules lifted Antæus high up into the air, where he could easily strangle him.

These old myths, as I have already observed, especially the folk-lore traditions, contain the profoundest truths.

Long after men had turned their back on nature, and were living in unhappiness and misery, there still lingered in the soul of the people an intuition, an impression of the correct life, of past and future conditions,—especially how men originally lived in nature without sickness and want, what an unhappy state followed the violation of the laws of nature, and in what way salvation will come. This intuition, this impression has found expression in poetic form, embellished by the imagination, in the myths which are often the creation of entire generations. These myths convey the truths of the past in quite a different way from history, which is written by individual men and which every one in his diseased condition has altered and fixed up according to his views and wishes.

> "What you the Spirit of the Ages call
> Is nothing but the spirit of you all,
> Wherein the Ages are reflected."
> —Goethe, "Faust."

The Bible is interwoven and embellished by a wreath of the most beautiful and most sacred myths. It contains the most sacred, and the profoundest truths concerning the past and the future of man, it is the Book of books. The Bible tells of the original perfectly happy state of man in paradise in the bosom of pure nature, of man's fall, the transgression of the laws of nature in respect to food, of the consequent misery, and of salvation.

Jesus, as I have already stated, founded His theory of salvation on the closest approach to nature, on a perfectly natural mode of living, without which there is no happiness for man. In the course of time many passages in the Bible have unfortunately been falsified, both consciously and unconsciously, and it is to-day often wrongly understood and wrongly interpreted.

From the classical myth of Antæus I inferred that the earth has a most refreshing, invigorating, and salutary influence upon man, her son, as soon as he comes into direct touch with her.

Animals and man are as much products of the earth as the plants; in consequence of their higher development the former have only become separated from the earth, have become walking nerve-plants. But animals and man are still as much subject to the laws of nature as plants, they still draw their strength and vitality from the earth.

After this I attached still greater importance to going barefooted on the earth (without sandals), and became more than ever convinced of the great curative effect of going barefooted. But I also asked myself if this influence of the earth could not be utilized on behalf of man in a still greater degree. For the first thing, I no longer had the patients sleep in high bedsteads, but on strawticks or quilts on the ground in the open or in light-and-air cottages. They were thereby brought closer to the earth during sleep. This was at once felt as a gain; sleeping became pleasanter and was more invigorating.

But soon the patients lay down on the soft grass entirely naked, even without a shirt, and covered themselves with quilts. They soon broke out in enthusiastic exclamations over the wonderful effect of the earth upon the body during the night's rest The opinion was often expressed that *all* diseases, but especially the score of serious nervous troubles of our age, would entirely lose their terrors if only sleeping and lying on the earth at night once became customary in the curing of diseases. It is indeed a fact that the effect which the forces of the earth have upon man during the night is quite incredible. Whoever has not himself tried it and convinced himself of it, can have no conception of how refreshing, vitalizing, and strengthening the effect of the earth is on the human organism at night during rest.

The chief end of all healing art must be to aid and strengthen the digestion of the patient. Nothing accomplishes this end better than lying on the ground during the night,—however much the natural bath and the light-and-air bath may facilitate the movement of the bowels.

By sleeping on the ground, consequently, more than by anything else the entire body is aroused from its lethargy to a new manifestation of vital energy, so that it can now effectively remove old morbid matter and masses of old fœces from the intestines, and receive a sensation of new health, new life, and new unthought-of vigor and strength.

Whether it is because the body at night, especially during sleep, is lying perfectly quiet, or because the influence of the earth on the body is more powerful at night than in the day time, the fact certainly is that one does not experience the extraordinary curative effect of the earth nearly as much in going barefooted or in lying naked on the ground during a light-and-air bath and sun bath as at night.

I have already mentioned the fact that animals, especially hares and deer, when they prepare their lair, carefully remove all leaves, bits of wood, etc. They evidently do this to be more directly in touch with the earth, so that the forces of the earth may exert the strongest possible effect.[1] The animals do not scrape together grass, leaves, wood, and the like for their beds—birds only do this in order to prepare a warm nest for hatching. It is a very striking fact that the animals of the woods always remove all the wood and leaves, and even the snow, so as to make an entirely bare spot on the earth where they may lie down and rest. Sometimes they also roll on the bare ground. In the case of deer, German hunters call this habit "plætzen."

The fox and badger drag many things into their dens, but their resting place is kept perfectly free. It is always on the bare ground. Wild boars will indeed creep into heaped-up leaves and under brush, but they tolerate nothing under them and lie on the bare ground; generally they even dig themselves into it to some extent.

I once observed a domestic hog that was sick and was let out of its sty. On my advice it was left entirely alone, so that it might do what it wanted to. It went into the vegetable garden, grubbed itself somewhat into the ground in a cabbage bed, and remained quietly lying there. After a few days it returned and—was perfectly well. Of course, the animal left off feeding while it was sick. Thus the animals, although they are constantly in close relation with the earth in their normal activity, walking, and running, strive to get into especially close and direct touch with the bare earth when they rest and when they are sick.

The agitation for a bed reform will be in order among men as long as there are beds, and the defectiveness of beds will be felt as long as men shall decline to sleep on the bed which kind nature herself has created for her creatures, and which she has endowed with a magic power by which man receives a greater enjoyment of life.

Following the lead of nature, man lived originally in perfect sinlessness in the enjoyment of the purest happiness, in a state of unclouded bliss, such as the myths of paradise current among all civilized nations tell us about. But reason—the serpent in Paradise—held out to man the alluring prospect of reaping still greater advantages and pleasures for body, mind and soul if they would no longer obey the commands of God, the laws of nature [which God communicated to them through the organs of sense (smell, taste, etc.), instinct, and conscience], but would pursue their joys and happiness in their own way.

Out of this false use of reason, out of this abuse of reason, as I remarked in the beginning of my book, grew science, the daughter of that serpent, not only the science of medicine, but also the other sciences (pedagogy, theology, philosophy, jurisprudence, etc.). Science does not observe the laws of nature in order to make mankind prosperous and happy. Medical science even declares that living strictly in accordance with nature would prove very injurious to man. Eating exclusively natural food

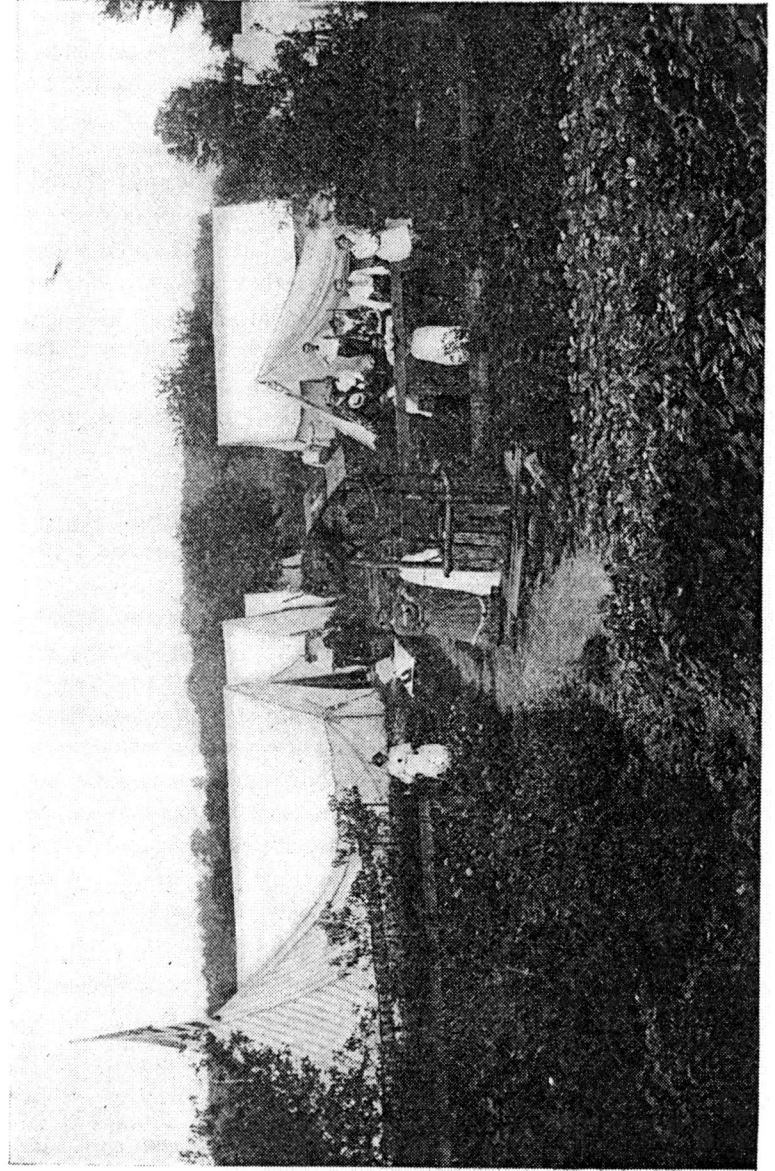

Camp in the "Jungborn," Butler, N. J.

(fresh fruit) does not give sufficient strength and injures the health, and the more intimate contact with light and air is very dangerous (colds, etc.), it declares. Moreover, the natural mode of life would deprive us of many joys. On the basis of anatomical, chemical, and other researches, it then goes on to prescribe an artificial diet, of which it says that it is at once enjoyable and strengthening to man, and thus lays down hygienic rules which leave instinct, taste (in its correct use), and conscience entirely out of consideration. Other departments of science, such as pedagogy, theology, philosophy, jurisprudence, etc., would also make men good and noble, and lay down precepts which in other ways than through close communion with nature promise to guide men to happiness and contentment.

In this way men came to put on shoes, to turn from the earth as their resting-place, and to make themselves bedsteads. They fancied thus to gain for themselves well-being, comfort, and joys which nature did not offer them. But men gain neither comfort nor enjoyment, neither health nor happiness, neither virtue nor nobility of following the false allurements of their reason and the teachings of science, but only disease and pain, disgust and vexation, vice and crime, misery and despair—the very opposite of what they wished to attain, for thus nature always avenges herself.

"Life somewhat better might content him
But for the gleam of heavenly light which Thou hast lent him:
He calls it Reason—thence his power's increased,
To be far beastlier [more unreasonable] than any beast."
—Goethe, "Faust."

Reason, this sublime gift of heaven, has become to man a snare and the cause of all his woe.

A certain bodily vigor, mental clearness, and joyousness of spirit,—true, complete health of body and soul, is not to be attained in any other way than by once more getting into direct relation with the earth, both when we are moving about and still more when we are at rest.

The late venerable prelate, Kneipp, of Woerishofen, deserves immortal fame for once more having made BAREFOOT-GOING popu-

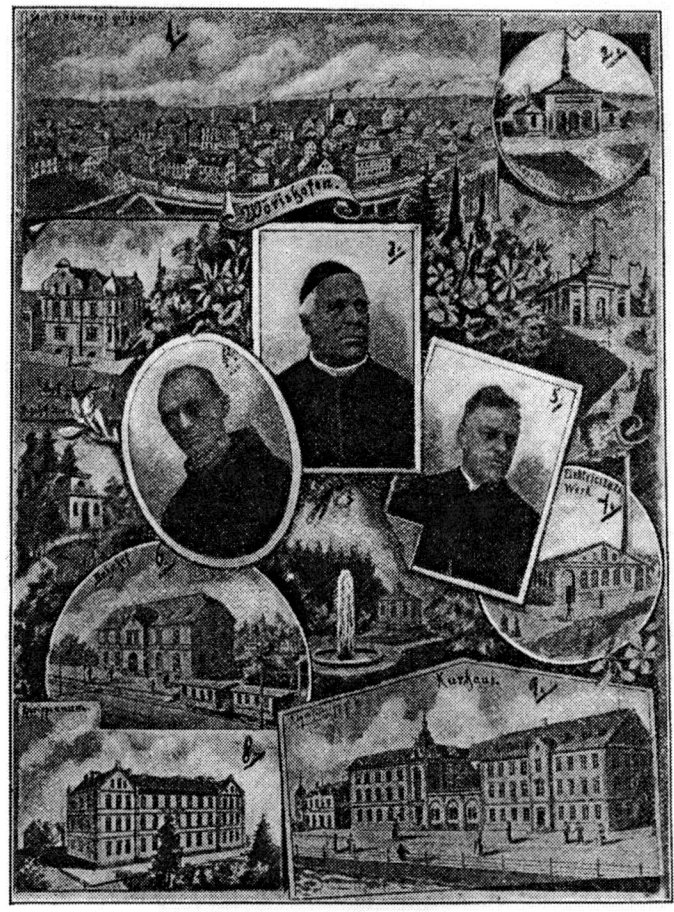

FATHER KNEIPP,
His Assistants and Woerishofen.

lar, at least in southern Germany, so that a return to nature in this respect is there no longer looked upon as comical and ridiculous. It is to be hoped, in behalf of the well-being of mankind, that this point of view may force its way also in the north of our Fatherland. It is not to be expected that men shall all at once abandon their clothes and go naked all day long, there are still too many difficulties in the way of this health-giver to be overcome; or that they shall suddenly resort to the natural diet, and live exclusively on berries, fruit, and NUTS: but they can at once begin going barefooted all day long, excepting a few very cold weeks in Winter, even in our climate, without ever feeling the custom as a torture or a burden, but rather as the greatest delight and pleasure. Going barefooted is no asceticism, but an augmentation of the enjoyment of life. For the earth has her son again, as soon as man goes barefooted, and can again shower on him fresh health and true happiness. The true regeneration and rejuvenation of to-day's sick, miserable, sinful, and wicked mankind will take place as soon as men shall again learn to go barefooted, not only for minutes and hours, but continuously at their daily work.

The feet are in a certain sense for man what the roots are for plants. Man draws vital energy and strength out of the earth through his feet.

Jesus also attached a great deal of importance to the practice of going barefooted; He Himself was also barefooted, and He gave to His disciples the command:

"Carry neither shoes."—Luke 10:4.

The order of barefoot monks, who always went barefooted, well knew that the blessings of Jesus' doctrine of salvation and happiness were not to be had without obeying the precepts with regard to a natural mode of life and the care of health which He impressed on His disciples, and through them on all Christendom, but which are unheeded now.

Going barefooted, without sandals, if possible, ought to be the foundation of every nature cure.*

---

*People ought to go entirely barefooted as often as possible, especially on the bare ground. But in rooms with painted floors it is better to wear sandals or straw slippers or similar footgear, since the painted floor affects the body injuriously if one walks on it with bare soles.

The people will then begin again to more and more regard bare feet, which nature has created, and which will soon regain blood and fine shapes, as more beautiful and more æsthetic than miserable, ragged, patched-up shoes; and the practice of going barefooted, which even Christ, the Saviour, prescribed to Christendom both by precept and example, will no longer be a matter for ridicule and scorn to them. To prefer to the bare feet of the masterpiece of creation some miserable footgear, which often presses and tortures men so as to contort their faces, is an insult to nature.

If the importance of sleeping on the ground is but once fully recognized and has become the common practice, the spell in which a diseased body and an unbalanced mind now hold mankind will soon be broken. The natural bath, the light-and-air bath, and a natural diet can of course also do much to shake and weaken the spell.

In acute as well as in chronic diseases this remedy will soon show its wonderful effect.

Jesus also avoided the cities with their foul air, their luxury and effeminacy, their moral degradation; he took up his abode mostly in the desert and in the mountains.

Here, moreover, he did most of his preaching, and if during the day He preached in the temple of Jerusalem, He tarried at night on the Mount of Olives,* where He certainly also made His bed on the bare ground. Only ONE flowing robe, such as the members of the sect of Essenes wore, was probably His entire covering in the lap of nature.

In order to sleep again on the earth it is best to select a nice grass plot; if there is no grass plot at hand, a *thin* reed matting, such as gardeners use, may be placed on the ground. In that way, of course, the earth power will fall very short of its full effect. Any thicker covering of straw, wool, cloth, or the like, to

---

* "And in the daytime he was teaching in the temple; and at night he went out and abode in the mount that is called the Mount of Olives."—Luke 21:37.

lie on must not be thought of, for the connection with the earth would in that case be markedly interfered with. No head rest is necessary, for it is of especial benefit for the head to lie on the cool, refreshing earth.

We must not be discouraged if the first nights spent on the earth should prove uncomfortable.

I have made the experience that patients, after the first few nights, were actually attracted to their bed on the ground, and strongly refused to tolerate anything under them. In rainy nights I was often concerned about having the patients come into the huts to sleep, so that the quilts should not get so wet, but it was with difficulty that I could induce the sick people to leave the ground. Soon, also, the hardness of lying on the ground is no longer felt. Nor need we fear that the earth is too cold nights to lie on entirely naked under covers; we shall only experience the sensation of a delightful coolness. Some perspire more easily lying on the ground than in a bed. Of course, beginners and those persons who have not yet regained sufficient animal heat through a natural mode of life, can only lie naked on the ground under covers in warm Summer nights, or in very mild or not too cold Spring and Autumn nights in our climate.

During the first nights one generally sleeps worse on the ground than formerly in bed. After that, and sometimes even in cases of protracted and obstinate insomnia, a long, exceedingly refreshing and strengthening sleep will set in, which state of affairs will last for some time. But generally most persons will soon begin to sleep less and less, sometimes only from one to two hours, and the less they sleep nights lying on the ground, the brighter, fresher and stronger will they feel the next day. I myself have not slept a wink for weeks at a time on the ground, but during that period I never felt the least discomfort or trouble of any kind, as was formerly the case in sleepless nights during my long and severe nervous suffering while lying in a bed. On the contrary, those nights were particularly delightful and free from *ennui*, and during the day I was never so entirely without any trace of weariness and languor, and I never felt more refreshed than at that time.*

If we look about in free nature we nowhere find that deathlike, leaden sleep which falls on men throughout every night and holds them for six or eight hours or longer.|| The time which a man spends in such a condition is actually wiped out of his life. Animals move about almost all night. They indeed sometimes rest, especially during the day, so that it seems as if for a moment all their physical and mental activity had stopped, but they do not sleep the way men sleep, not even our domestic animals, for instance horses, after the hardest labor, sink into a deep sleep lasting for hours. But the animals, though they do not sleep, are always fresh and lively; they never yawn and never show a sleepy, weary demeanor like man who sleeps so much. Therefore, in order to be bright and not grow tired, we must strive to live again so closely to nature that we shall at first sleep less and finally perhaps no more at all. But I wish to observe that I distinguish between sleeping and resting There is also in nature an alternation of activity and rest. Complete rest of mind and body, to which man with his inner unrest and excitement hardly ever attains in these days, but which might be one of his sweetest joys and most beautiful pleasures, will again come to him the more he regains his health.

---

*The more closely man will approach to nature again, the more will that morbid phenomenon called "ennui" disappear. By nature's design every moment ought to be filled with joy and happiness for man, more than for the animal, for he is gifted with reason and imagination. This noble gift enables the healthy man to live in a world of poetry. Where ennui makes its appearance in a man it is only the sign of native shallowness and barrenness, which also is a diseased condition.

||The Winter sleep into which some animals sink, cannot be compared with the sleep of man. The former is a peculiar arrangement with some animal species in whom the circulation is very sluggish during the Winter months, and whose digestion is almost completely at a standstill, so that the animals during this whole time require but little food or none at all.

But this is by no means a sinking into unconsciousness; it is not mental death.

Animals hear and feel everything during their complete rest.

With a strictly natural diet, and the use of the natural bath, people will soon experience a lessening need of sleep.

Even in the warmest Summer nights one does not fall asleep lying naked and uncovered, even when not lying on the earth, just as one never falls asleep taking a sunbath naked, even when lying on a blanket. Therefore the more closely we approach nature again, especially by lying on the bare earth with enough covering to be comfortable, the more shall we be strengthened and refreshed without relaxing into sleep.

In order to produce sleep, the nerves and the entire organism of man must be artificially relaxed. This is done by poisons, such as bromide, morphium, opium, etc. By this method, the relaxation is so powerful and violent that the injury to the health is plainly felt afterwards. The sleep caused by alcohol, unnatural food, heated rooms, warm clothing, warm beds, etc., which people consider exceedingly strengthening and beneficial, is likewise only a consequence of artificial relaxation and is also injurious to the organism, only the injury is not great enough to make itself plainly felt.

But after all, people experience a certain feeling of confusion and consternation after their sleep; and it is just this uncomfortable, disagreeable sensation that they will get rid of when they lie on the bare ground and sleep only a little or not at all.

Of course those people are in a sad and serious plight who in consequence of the present mode of life, nervous excitement, warm beds, etc., never relax at all and never get any prolonged sleep, as is the case with many sufferers from nervous troubles.

It would be a great mistake in people who use alcohol and other unnatural food, live unnatural lives, wear warm clothing, etc., and who do not sleep on the earth nights, not to wholly abandon themselves in warm beds to the feeling of weariness that will come over them. First to create weariness and then struggle against it would consume the body too rapidly. If, for instance, on taking opium or morphium, we should fight against the sleep that would set in, we should only very much increase the bad effect of these poisons on our health, and after all our pains would prove futile.

If I have here set down my ideas concerning sleep, it is not because I take pleasure in advancing claims which are directly opposed to the old views and prejudices on the subject, and which call out either the applause of the masses, or, in case they prove inconvenient and burdensome, their derision and indignation. I only wished, in case anyone should try the experiment (perhaps in beautiful Summer nights) of lying on the bare earth with the naked body, to guard against his being discouraged if his sleep should grow less, and against his abandoning a cause which would prove of unprecedented advantage to his health and his well-being. Such a person would thereby forego a remedy which was not brewed in any swill kitchen, which did not originate in a sick brain, but which nature herself offers, and to which healthy creatures are directed by instinct, the only sure guide of life, the prime minister of health.

No one who seriously desires to go barefooted need to-day be in any anxiety as to a place where he can do so. Fields and woods, meadows and paths offer ample opportunity for going barefooted, a sound view of the matter is spreading among the people who are becoming indifferent to the unusual sight, so that the devotee is less and less liable to annoyance and ridicule.

But many a one may like to ask where he is to go at night with his blankets to lie on the earth without clothes. In sanitaria the opportunity is easily provided in parks surrounded by high board fences (men and women separated), which contain also light-and-air cottages, so that a patient, according to his inclination, may at any time take a light-and-air bath or sleep in the open air on a rug (strawtick or quilt) or on the bare ground.

Here, likewise, the opportunity must be afforded for the

natural bath in the open. Little bath cells should be constructed for the natural bath.

However, I do not wish to persuade any one single-handed to completely and suddenly break away from all the old, deep-rooted views, false and harmful as they often are, and thus to enter a state of open and violent opposition and warfare with those with whom he has erred and suffered, and with whom he is still united by many bonds of friendship and love.

We ought at least to try and avoid such an open rupture as far as possible. We must never renounce the great cause; that would be dishonorable and cowardly. And we must also, above all things, bear in mind the importance of regaining health, upon which all happiness on earth depends.

Neither must anyone get into conflict with the authorities who care for the public welfare in good faith. The laws of the State, which have been made by the representatives freely elected by the people themselves, must not be transgressed, even when they are recognized as wrong.

But everybody should see to it that such laws (vaccination laws) shall do as little harm as possible, and agitate for their modification or abolition in the course of time.

Many are the causes which prompt people to ridicule and place difficulties in the way of those who lead a strictly natural life. In the first place there is the instinctive consciousness of their own false mode of life with all its disastrous consequences, and the involuntary grudge they bear against the great advantages which others derive from a natural mode of life. There is, moreover, not sufficient strength of mind, opportunity or encouragement for them to abjure all unnatural food and the like, to which man is enslaved as to every poison and vice, and above all they are not sufficiently informed as to the right course they should pursue.

But when once individuals shall recognize these great truths more and more clearly, and order their lives accordingly in a quiet, sensible way, so as to obtrude themselves as little as possible upon the great masses and give no offence, the natural mode of life will gain more and more vantage ground, and there will be fewer and fewer obstacles placed in its way—the trend of the time is already powerful in that direction.

Then also many men, God's favorites, will find their opportunity to rest in magic union with mother earth, and procure for themselves and their health and earthly happiness an inestimable advantage,—just as the earth is at all times free to the glad enjoyment of life and as a resting-place to all creatures, frog and mouse, hedgehog and hare, deer and elk, fox and badger, who certainly range below man in God's love.

When not so very long ago the rumor spread that in some places people were beginning to go barefooted even in the snow, for the improvement of their health and the curing of diseases, it was met only with ridicule and scorn.

People shrank from the mere thought of exposing the tender feet, which had hitherto been treated with especially great care and had always been kept warm, to the cold air, the rough ground, and in Winter even to the snow. Had not grandmother often said: "Be sure always to keep your feet warm!" and had not physicians always warned against wet feet? Afterwards a few tried the thing, and convinced themselves that besides being of great advantage to health and the entire well-being of man, going barefooted was a pleasant exercise; and since then the opinion concerning this purely natural remedy for the restoration of health has undergone a great change.

Lying on the ground will make its way in a similar manner For a time it will still appear hard and cruel, more so than going barefooted. But upon the trials that will be made with it, people will become convinced of its entire harmlessness and its exceedingly great curative qualities still more readily than was the case in the matter of going barefooted.

The sun has the greatest curative effect upon the sick body. This effect is very considerably increased if instead of walking the patient lies quietly in the sunshine. The earth power, likewise, can affect the body more directly when lying in complete rest than in walking. The earth power stimulates the body toward a curative activity in the same way as the sun; but if the body must spend its energy in walking and other like exertions it cannot manifest its full curative activity, in spite of the influences of sun and earth power.

However, out of regard for the prevailing opinions which no one can at once overcome, we ought to exercise the greatest caution, especially in sanitaria before advising others to lie or sleep upon the bare ground. This must be left entirely to the option of the patient. The success of here and there an individual will suffice to cause others to follow his example. It may be well in the beginning to sleep one night on the ground, the next night in bed.

When I first attempted to introduce lying on the bare earth at the Jungborn, I also encountered many prejudices. There was no great desire to try the experiment. Then several of the patients made an energetic effort; they soon became greatly pleased with it, and in their enthusiasm induced most of the others likewise to sleep on the bare earth. The success achieved by all of them was of course surprising.

Water applications have been long in vogue since Priessnitz, Kneipp, Kuhne, and others. To combine rubbing with the bath has also already been taught. But thes methods are not yet fully in accord with the precepts of nature.

Going naked was preached long ago by Rikli. But it was by no means practised by him with a complete understanding of the laws of nature concerning light and air. Therefore Rikli could not make a general practice of going naked for both the sick and the well.

But the earth power and its application has been overlooked entirely. When in the first edition of my book I for the first time called attention to the earth-power, many were surprised. But soon this subject of the earth-power elicited the greatest interest and attracted everywhere the most lively attention.

And there is indeed nothing of greater interest and greater importance than the earth with its manifold and powerful curative effect. I wish, therefore, to treat of it more in detail in this edition.

Our globe is a body in which a powerful life has been stirring from the very beginning which no amount of human unreason could disturb. Of this powerfully pulsating life the earth is most willing to give a share to man, as soon as he will but enter into direct communication with it again.

We can frequently make use of this earth power. And men draw upon it the more, the more they lead a natural life. Whenever opportunity offers one ought to sit on the ground, even with clothes on. In taking walks and making tours, we ought frequently to rest by sitting or lying on the bare earth. Naturally the earth power influences men even through their clothes. Every one may experience this who will stretch himself quietly upon the bare earth for a time.

I have often observed that persons in an excited frame of mind, in melancholy and despairing moments, in hysteric fits and convulsions, and other morbid conditions, were most speedily quieted, relieved, and cured by sitting or lying on the ground.

We need not fear the coldness and dampness of the earth. The curative effect is even most potent under these conditions, which is proved by the fact that colds are often caused thus, a most favorable and not at all dangerous symptom, as I have repeatedly shown.

A peculiar life exists in nature during the night. If we go into a forest at night we get a feeling as if the whole spirit world were abroad. Grass is said to grow at night, not in the day-time. It is probably for this reason that the earth power is of especially powerful effect at night.

I have made various attempts at the Jungborn to make sleeping on the bare earth during the night more and more agreeable. Finally it occurred to me to construct sand beds, upon which it is much more comfortable to lie than on the ordinary ground. They are somewhat softer than the earth.

A layer of sand from four to eight inches will serve as a sand-bed. This may be covered with a coarse, porous piece of burlap or linen without essentially weakening the effect of the earth power, while the quilts used for covering are at the same time kept clean thereby. There may be still other advantages. The layer of sand may be surrounded by a border of sod, at least it is very desirable to have a somewhat elevated soft strip at the head as a head-rest.

It is of the greatest advantage, of course, to have the sand-bed in the open air, for man is also influenced by a wonderful, mysterious curative power from above that seems to be especially active at night, invigorating and strengthening his entire organism while he is resting under the starry sky, under the great dome of heaven.* This power, in conjunction with the earth power, produces the most wonderful curative effects.

In unfavorable weather, to be sure, the bed must be prepared under a roofed space (perhaps a tent), which ought to be as roomy as possible.

Moreover, a large, longish receptacle, a box or the like, may be placed in any room, and filled with earth and sand for sleeping purposes.

THE FEAR OF COLDS.

When I was speaking of sleeping in open light-and-air huts and cottages and upon the bare ground even in cold weather, and especially in days of sickness, many a one may have seen in his mind's eye a whole army of colds, rheumatism, gout, typhoid fever, influenza, pneumonia, etc., accompanied by terrible pains and tortures, to be succeeded even by the certain dreadful end, death; and many others, among them adherents of the current nature-cure method, may have felt their hair stand on end in fear and trembling.

I have already tried to dispel the fear of colds. I shall try once more to deal it a death-blow, although I well know that

---

*Plants covered with a large, wide-meshed wire screen have been observed not to thrive as well as plants that grew entirely under the free sky.

while it stalks abroad like an uncanny ghost among mankind, its full danger and malignity have as yet nowhere been recognized.

Here I shall be obliged, of course, to repeat some things that I have already spoken of.

The digestive organs of the body are by their functional activity adapted only to the food which nature has intended for man, that is, the food which the earth yields freely without the aid of horticulture or agriculture, and which man can relish in its natural, unchanged state (nuts, berries, fruit, and several other things). Now if man eats this natural food in a changed form (changed by cooking, etc.), or partakes of other things which nature has not intended for him and which merely resemble the natural food in a greater or lesser degree, the digestive organs will digest them only with difficulty, partially, or not at all. The body cannot fully utilize these unnatural foods, if it can utilize them at all (in building up the blood, muscles, bones, etc.). With unnatural nutrition, therefore, the body does not receive the material which it requires for its growth, for its normal physical and mental development, strength, and vitality. Food remnants will moreover lodge in the stomach, and penetrate from the abdomen in solid, liquid, and gaseous form into all its parts, to the very extremities, and change the whole shape of the body. This matter does not belong to the body; it is foreign matter, which may get into the organism in still other ways, by breathing and through the skin; for instance by vaccine and other poisons.

The foreign matter now lodges between the organs. According to its kind it will injure and destroy the organs, some sooner, some later. It also passes into a state of fermentation, producing heat which has a particularly injurious and destructive effect upon the entire body. In this manner it causes distress and pain, now here, now there, and disturbs all the organs of the body generally in their normal functions, including those which mediate between body and soul, and likewise brings about untimely death. The formation and deposition of foreign matter, the cause of disease, goes on the more readily in these days since by wearing heavy shoes and clothing, by avoiding cold water and separating ourselves from the earth, by shutting ourselves off from light and air, by breathing foul air, and by other crimes against nature the vitality and digestive power of the body are increasingly interfered with and paralyzed.

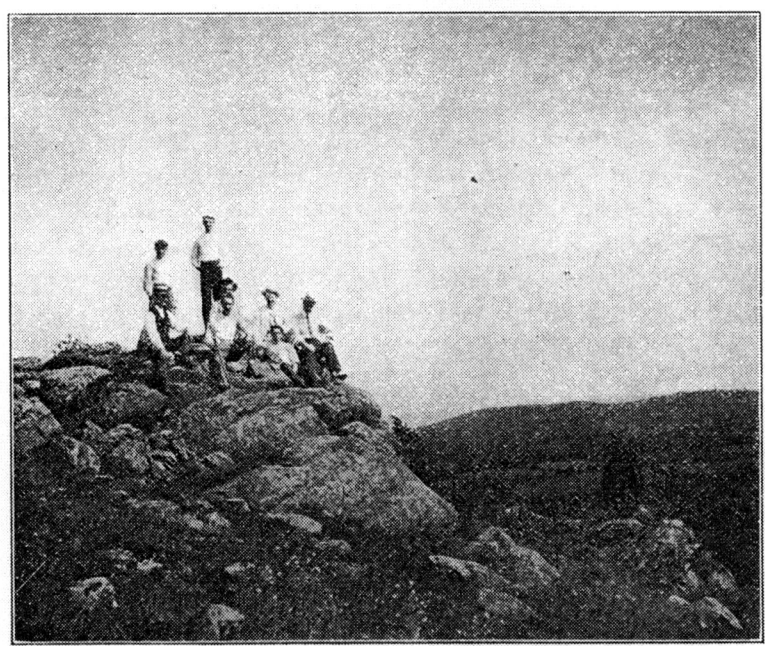

Summit of Keckout Mountain, 1,400 feet high, near the "Jungborn," in Butler, N. J.

But as soon as men shall cast aside their thick shoes and wear lighter garments, so that water, light and air, and especially the sharp, cold wind may reach the body more easily, nature will at once seize the opportunity to stimulate the vitality to a wholesome activity and bring on a curative crisis for the purpose of loosening the foreign matter and expelling it by force.

This manifests itself naturally most promptly and violently among the weak, effeminate and spoiled. But these are also most in need of this sort of help from nature, for in consequence of their great dread of cold water, light and air and moist earth, and their many protective measures against the beneficent remedies of nature, their vitality has become very sluggish, and has favored in a special degree the accumulation of foreign matter within them.

Colds and catarrhs now set in, also such acute diseases as measles, scarlet fever, pox (children's diseases), diphtheria, typhoid fever, pneumonia, influenza, etc., according how the organs (lungs, nerves, etc.) are most active in ridding themselves of the foreign matter. Acute diseases (typhoid, cholera, etc.) are of course also brought on by other causes than dampness, air, and cold, for instance by a sudden change of temperature, by great mental excitement, etc. Sometimes the body starts them of its own accord, with no recognizable external cause to account for them.

These acute diseases are always accompanied by acute fever. The first symptom often is a chill; the violent commotion of the foreign matter, the friction of the particles against each other cause the inner heat to increase; the blood is therefore withdrawn into the interior of the body, the external skin becomes cold, and the patient feels cold. But soon the heat extends to the external skin, the patient becomes hot, for the body begins powerfully to force the foreign matter, now in motion, outward, in order to expel it through the skin. In diphtheria the throat is the chief sufferer. The foreign matter, whose volume is moreover increased by the rising heat, is stopped on its way from the abdomen to the head, and danger from suffocation is imminent.

Now if we work against nature by shutting the patient off from light and fresh air, and by giving him poisonous medicines, antifebrin, etc., whereby the vitality of the body is again weakened, poor, foolish man must of course always succumb in his struggle with powerful nature. The patient will now have to endure horrible pains and tortures, and it may easily happen that he will die in the struggle against nature; or he may be apparently cured, that is, the body will suspend its curative activity, and the symptoms of the disease will disappear, but only in order to enable the body after some time to again seek to free itself of the foreign matter in a still more difficult manner, in a still severer crisis. Influenza, for instance, may be apparently cured by antifebrin, but soon inflammation of the lungs will set in. The vitality of the body may also be permanently at such a low ebb that the latter can no longer forcibly throw off the foreign matter through acute diseases.

Chronic disease appears as soon as there is foreign matter present in the body that has begun to ferment, which produces heat, injuring the body.* The chronic disease now becomes increasingly dangerous; in the course of time serious troubles may set in, such as nervous affections, consumption (in consequence of influenza and inflammation of the lungs), cancer, gout, diabetes, open sores, etc., which drag the patient through long years of invalidism slowly to his grave, unless indeed the vitality of the body is once more strengthened by nature's remedies, which can now be done only slowly and gradually.

As we have seen, medical science can with the aid of its poisonous remedies cause acute diseases to disappear, but of course only to the greater injury of the body. However, it is entirely powerless in regard to chronic diseases.

---

*The internal heat in chronic diseases, which leaves the patient outwardly chilly and cold, constitutes the chronic fever. But as the patient's condition progresses, this fever extends to the exterior of the body, so that the patient in an advanced stage of chronic disease has a very high temperature. When the patient has reached this stage, the body seems to have become completely powerless. It appears that here the fever did not arise to expel the foreign matter, as in the case of acute diseases, but as if in consequence of the sinking and cessation of all the vital impulses of the body, which had confined it to the interior organs (except in times of that violent revolution, the acute diseases), it had now spread over the entire body. To reduce and temper this chronic fever in these last stages, it is clear that only the remedies of nature, light, air, water, earth, and a natural diet, can be successfully applied.

Here, too, by means of operations and poisons, such as arsenic, creosot, etc., changes may be produced in the condition of the patient, isolated symptoms of the disease may be made to disappear, and manifestations of the disease in individual organs may be suppressed. But hardly any one will be deceived thereby, for a little thoughtful observation will easily reveal the fact that in reality the general diseased condition of the patient progresses all the more rapidly under such treatment, till everything that man, strayed from the path of nature, can accomplish in the struggle with her, is hidden in the grave and rests forgotten in night and darkness.*

The vital energy of the body may be paralyzed from the very start by vaccine poison, so that certain acute diseases, children's pox, etc., children's diseases, through which the young organism, still filled with vital energy, so readily rids itself of foreign matter, can no longer be contracted. But in their stead other, more serious diseases will appear, diphtheria, inflammation of the lungs, etc., and the whole grewsome array of chronic diseases, such as severe nervous affections, consumption, cancer, etc., become increasingly prevalent, as is most convincingly attested by the present age. Countless people are tottering to their graves on sticks and crutches as consumptives, nervous sufferers, scrofulitics, deaf, blind, deformed, and mishapen. Many of them are the pitiable victims of vaccination, the great health preserver legally prescribed by medicine and the State. But

---

*An open suppurating wound, for instance, may be healed with salve. But we thereby only close the outlet of a canal through which diseased matter (foreign matter) is carried away. The foreign matter is now stowed away in the interior of the body where it can do great damage, even cause death, before it has succeeded in finding another outlet. But if the formation of more foreign matter is prevented by a natural diet, and the vital energy of the body is strengthened by light and air, water and earth power, so that the digestion is improved and the foreign matter is disposed of in the natural way through the urine, feces, and perspiration, the wound will soon cease to suppurate and will heal in consequence of the increased curative powers of the body. No disadvantage will follow this sort of healing, and no harm need be feared for the health.

who recognizes the fact, and how long will it be before here, too, light will penetrate the darkest night?

Thus we see that the greatest disadvantages and dangers, misery and ruin come to man through the treatment prescribed by medical science of colds and acute diseases. Here, too, medical science disregards the voice of nature and misconceives her good intentions.

The more, however, we meet nature half way and assist her in her efforts to gain her ends in acute diseases,—the more we avoid the things which constitute the real cause of the disease, unnatural food, the foul air of cities and rooms,—and the more we introduce the body to light, air, water, cold, and earth-power, the more thoroughly and speedily will the dangerous internal heat be allayed. Then also the discharges (from lungs and nose) will be all the more prompt and copious, the kidneys and bowels will do their work, and when warmth is restored sweat will set in, rash will appear on the skin (measles, scarlet fever, and small-pox), and other excretions of foreign matter will take place. The patient will suffer but little pain and distress (in consequence of the lowering of the internal heat) and will soon experience considerable relief and comfort,—he will rise from his acute disease rejuvenated and invigorated like the phœnix from his ashes.

The failure of medical science in the treatment of acute diseases, and the disaster that follows in its wake in the manner indicated by me, are recognizable by all who are not dazzled by the glamour that surrounds science and who watch its ministrations at the sick bed with an impartial eye. In the same way any one may plainly observe, in nature cure institutions or perhaps in his own case, the favorable issue attending acute diseases under natural treatment and the benefits that accrue from them for the body. He may then also convince himself of the correctness of the observation that acute diseases are not at all dangerous, and are altogether favorable curative crises by means of which the body frees itself of foreign matter.

Yes, the acute diseases, typhoid fever, diphtheria, cholera, and what not, which are mostly brought on by taking cold, and which are to-day still terribly dreaded by mankind, are wholly without danger, and prove under correct treatment of the greatest benefit. They are a blessing to man, and ought to be hailed with joy on their appearance.

Through all my most careful observations of nature in the case of numerous patients and myself, I have been more and more firmly convinced that nature has only the very best of intentions when she visits us with colds and acute diseases; and I will give practical proof of this to any one who will observe my methods or trust himself to it.

I do not in the least doubt, however, that most people will regard me as a fanatic on account of the claims that I have made, and the convictions I have expressed with regard to colds and acute diseases; and that from the cothurnus of their mistaken way they will look down upon me with a pitying scientific smile.

But the acute diseases are only a sort of makeshift of nature. They are not altogether necessary and may be entirely avoided by returning to nature. When a cold or some acute disease has made its appearance and the patient submits early enough to the natural treatment, that is, if he takes the natural bath, and frequently and for a long time, according to the temperature, remains without clothes (entirely naked) in a room in which *all* the windows and doors are open, or better still in the open air. and brings himself into contact with the earth in walking, resting, or sleeping as often as possible, even the most dreaded acute diseases, such as small-pox, diphtheria, typhoid fever, cholera, etc., will entail almost no suffering, and those about the patient will scarcely find any cause for anxiety during the various phases of the disease. But if so-called healthy persons, or chronic patients, before acute disease sets in, will return to nature as far as possible with respect to water, light, air, and earth in the manner already described, and with respect to diet as I am going to explain, phenomena like colds and acute diseases will not appear at all.

Not in a single case, neither in my former practice, nor at the Jungborn among the numerous patients who took a course of treatment there with perfect confidence in my prescriptions, did a cold or an acute disease set in. A curative crisis of this sort, after all, still has some disagreeable features and interferes with our enjoyment of life, but among the many young and old people who without any transitional expedients or caution whatever at once started in going barefooted, taking the new bath in the open, sleeping in an open light-and-air hut or entirely in the open air and on the bare ground, and walking about naked, not one such crisis appeared, although the natural mode of life was adhered to in good and bad weather, in rain and sunshine, and sometimes partly even in the coldest winter.

Such complete return to nature stimulates the vital energy of the body enormously, and the latter at once begins to work with all its might to eject the foreign matter it harbors. In consequence of this a severe griping is often felt throughout the body, and sometimes more or less sharp pains (boils may also appear), but at the same time, and more than usual, the internal heat which is being developed, and which is the principal cause of acute disease, with its suffering, its excitement, its exhaustion, etc., is always immediately lowered and carried off, and thus acute fevers and in general colds and acute diseases are avoided. Even in ordinary life, the more man again boldly exposes himself to cold water, cold air, wind, and weather, without thick clothes and heavy shoes, and the more strongly he refuses to waver in his faith in the good intentions of nature, even if he occasionally takes a cold, the more harmless and lighter will such crises become and the more easily may they be wholly avoided by being continually drained away.

It is a well-known fact that those who have overcome their fear of colds, or who are too poor to buy many clothes and shoes, etc., very rarely or never are visited by acute diseases.

But may I now hope by these explanations to have dispelled the fear of colds in anyone? No! I am not presumptuous enough to think that I could in the least shake the fear of colds in its dreadful stronghold. You may adduce every proof, show men how others expose themselves fearlessly and with impunity to wind and weather, to wet and cold, and they will only advance every possible objection: he is still young, this one has a particularly strong constitution, that one has become hardened, therefore he can stand it. Such are some of the many palisades with which the fear of colds strongly fortifies itself.

We are so ready to have confidence in a physician, and expect to regain our health through him even if he himself is afflicted with disease and suffering. We so readily and blindly trust in every remedy that comes from the apothecary's shop, even if it is a poison, and consequently always detrimental and ruinous to health, and through some oversight of the apothecary may even cause instant death. People put their trust in these dangerous remedies, if they are only written in Latin on a prescription blank, so that they cannot understand them.

But everybody fears nature, and withholds from her his confidence,—nature, all of whose remedies, water as well as light and hair, heat and cold, form a part of the harmony of the world, for the welfare and happiness only of all living creatures,—nature, in whose bosom everything was sound and happy as long as man did not interfere with her, and who speaks plainly and distinctly to all. Medical science in good faith eagerly fosters this distrust.

However, the whole universe sprang from the fountain-head of eternal love; from this source only good, nothing harmful and nothing bad could come. In nature, therefore, there is not the tiniest atom of a drop of water, not the gentlest motion of the mildest zephyr, not the smallest degree of cold that was not created for the welfare and happiness of animated beings.

When man had fallen away from nature, it was a part of his character to look for the cause of his afflictions not in himself, but outside of him, in nature. Nature was therefore regarded as something full of dangers, something cruel. Out of this arose the distrust of nature, from which in turn came the misunderstanding of nature and her processes, in consequence of which man often employs the means that nature offers in a harmful and dangerous manner and brings much affliction and pain upon himself. But in one respect a breach has already been made into this fatal misunderstanding of nature.

Even as late as the last century cold water, as it is found in nature and as it is used by the animals that follow their instinct, was entirely rejected and condemned in the treatment of the sick. The physicians even cleansed and washed wounds with warm water, until the patient died half decomposed and in a nauseous condition.

Not a long time ago physicians forbade every patient, even when in a high state of fever, to drink cold water, even when in his excessive thirst he was suffering the most cruel torments and was actually burning up with internal heat. No one was allowed to drink cold water while in a heated condition, anyway. Soldiers were forbidden on severe penalty to drink water while marching, even if they sank down exhausted with the tortures of thirst. It was considered very dangerous, indeed, to take a bath in cold water while the body was in a warm and heated condition.

To-day, however, if somebody is wounded, recourse is first had to *cold* water, cold water is willingly handed to the fever patient to alleviate his suffering, soldiers on the march must to-day everywhere be supplied with cold water for their refreshment, except, indeed, where the bacilli craze, which is rampant in modern times, has frightened people here and there.

It has been observed that the bath is the more effective the warmer the body is when it touches the cold water, indeed, people even go from the steam bath dripping with perspiration into the cold water.

Mankind seems to desire a return to nature, there are unmistakable signs of this, but strange to say, it is cold water to which people first turn again. Everywhere cold-water cures have been established which are very much frequented by sick people.

Nature is indeed wonderfully kind; if but one step is taken in her direction, she hastens towards us with open arms and extends the hand that is always ready for beneficent deeds. It is an established fact that cold water alone, although it is only partially applied in the form intended by nature, has already achieved most excellent curative success. And if these happy results from cold water are compared with the successes, or rather failures, of medical science, they must really astonish mankind. Cold water, however, can always be applied only for a few moments at a time and to a very limited extent.

But pure, fresh air, on the other hand, is the very life element of man. Exactly in the measure that man is supplied with pure air through skin and lungs his well-being, his entire physical, intellectual, and spiritual life rises and falls.

If we deprive man of air entirely, even for a moment only, his life immediately goes out. And, if we were to cover a man with an air-tight substance, only for several hours, so that he can take in air through nose and mouth, but not through the skin, he likewise dies.

In pure air, otherwise than in water, the patient can remain and move about permanently, and even for a long time without clothes. The further development of diseased matter is at once arrested by a natural diet, from which the entire substance of the body and the nerves is built up. When air, and cold, and earth-power, and a truly natural diet, which the present vegetarian diet by NO means really is, once begin to be employed for the maintenance of health, and the healing of diseases, then all the brilliant successes which cold water has already achieved will fade away. But this must all be done according to my method, as I have already described it and shall further describe it.

Water employed in a wrong way, or for too long a time can do harm, but air will in no case do harm, and always does much good. But nevertheless air is always looked upon with especial distrust. We no longer hesitate when very heated, and even dripping with perspiration, to take a cold bath, and fever patients are also put into cold water. But what tourist would venture to-day, when very heated from rapid walking so that he is perspiring violently, to expose himself in an open place, or on a rocky projection, half undressed (with bare breast, bare feet and bare head) or entirely naked, to an icy cold draught for a time? Or in the case of a child sick with diphtheria, or measles, or an adult in a high state of fever from typhoid or pneumonia, tossing to and fro under thick feather beds, and protesting frantically against the cruel burden, who would to-day, in any such case, venture to take the patient in cold weather (even in Winter) entirely without clothes into a cold room, in which all the windows and doors are open, or even naked into the open air?

Who would to-day take such a patient out of the house, and out of the city, with its fumes and evil odors, and its poisoned air, and lodge him, even when it is cold, in an open hut in a garden or in the woods, and even in but moderate temperature let him rest or sleep in the open air, entirely naked, on cool, even damp ground?

At the very thought of this even our nature-curists and the adherents of the present methods of natural healing would quake and tremble with fear; and those who would openly advise such a thing, would simply be declared insane by the rest of the people.

Yes, if the law were to-day what it was centuries ago, we should lock up these rash people in insane asylums and prisons, as was done with Galileo for declaring that the earth revolved around the sun, and not the sun around the earth, and as then so to-day scientific bodies would sit in judgment over them.

But for all that, fresh cold air would prove particularly beneficial to the warm heated body, as much so as cold water, and would refresh and invigorate it. The cool night follows upon the warm day, the cold Winter upon the hot Summer; nature provides the change between warm and cold for great purposes. In the open air, in the garden, or best of all in the woods, where the patient breathes only pure fresh air, where the cold air which plays about the naked body, and the earth take all suffering from the fever-stricken and rob diseases of all danger, the acute patient would quickly recover, and the chronic patient would be gradually led, by the hand of nature, along a beautiful flowery path to new and unexpected health and happiness.

If we only mention employing water, light and air, and earth-power, in the manner I employ it in the healing of diseases, people will cry out horrified, "horse-cure." By this appellation they mean to signify a cruel, hard, dangerous form of treatment, which a few can live through, in spite of great dangers, and probably by accident, and get well as if by a miracle, but which would kill most people.

In point of fact, however, it is the very acme of all carelessness, all cruelty, all danger, all hardness, and all unreason, if a weak patient is deprived of water, light and air, and treated, moreover, with medicines, especially with poisons.

On the other hand we cannot treat a patient more gently, with less danger and with greater hope for his recovery, than by putting him into the charge of nature.

In her care his sufferings will soon be alleviated, he will feel relieved, and experience new vigor and happiness.* If diseases

---

*Cases are often cited where men were frozen to death in the open, in order to prove that nature is harmful and dangerous. But what kind of men are most likely to freeze? Those that have partaken freely of alcohol. There is a prevailing belief that meat eating and alcohol drinking are necessary in our part of the world, to endure the climate, but those who eat the most meat and drink the most alcohol are just the ones who possess the least animal heat, and who suffer most in a cold climate, and are eventually most likely to be exposed to the danger of freezing to death. The most tender animals, little birds, the dainty hare, are out of doors in the severest cold, and when we touch them we find they are thoroughly warm. They never even look as if they were cold. If it does happen, in very rare cases, that an animal freezes to death, during an unusually cold snap, it is generally an old animal, whose time of life has expired and whose dissolution takes place in the cold Winter time. Moreover man has interfered so powerfully with nature that even animals are suffering from his interference, so that if it should really happen that a young animal is found frozen to death, this might be

were treated in the way indicated, by means of water, light, air, cold, and earth-power, surely incalculably fewer children would be torn from the hearts of despairing mothers and from the arms of disconsolate fathers, to be laid away so young in the cool earth; and there would be fewer orphans and widows, living forlorn in sorrow and want; and fewer men who have lost all that was most precious to them, and who must live on without love or joy.

My mind is unable to grasp how much less sorrow and want, how much less misery and despair there would be in the world, if we should once more trust ourselves wholly to the air, to the earth, and to a natural mode of nutrition (BY WHICH IS NOT MEANT THE CURRENT VEGETARIANISM).*

But to-day the fond mother still dresses her children in heavy clothes and cloaks, and wraps thick bandages about their limbs, and especially the head and throat; she runs after her husband to fetch him an extra wrap. If a crisp wind and bracing air reign outside, inviting human beings to be refreshed and strengthened by them, the mother takes care that her own dear ones remain inside in the warm stuffy room. The fear of colds will not give her a moment's peace. From sheer anxiety

---

a sufficient explanation. Man is the most highly developed creature; he originally surpassed all animals in strength and the power of resistance, otherwise he could not so long have endured his unnatural mode of life. His present delicate and weak constitution is only the result of his sins against nature. As soon as man shall return to nature only in a measure with regard to his mode of life, he will at once perceive that everything in nature, even the severest cold, exists only for his good.

*Of course, light, air and earth-power, as well as the natural bath, or light and air without earth-power, may be employed in the manner set forth, unaccompanied by the natural mode of nutrition, and yet very important results be achieved in the way of health and happiness. But the gain may obviously be greatly increased if the natural mode of nutrition that I shall describe in the second part of this book is added.

for the health and welfare of her loved ones, she works incessantly in her untiring love to dig their early grave.

In consequence of false nutrition an ever greater quantity of disease matter accumulates in the body, and nature is not given an opportunity to augment the vital energy of the body by means of air and earth-power so that it can free itself of this burden. Should she, after all, succeed for once, the physician is at hand with his poisons to beat down every vital effort of the body. Then after a coffin is borne from the house, it contains so much love and hope, death has claimed his own. In reality this is only a natural phenomenon which in itself is nothing bad or unpleasant, but still the people sob disconsolately after the coffin. The bells toll with such a dull sound, one feels oppressed and afraid, as if a crime had been committed. Human ignorance has once more cruelly murdered a human being. But at the open grave the voice of the Church is heard: "What God does is well done."*

However, we have already again taken to cold water, and the day will surely come when we shall also give our confidence to air, earth, and a truly natural diet; these deserve it still more than water. The day is already dawning in the distance.

Then men will drink in new health, serene enjoyment of life, and the freshness of youth to a ripe old age at the fountainhead of all life and happiness. Then they will no longer walk in pain and sickness, in sorrow and melancholy, in want and despair. Then death will no more come among men unexpectedly, like lightning from a clear sky, to tear asunder the tenderest bonds of love, and to destroy so much happiness upon earth.

---

*It is one of the greatest and saddest errors into which men fall when assuming that God sends disease and premature death out of love This is making a caricature of God's love and wisdom. All the diseases and all the misery in the world are nothing but the necessary consequence and punishment for our offences against the laws of nature in our mode of life.

EARTH BANDAGES AND EARTH COMPRESSES.

In the Bible we read, Gen. 2:7: "And the Lord God formed man of the dust of the ground, and breathed into his nostrils the breath of life; and man became a living soul."

Man then is made of earth.

For wounds and all skin diseases, therefore, moist earth is the only truly natural bandage. The body is thus repaired, so to speak, with the element from which it is created.

Savage nations (in India, etc.) always use moist earth for wounds and skin troubles, as I have been repeatedly informed by travelers, and thus achieve wonderfully rapid cures.

Animals, too, employ earth for wounds. If an elephant, for instance, has been cudgeled, and has received skin wounds from it, he at once moistens the earth with his saliva, stirs it into a soft mass, and covers his wounds with it.

The bandage with moist earth or clay has frequently been used for animals, for instance, for horses in diseases of the legs.

The bandages with moist earth which we are led to adopt when we once more attend to all the arrangements and voices of nature, is one of our greatest achievements. All wounds, all dangerous inflammation of wounds, all wound-fevers, and all skin diseases have through it lost all their dangers and horrors. All the many amputations and operations could be prevented, and endless evil could be avoided. The curing of all wounds and all skin troubles is accomplished through moist earth in the shortest possible time without any pain and any distress whatever. This truly natural bandage is so very excellent that it is mere play to cure wounds and skin troubles with it. In times of war, especially, this earth bandage must acquire the very greatest significance.

For every injury of the skin, wounds of cutting, stabbing, burning, shooting, etc., for every boil or ulcer, every inflammation, stings and bites of animals, blood-poisoning, for all skin diseases, cancer, lupus, tetter, dandruff, eruptions, leprosy, for

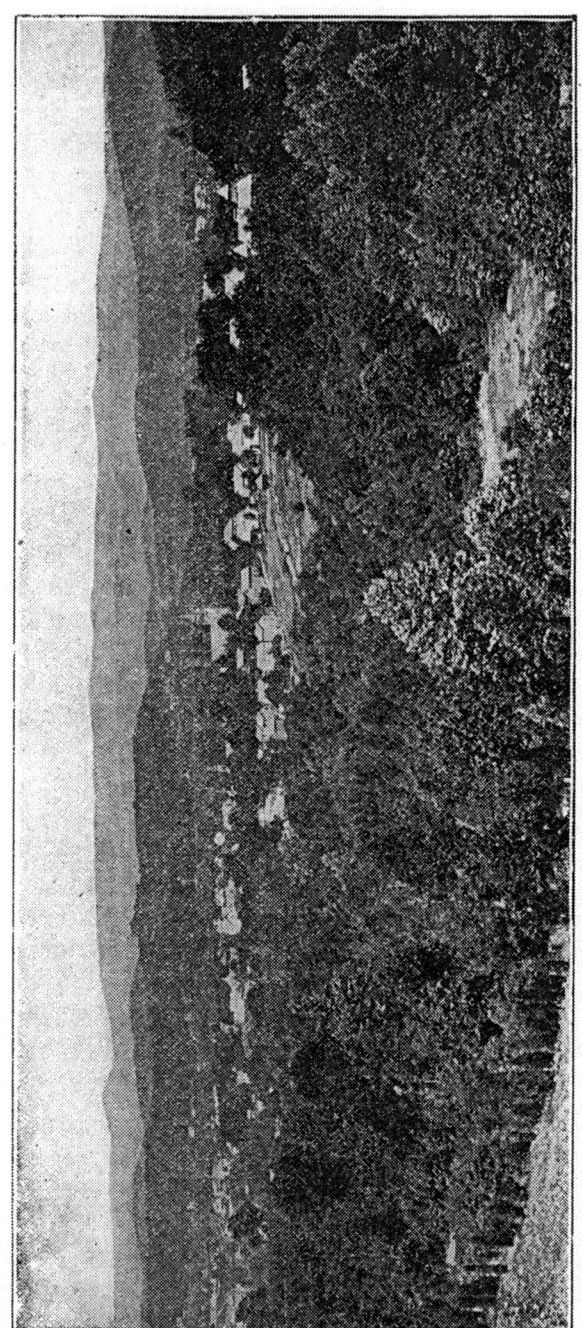

View from American "Jungborn" Sanitarium, Butler, N. J.

broken bones, etc., the affected locality ought to be bandaged with moist earth or moist clay.

The earth is moistened with water, but saliva may also be used.

One will soon feel the coolness and the great comfort of such a bandage, and will be amazed by the striking curative effect of it.

Yes, the earth, indeed! How many are there who recognize its wondrous curative power?

The earth bandage is made by taking the earth (or clay) as moist as possible, and placing it directly on the wound (if possible into it). A linen bandage is then tied around it to keep the earth in place. The wound must not first be covered with a linen rag to prevent the earth from directly touching the wound.

Of course, people to-day will think an earth bandage much too simple. Their restless, unstable mind tries to concoct salves, by means of great scientific researches, and with the aid of complicated apparatus, although a simple bandage with earth will heal the wounds exceedingly well, and without any danger whatever, while salves are often most dangerous.

Many fear that blood-poisoning may set in from a bandage with moist earth, because the earth might be contaminated. No one will be likely to take the earth from a place where refuse and other impurities have been deposited.

But no one seems to think to-day of the impurities which are introduced into the body through unnatural food, through meat and alcohol, which cause so many diseases, and on account of which wounds often become so dangerous. One never fears the poison within, but thinks always of those that may penetrate the body from without, without the knowledge of man, although no danger whatever threatens from the latter source (not even in a bandage with moist earth).

When the earth bandage is taken off a fluid of an offensive odor generally flows away. The earth has drawn this impure matter from the vicinity of the wound; it has, therefore, kept the wound itself, and the surrounding parts, free from impurities and decayed matter, etc., and this explains how it is that a bandage with moist earth heals so remarkably fast and well.

How can one fear that wounds will receive dangerous impurities from the earth? If some impure matter should find its way into the wound through the earth the latter would at once draw it out again and destroy it.

Some object, too, that the earth might contain manure. But it is a well-known fact that country people, for instance, will place cow dung directly on the wound, and so heal it without blood-poisoning setting in. Therefore the dung in the earth of the earth bandage need not frighten us.

The fear of bacilli, however, which, according to modern researches have been found in the earth, is so great to-day, and every calm reflection is so entirely wanting in the matter, that one can hardly venture to advise anyone to try the moist earth bandage. One might actually get into conflict with the police in doing so. But we need not be intimidated by such old and deep-rooted views and prejudices.

It goes without saying that I have always observed only the most conspicuously favorable results with all the many moist earth bandages that I have applied. Never was there any damage done to health, or a single case of blood-poisoning.

We have seen that instinct leads savages and animals to cure their wounds with earth. But instinct never misleads; we can always follow it without misgivings. It can never harm us.

A natural mode of living (abstention from alcohol, tobacco, meat, etc.), is, of course, strongly to be recommended, or rather necessary, especially in the case of large wounds, as I have already demonstrated.

I have now still a few words to say about EARTH COMPRESSES, which are used in a variety of ways.

The earth has, as I have already said, the power of dissolving and absorbing. It dissolves the foreign matter and absorbs it, so to speak.

It is well known that earth has been instinctively applied to the sting of bees, and the bite of snakes.

In John 9:1, 6, and 7 we read: "And as Jesus passed by He saw a man which was blind from his birth."

"When he had thus spoken He spat on the ground and made clay of the spittle, and He anointed the eyes of the blind man with the clay.

"And He said unto him, Go wash in the pool of Siloam. He went his way, therefore, and washed and came seeing."

Through the wonderful healing power that inheres in the earth, earth compresses, too, become of the greatest importance. Many a local trouble will flee from an earth compress as if by magic. It is nature's power again that works the wonder here.

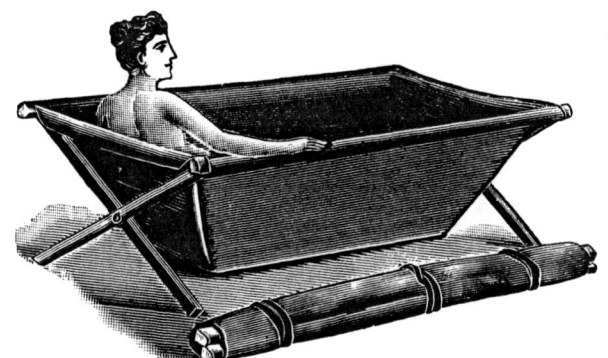

Folding Bathtub for the Natural Bath.

In the case of ALL diseases the general treatment of the body with water, light and air, natural food, etc., is very important. It is through these measures that health may be permanently restored. But great advantages attach also to local treatment. If prompt results are to be achieved, direct treatment of the affected spot is sometimes even very necessary. But for this purpose the only truly natural and really effective remedy is EARTH.

Hitherto water compresses have been employed in such

cases, the Priessnitz compresses and packs, which consist in applying a wet linen cloth to the sick spot and covering it with woollen bandages to produce warmth.

The earth compresses, however, are much more in accordance with nature and much more effective, since the earth will hold more water and retain it longer, and possesses moreover a dissolving and absorbing power of its own.

The entire list of Priessnitz water compresses, including the compress on the abdomen, and all the different kinds of packs, are far surpassed by the earth compresses, and will soon be entirely superseded by the latter.

These compresses are made of moist earth in the same way as the Priessnitz compresses and packs, only that moist earth is used instead of water. The earth must be as moist as possible short of being thin enough to run.

In order to make an earth compress, the moist earth (or clay) is spread over the affected spot, on the abdomen, the chest, the eye, around the throat, on the neck, the cheek, the leg, the calf, the foot, the hand, the sexual parts, on the region of the kidneys, the liver, the spine, etc. It is then first covered with a linen cloth, somewhat larger than the spot covered by the earth. Then another covering of cotton or wool is placed over the linen, and the whole wound about with bandages, so as to remain in place. Strings may be sewed to one end of the bandage to facilitate the operation.

Every thinking, skillful person will soon find out how the earth compress may best be put on in each particular case. The point to be considered is chiefly this, how the moist earth may be made to stay securely in place.

The bandage may be made of cotton or wool. Wool, however, is not as necessary as it is in water compresses, since the earth warms itself. But in the case of patients who have little animal heat, it is always best to use woollen bandages.

In these earth compresses we possess a remedy which we may AT ONCE apply in all the cases of sickness that occur in daily life, and for all manner of pains. It will always prove most effective. In most cases it will produce instant relief and improvement. In difficult cases the compress must be continued for some time. Earth is, so to speak, a universal remedy.

Whether the affected part is internal or external, the earth compress will at once draw out the heat. If the disease is in the chest, the earth compress is naturally put on the chest; in kidney and liver trouble on the region of the kidneys and liver; in diphtheria around the throat, etc.

Since the abdomen is the seat of all diseases, an earth compress on the abdomen is of the greatest advantage in all diseases. This is especially the case in diseases that are not local, but which may be described as a general illness of the system, nervous disorders, melancholy, etc.

The earth compress on the abdomen is of the greatest consequence in reducing fevers, and may, therefore, be relied upon in acute diseases: typhoid fever, scarlet fever, measles, influenza, etc., and in the case of the impairment of the general health.

More heat is, of course, drawn from the abdomen by an earth compress, which remains on the abdomen for several hours, than by the natural bath, which can be taken only for several minutes at a time.

But since the abdomen will have to be washed to rid it of the earth after the compress, a natural bath of short duration may always follow the application of an abdominal compress. The bath may, however, sometimes be dispensed with, as I have said before.

One can always become convinced of how much heat the earth compress draws from the body or a wound by occasionally placing the hand over the compress.

It is very grateful to the body to cover it all over with wet earth or wet clay and then lie down in the hot sun. By doing this the skin will not become sunburnt.

Merely washing the body with clay water will prevent its burning during a sun bath.

The earth compress may be kept on for several hours, according to circumstances, and may be repeated several times during the day. In serious cases the compress must be repeated oftener in the beginning. It may also be applied in the evening, on going to bed, and if not uncomfortable, be kept on during the night. In case the compress becomes too heated, it may be taken off and renewed after a time.

Any kind of earth which the region where one lives happens to produce may be used for an earth compress or earth bandage. Clayey earth adheres readily and has some advantages. If obtainable, it is well to use clay.

The earth compress may be relied upon in countless cases that occur in daily life; for swellings, lung troubles, diseases of the throat and larynx, eye and ear troubles, gout and rheumatism, tetter, dandruff, abdominal and sexual complaints, kidney and liver complaints, diphtheria (compress around the throat), for every variety of pain, neuralgia, headache, toothache, etc.

It is the surest remedy for soothing PAIN and truly harmless, for it draws out the cause of pain, the foreign matter, and thereby removes the pain permanently.

Just as unnatural means are often employed in the case of inflammations, boils, etc., which, while they affect a cure, are all the more dangerous because they actually drive the foreign matter back into the body, so harmful and dangerous remedies are often used for soothing pain.

Dentists to-day often destroy teeth with their pain-killing remedies, which ought in all cases to be avoided. If the toothache can be cured without pulling the tooth, the gain, naturally, is very great.

For toothache the earth compress is applied externally at the spot of the pain, on the cheek, the chin, etc.

If one application does not stop the pain, the compress must be repeated till the desired effect is produced.

Earth compresses on the neck are of especial advantage in the case of headaches.

Persons struck by lightning, or poisoned by snake bite, or taken dangerously ill otherwise, have been buried in the ground with their whole body excepting the head; or with single limbs, especially the legs and arms; and have thus been quickly healed and saved. Burying of the whole body or single parts in the earth may be done at a proper season of the year in particularly dangerous cases. In severe cases of cholera or typhoid fever this would be an excellent method. But the earth must not be too dry for this purpose.

The great curative effect of the earth becomes apparent when one sees how invigorating and strengthening its influence is upon the affected parts of the body that have been treated with earth compresses, or upon the body or parts of it when buried in the ground. Persons suddenly struck dead have been recalled to life by this latter process.

Burying one's self in the sand in the sunshine is also to be recommended. The effect is heightened by the warming of the sand by the SUN.

But the earth ought always to be applied cold, and must never be ARTIFICIALLY WARMED BY FIRE. In drinking warm water we can at once feel that it has lost its freshness and its invigorating effect. So, also, the water that is used in bathing, and the earth that is used for compresses, lose their real healing and invigorating quality by being artificially warmed. It is indeed possible to dissolve diseased matter and achieve so-called cures with warm, even hot, water (for instance, by hot moor baths). But on the other hand the body is thereby debilitated and very much injured, so that the harm done is in truth much greater than the good. To be sure ,the evil often does not appear immediately, but comes limping on behind later on.

Cold washes, cold douches, and other cold baths directly after the application of warm water or warm earth cannot neutralize the great harm that has been done.

In this place I should once more like to call attention to the injuriousness and disadvantage of hot steam baths.

Earth or clay are also most excellent means for cleansing the skin. Frequent washing and rubbing of the body with clay cleanses the skin perfectly and makes it at the same time smooth and pliable.*

The successes achieved by this wonderful remedy, earth, in curing diseases in such an easy and agreeable manner are of such a nature as to call out the greatest enthusiasm and applause in behalf of earth-applications. The use of earth in the form of bandages and compresses had also been almost entirely overlooked (only the late venerable Prelate Kneipp occasionally employed clay). But already in the first edition of my book I expressed the conviction that earth as a remedy had a great future, and that it would soon be generally introduced as a household remedy, which would be always on hand and never fail. Facts have already justified this conviction.

Already the most wonderful and brilliant cures are continually being reported to me as the result of earth bandages and earth compresses, and the greatest enthusiasm has been expressed for these applications on all sides.

Many, too, have written to me that my ideas have met with their most heartfelt response.

The well-known Pastor Felke has become one of the chief champions of earth applications. ·He has been at the Jungborn, and has become deeply interested in my methods.

It is my ardent wish that this old, simple, popular, and natural remedy should soon again receive its due meed and be appreciated at its full worth.

Mankind will then be once again in full possession of the greatest natural remedy.

---

*To-day we use soap made of the fat of animals that have perished from all sorts of diseases; that is the filthiest material conceivable, to cleanse our skin. But strictly speaking, the skin is not cleansed by the use of soap, but rather defiled. The corrosive substances contained in soap always injure the skin. If men were to discard the use of soap in their daily ablutions they would be much cleaner. Those who wash themselves with pure, clear water will be as clean as they need to be. Besides, clay and also sand is a natural cleansing material.

HOW ARE WE TO BURY OUR DEAD?

Death takes place when the soul is separated from the body. The body is then nothing more than earthly substance that immediately begins to disintegrate.

Men have become very material-minded nowadays; they cling to matter. They are no longer conscious of their higher significance; their thoughts and aspirations are not directed towards their soul life that continues also after death.

If a man has died, our thoughts do not follow the soul of the deceased, which is now seeking in higher spheres the perfection it did not find here on earth.

Our first impulse is to cling to the corpse. We still try to honor it by solemn burial, costly coffin and monument.

But in burying the dead the intentions of nature are again entirely disregarded. For us burial ought to mean nothing but "Earth to earth, dust to dust."

The body must become earth again as soon as possible.

In the coffin, however, the body must first undergo horrible processes of corruption. It is for the most part eaten up by worms, and in this gradual decay offensive gases are produced, so that our cemeteries poison the air round about, and make it unwholesome. We must not allow ourselves to fully realize the condition of the bodies in the coffins; it is too horrible. This has been sufficiently shown where bodies have been exhumed.

But why must we bury our dead in a manner that is so disgusting to our imagination and so productive of pestilential gases and the like?

Men have been known to have been buried in a state of apparent death. The reawakening of such an apparently dead person in his coffin, where he is at once doomed to suffocation, is one of the most horrible things imaginable.

Much has been said in favor of cremation. Most expensive apparatus has been constructed for the purpose. Costly silver vases are made to receive the ashes of the cremated body. In these the relatives preserve all that is left of their beloved,—

ashes. The advantage here is that one can always carry this earthly remnant about with one, wherever one goes.

This again is of a nature to dazzle many people, just as many another grand contrivance of our civilization. But after all, it only takes us still farther away from nature.

Why do we not, in burying our dead, also do the most natural, the simplest thing?

In nature dead animals are devoured by beasts of prey. The bodies thus serve as food for other creatures. On the other hand one may assume that beasts of prey had originally no other purpose than to devour the corpses, that would otherwise have contaminated the air with their decay. Beasts of prey, therefore, likewise serve a good purpose in the economy of nature.

There also still are people whose religion bids them to give the bodies of their dead as food to the beasts of the wilderness. They strictly adhere to the designs of nature, thinking that they thus come nearest to doing God's will.

It is not to be thought of, under present conditions, that we should dispose of our dead in that way, and I need not say anything more about it.

But, as for the rest, I think that we should be acting most in accordance with nature if we should simply return the bodies of our dead TO THE EARTH WITHOUT COFFINS. They would then re-combine with the earth in the simplest and quickest manner, without the products of decay, offensive gases and the like.

We have long ago been compelled to this mode of burial, in times of war, although here, where great numbers of bodies are put into one grave, it may be that the gases are emitted through the earth.

By the above mode of burial the reawakening of the apparently dead would be avoided.

It is God's highest commandment that we should love and honor our fellow-beings more during their lifetime than we do to-day. After a person is dead, his body has no longer any value.

But among our contemporaries it often seems that it is only

after a person has died that the desire awakens to show their love for him.

> O, lieb so lang du lieben kannst,
> O, lieb so lang du lieben magst.
> Die Stunde kommt, die Stunde kommt,
> Wo du an Græbern stehst und klagst.

When those we loved die, our love must be directed toward the soul of the deceased that is now seeking its way to the throne of God.

Not that we should ask God to return the soul to earth, but we should sincerely pray for its acceptance in grace and forgiveness, and that when our time comes, we may be reunited with the departed one in the arms of God. Till the time for that reunion comes we must be patient.

We need, however, not to break with old customs and usages, or do violence to the sentiments of anyone. The burial could take place with all the former solemnity. The coffin might be so contrived that it could be easily taken apart and removed, after being lowered into the grave, and the body thus given directly to the earth. The grave could be adorned with flowers and cared for, just as well as before.

To be sure, all expressions of love and honor for our dead, when they are sincere and heartfelt, are pleasing to God and helpful to the souls of our beloved dead. And love is its own reward. Therefore, such veneration redounds to our own good.

This mode of burial does not in the least militate against the belief in the resurrection of the body, as taught by the New Testament. As for the rest, it is entirely immaterial how we conduct our burials. The resurrection of the spiritual life is the only thinkable one.

"It is sown a natural body; it is raised a spiritual body. There is a natural body and a spiritual body." (1 Corinthians 15: 44).*

---

*I cannot here develop my ideas of the spiritual body; it would lead me too far.

Since the question of a new mode of burial has been frequently raised in our time, and cremation has received much consideration, I merely wished to call attention to the most natural way of disposing of our dead. This article has no other object.

NATURAL FOOD.

Since thousands of years science has endeavored to ascertain what substances man required for his nutrition: what, indeed, constitutes the right food for human beings. Physiology, chemistry, anatomy, histology, anthropology, and still other branches of science are pursued for this purpose.

But what has been the result of this research of a thousand years? One very prominent and celebrated professor declares that a truly scientific dietary is still impossible to-day; that science after long labor and research still does not know what men ought to eat and drink. He thereby gives science a certificate of incompetency, which is unfortunately not yet recognized as incompetency.

Science to-day does not even know what men originally knew without any study or research, but continuously promulgates the greatest errors without ever realizing it.

We might apply the words of the apostle to the great scholars of our time:

"Professing themselves to be wise they became fools" (Romans 1:22).

To him who again turns to nature, and thus learns in a simple manner and as it were from himself what he needs to know in order to be well and happy upon earth, to him those men, who are forever studying and experimenting with great pains and labor, in order finally to arrive only at absurdities, appear in a high degree comical.

In spite of all their scientific researches, that which really furthers men's health, welfare and true happiness has become more and more obscure to them. But whoever again follows the voice and dictates of nature, in his mode of life, perceives that all plants and animals, in fact all creatures that remain under the tutelage of nature, are not tormented by diseases, want and misery. He reaches such a firm conviction that he is upon the right track to health and salvation, that he remains entirely untouched by that restlessness and uncertainty about the right, in which men to-day are tossed to and fro and incessantly tortured. He looks out upon that turbulent and mean-spirited strife of men concerning the good and the bad, the harmful and the beneficial, from a safe harbor with complete inward calm and cheerfulness, and his unshakable consciousness of doing that which is really right is in itself a great happiness and curative power.

Man is to-day exposed to the especially grave danger of being misled and confused on the question of nutrition. The body, it is claimed, must have albumen, nitrogen, nutritive salts, etc.

We know, however, that only that is the true food toward which *in pure nature* instinct and taste direct us. Moreover, we know nothing definite, strictly speaking, of the necessary substances of our food-stuffs and of the processes of digestion. This is in the main a secret to us, and always will remain one.

The theories which science has advanced concerning nutrition and the substances which the human body requires can well be described as the most absurd of all the absurdities that the misguided human mind has produced. This is also the reason why these theories change almost every day.

Therefore we must be especially firm in this matter and allow ourselves to be guided only by the voices of nature as the only true guides of life.

Is the young animal that leaves its nest and gets out into the open air for the first time in the least doubt as to what it is to choose for its food? It is guided by instinct, and finds its food without any ado.

The young fawn eats grass, the little squirrel looks for nuts, the young fox immediately chases a mouse or some other animal.

The young animals from the start avoid everything that is harmful,—poisonous plants and the like.

Man who originally followed the voices of nature unerringly, guided by instinct and taste, chose the noblest and most beautiful products of the vegetable world, the *fruits*. Man probably could not eat grass, and he probably did not care to catch an animal and bite into it.

We also read, Gen. 1:29: "And God said, Behold I have given you every herb bearing seed, which is upon the face of all the earth, and every tree in the which is the fruit of a tree yielding seed; to you it shall be for meat."

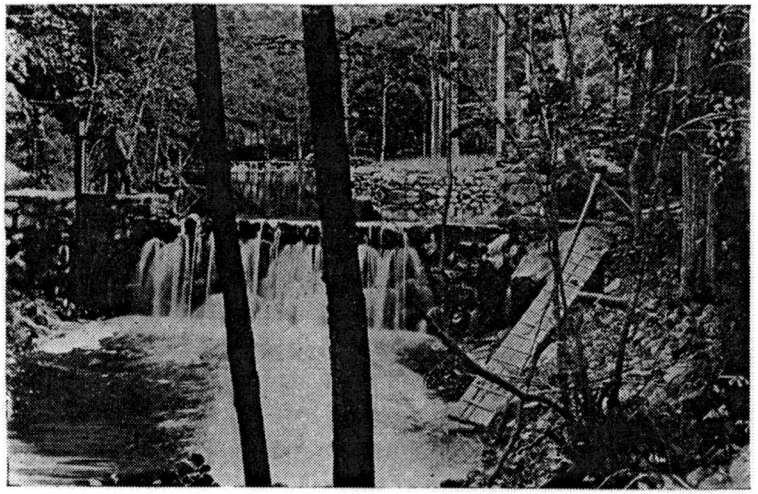

Scenery in Woman's Air and Sun Bath of the American "Jungborn," Butler, N. J.

"Herbs bearing seed" and "trees yielding seed" are here specified; that is to say bearing fruit which is to be the food of man. To the beasts of the earth it says are given "every green herb for meat" (Gen. 1:30).

We certainly cannot assume that the trees themselves were to serve men as food.

Wherever men lived nature originally produced fruit abundantly, and spontaneously, without the labor of man. But the fruits differed according to the country, according to the warmer or colder climate.

In our part of the globe the berries of the forests were the original food of man; later he added the fruit of trees, and chief of all the *nut;* everything that tastes good in the raw, pure, unchanged state of nature.*

The nut could be found during the greater part of the year, for nature has so arranged it that the nut will keep perfectly for a long time after it has dropped from the branches on the ground or in the dry leaves.

As long as the forests had not been cleared, and nature was everywhere still undisturbed, nuts and berries grew in such abundance, even in our parts, that they afforded sufficient nourishment to man. Nature in her infinite goodness has provided for all her creatures from the start, but most lavishly for her darling, man.†

In this way we have easily and surely arrived at a knowledge of our proper food. But we must not allow ourselves to be led astray again, for objections are at once made on all sides, and there are always men who think they can teach us better than nature and her voices.

People are generally very much alarmed when they hear of man's proper food, for the first time, and think that they must at once adopt it. We touch men's sorest spot when we question their present mode of nutrition.

I shall therefore try to be very considerate in speaking of food, and not discourage anybody.

---

*Only the things that taste good to us in the raw, natural condition can be considered as our natural food, for by artificial preparation the most unnatural nauseating things can be made to taste good, for instance, the excrement of snipe. It is very easy to deceive the tongue.

† It is a well-known fact that the old Germans in the beginning subsisted exclusively on the fruits of the forests. Hunting did not begin till later. But even then berries and fruit remained for a long time their chief food.

Let everyone, in the first place, turn again to water, light and air, and earth in the way pointed out. Whoever cannot follow this up at once with a natural diet can at least simplify his mode of feeding as much as possible, and especially avoid harmful dishes and luxuries.

Above all things one ought to control himself as far as possible in the matter of meat-eating.

Salted and smoked meats are the most injurious. Pork and the various kinds of sausages are the worst of all.

Instead of meat more milk might be taken, uncooked sweet milk, sour milk, cottage cheese (curds), etc.

I cannot recommend eggs and dishes containing eggs.

Potatoes, leguminous seeds, and bread as food for man are contrary to nature, as I have repeatedly indicated. We ought, therefore, to eat sparingly of these food stuffs.

Instead of potatoes and leguminous seeds we ought to choose green vegetables and salads. Of the young vegetables some may well be eaten raw, for instance young peas, carrots, spinach, turnips, etc.

It is less hazardous for laborers, who daily perform severe physical labor, to eat leguminous seeds, potatoes and bread. Persons who do no physical work must take these foods in limited quantities if they cannot avoid them altogether. In times of sickness this is of course especially necessary.

Nuts and fruit ought to be always on the table.

Cake and other sweetmeats, chocolate, cocoa, pudding, etc., always disturb the digestion, and are therefore injurious to health.

Alcohol is the dangerous demon that is raging incessantly in the world to-day, and is everywhere cruelly destroying health and human happiness. One ought therefore to partake very sparingly indeed of beer, wine, etc., or better still, avoid these so-called luxuries altogether.

But tobacco, too, is a false friend. I cannot warn against it sufficiently.

Other stimulants, like coffee and tea, are likewise undermining men's health everywhere at present. These, too, are slow poisons whose dangerous character is not recognized.

I wish especially to warn against coffee on account of its being in such general use at present. Instead of the real coffee cereal coffee (malt coffee) could be used. But of course the only natural drink is water. The deer of the forest drinks only water.

On the whole, people ought to drink as little as possible. Soups, too, ought not to be served so often, nor much liquid food. Nature prescribes solid food which requires chewing.

But if drinks and liquids are to be avoided, food must not be too highly seasoned. Salt and all spices are very deleterious to health, they are directly responsible for many diseases (cancer of the stomach, etc.).

I have now been sufficiently regardful of people's weaknesses in respect to diet. We must let well alone if people will only begin for the present to simplify their tables, to avoid a part of their unnatural food, to learn to appreciate fruit and nuts, and to give them a place on their table again.

But I now want to point out the way to those who are already desirous to come into full harmony with nature, who do not wish to make fruit a side-dish, but the staple article of their diet, or even their exclusive diet. I know how many there are even now, who would become willing and enthusiastic followers. The time is at hand for a return to nature.

If the integrity of nature were undisturbed, man's instinct, taste, and conscience would lead him to choose only *nuts* and berries (preferably and chiefly nuts) for his food.

Besides nuts, *berries growing* in the woods, in free nature are the most appropriate human food. The berry especially to be considered here is the huckleberry, since that still grows in great abundance in our forests, and in its season is brought to market in great quantities. Would that the huckleberry would soon again receive the appreciation it merits.

As complementary to the berries we have our splendid fruits, apples, pears, plums, peaches, apricots, grapes, to choose from, to which we may add tropic fruits: almonds, figs, dates, oranges, melons, bananas, etc.

O man, how richly God has spread the table for you!

Fruits are the food that God offers us, his sun has ripened them. Would that men no longer refused that divine gift.

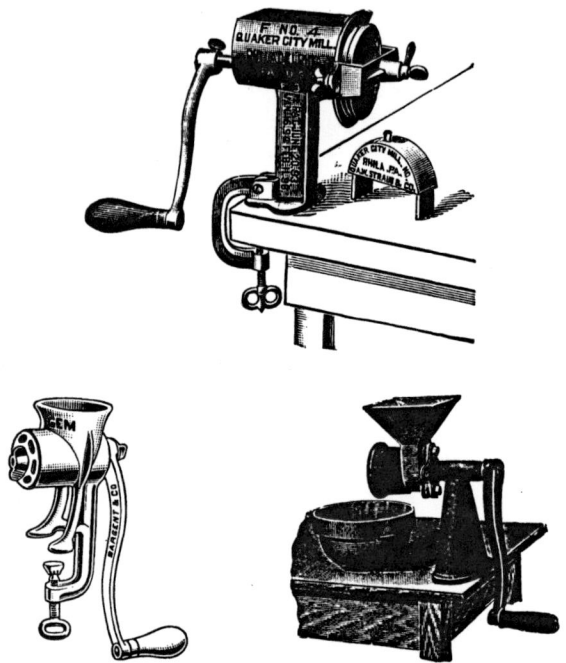

American Handmills for Grinding Nuts, Cereals, Malt-Coffee, etc.

In refusing it they gravely sin against nature and God, and the penalty is inevitable: sickness and misery in a thousand shapes.

Does not your heart rejoice within you when you see a fruit-tree laden with magnificent fruit? Do you not recognize in this the voice of nature?

Cooked potatoes, leguminous seeds, bread, corpses of animals, etc., what are they in comparison to magnificent fresh fruit? These cooked foods are dead and insipid; salt and other spices must be added in order to make them at all palatable.

Fruits are delicious to the taste, possess a splendid aroma, in them there still is freshness and life.

The unnatural cooked foods oppress our intestines; they make us languid, dull, and tired of life. Raw fruit again brings pure blood, life and strength, joy and gladness into our weak, sick body.

Why does man seek after healing draughts? *Fruit alone contains healing draughts for man;* nature offers them ready made, they taste deliciously, and are sure to cure all his suffering and disease. Fruit contains nectar and ambrosia. Why does man reject these healing juices of nature, these most delicious potions, and brew instead horrible drinks, mixtures, herb lotions, teas, etc., forcing himself to swallow them in order only to bring unspeakable misery upon himself?

Medicines do not cure our diseases.

"In vain shalt thou use many medicines; for thou shalt not be cured."—(Jer. 46:11.)

It is a sad fact that men do not recognize the great harm that medicines, salves, etc., always do to health. The poisons, unfortunately, are often misleading in their effects.

Nature spontaneously produces fruit; or fruit grows without much interference on the part of man. In order to produce the unnatural food, men must incessantly toil at severe, hard labor, at horticulture and agriculture. Only with a great deal of trouble can nature be made to yield the present food stuffs, bread, leguminous seeds, potatoes, etc.

In the face of all this it is inexplicable why men should reject fruit, the natural food. Here again we stand before a great riddle and cannot comprehend the folly of men.

Fruit, too, ought to be eaten in the state in which nature produces it. If we dry, cook, or preserve fruit it naturally loses more or less of its original worth. The preparation of fruit juices, too, is not in accordance with nature, for the juice that is artificially withdrawn from the fruit is certainly not as wholesome as the juice eaten with the fruit in its natural state.

The nut must therefore take the most essential part in

human nutrition. It is the nut that imparts warmth and strength to man.

If some people cannot bite the nuts on account of bad teeth, they must eat them grated.

Machines for grating the nuts can be bought in any house-furnishing store.

I generally give hazel nuts the preference, because they are more likely to grow without artificial contrivances and culture. But walnuts will do very well, likewise other nuts.* Dates and nuts eaten together are delicious.

Raw, uncooked milk can be added to the bill of fare. Butter and very soft cheese (curds) may be tolerated; they ought both to be unsalted if possible. Hardly anyone can be expected to return at once to a purely fruit diet. We are therefore obliged to make the transition with milk, butter and bread (perhaps also some green vegetables). Among animals, young mammals likewise retain the mother's breast for some time, while making the transition to the food of the adults. It seems that the degenerate civilized stomach must in the same manner be gradually led to resume the natural food. Milk seems to me to be the best means for making the transition.

A little bread, as a necessary evil, so to speak, may also be

---

*Besides the hazelnuts, which are called filberts in this country, I would greatly recommend our pecan nuts, as this kind is growing wild without any cultivation, and is preferred as an original natural nut, containing still more oil than the hazelnut, besides the pecan being the finest nut in the world in taste and flavor.

A cousin to the pecan is the hickory, also a nut growing wild in the woods without any cultivation, and is greatly recommended also.

Our black walnut, also growing wild, contains more oil than any other nuts. The following list of nuts, composed by the translator, gives the principal kinds of nuts found in America and other countries: Almonds, Arhut, Bambarra ground, Brazil, Bread, Sonari, Cashew, Chestnut, Cob (Filbert or Hazel), Cob of Jamaica, Cocoa, Cola, Dika, Gingko, Hickory, Moreton Bay, Olive, Pecan, Pekea, Pine (Pignolia), Pistachio, Quandang, Rush, Sapucaya, Tahiti, Walnut, Water Chestnut. All of these can be used as food in their natural state.—B. Lust.

eaten. It is best to take wheat or graham bread. Our ordinary soured bread is very hard to digest, and can therefore not be recommended. Bread and butter with figs are very good.

Stewed fruit, preserves, but also fresh fruit, strawberries, huckleberries, raspberries, etc., are very good mixed with curds.

Such dishes are to be especially recommended to beginners, so that their table may not become too simple all at once.

The curds are prepared in the following manner: Set the sour milk in a warm (not hot) place until the whey separates from the curds, then pour them onto a fine sieve, and at last mix the curds (cottage cheese) with sweet cream or sweet milk.

Whoever cannot entirely dispense with cooked food may have one meal with vegetables cooked in butter (cocoa-nut butter is better) and perhaps a few potatoes.

With the combinations thus suggested (nuts, all kinds of fruit, milk, butter and bread, also some cooked vegetables, etc.), this fruit diet can easily be generally introduced. This mode of nutrition will insure to a family many gustatory delights and much health. A diet reform in this manner is most necessary at present. The upper classes especially ought to take the lead in introducing this sort of a table into their families, not only in cases of sickness but for general use.

The lower classes look upon the so-called delights of the table, which the well-to-do allow themselves in the shape of meat, wine, tobacco, and the like, as an advantage which the rich have above the poor. The poor, therefore, greatly aspire to gain this advantage for themselves likewise, but in this way they are striving for the diseases and the glittering misery of the upper classes. Therefore it would be very desirable that the upper classes in the first place should deny themselves these unnatural foods, and all pernicious luxuries, and thus set a good example to the lower classes.

But the true return to nature is the right way for both rich and poor, high and low, if they desire once more to obtain health and happiness. Nature knows no difference of class or rank. But under existing conditions a general return to nature, a so-called reaction after the extreme of unnatural living, must proceed, in the first place, from the upper circles.

Here, too, help is most urgently needed.

I have not only observed at Jungborn, how quickly people became enthusiastic over the fruit diet suggested above, with the proper helps and transition dishes, but I also know a number of families, who have already accepted this sort of diet in their homes, and consider themselves happy in the change. The members of such a family are always full of praise of their new diet, its pleasures and delights.

The table can, of course, be still simpler: nuts and native fruit are best and really all that is necessary. In some cases of sickness it is even necessary to simplify the table still more.

Many, too, will be obliged to live plainer according to their means. But I have intentionally allowed for as much liberty and scope as possible in furnishing the table.

This new departure in a meatless diet, in which fruit occupies the chief place, might be called the *new vegetarianism*.

Leguminous seeds, green vegetables, potatoes, cereals, rice, etc., were not intended by nature as the food of man any more than meat; for these, too, do not taste good to us in their raw, uncooked condition without any seasoning. Now if man discontinues the use of meat, as well as alcohol, tobacco and the like, he breathes more freely as it were, as if relieved from a great crime against nature. But a diet of fruit, bread, green vegetables, leguminous seeds, without nuts and milk, is wanting in the chief ingredient of human nourishment, i. e., fat, which the nut contains.* People thus fed generally look pale and thin, are always cold and often nervous, and other troubles, too, put in

---

*It is often said that our stable-fed cows are all sick, and that therefore we ought not to drink any milk. According to similar reasoning our babes ought not to drink their mother's milk uncooked, for our women are all still more diseased; and yet the children that are not reared on their mother's milk thrive but poorly. Of course, the milk of healthy cows, such as go out to pasture, is much better than that of sick animals.

their appearance more and more. They have neither warmth nor vitality.

The experiences that one has with regard to the health of old vegetarians are very bad.

There are among them a great many pale, bloodless, dried-up, emaciated individuals. Old vegetarians ought therefore to listen to reason.

It has been observed, however, that some persons can endure the unnatural diet of the old vegetarianism longer and better than others, and that the bad results do not appear alike in all cases.

All that is said against the nut as a food is of course entirely false.

It is claimed that the nut is hard to digest for man on account of the oil it contains. Those who make this assertion do not consider what a reproach it implies against nature, as if she had created an improper and indigestible food for the highest of her creatures.

Nature intended the nut for the squirrel as well as for man, and this little animal which so lightly skips from tree to tree in our woods does not in the least make the impression as if it were subsisting on indigestible food.

I should like to advise the vegetarians, who make the above statement, to seriously make the attempt to live chiefly on nuts, instead of nourishing themselves with green vegetables, leguminous seeds, potatoes and bread. They will soon find out how their sluggish digestion becomes vigorous and strong.

The immense strength that the ox derives from grass alone, and the elephant from rice alone, is also often cited to show how man, too, could become well and strong from only vegetables, leguminous seed, cereals (bread), and fruit. But I should like to call the attention of vegetarians, who make this claim, to the fact that the lion, and still more the whale, also receive immense strength from their meat diet. All creatures thrive only on the food to which nature has directed them through their instinct, sense of taste and conscience, and for the attainment, mastication, and digestion of which nature has arranged their organs. Thus the fox thrives on a meat diet and the ox on grass. Fox and ox would fare badly on nuts. The dung-beetle feeds on dung. What other creature could likewise subsist on dung?

It does not follow, therefore, that man can be healthy and happy on a diet of vegetables, leguminous seed, or *fruit and bread,* because the ox is strong and powerful on a diet of grass.

On the other hand, man receives strength and vigor when he lives chiefly on nuts, for the nut is the food that man can relish in the raw state, therefore it was intended for him by nature, and she keeps it in store for him during the greater part of the year.

It has frequently been pointed out in old and modern times that nature did not intend flesh but rather plants to be the food of man, but rarely has it been insisted on that nature's plan was not for man to eat green vegetables, leguminous seeds and bread, but raw fruit (berries, etc.), and it has been especially overlooked, so far, that nature chiefly intended the nut for man.

An Englishman, the late Dr. med. Densmore, was the first to publicly call attention to the dangers of our present fatless vegetarian diet, and to refer us to the nut as the chief food of man. For this he deserves great credit.

But Densmore was still entirely too much under the spell of science. Therefore his system had many faults. Densmore proves the correctness of the nut-diet scientifically, especially by the arrangement of the intestines. But scientific proofs have no value. All the absurdities of the medical art have been demonstrated as correct by scientific proofs. Everything, whatever it may be, can be proven right or wrong by the scientific method. The science that has not nature for a basis, and therefore has no basis at all, can be used in this manner. Therefore it has already been scientifically proven that the theories of Densmore are incorrect. But what is especially significant is that Densmore's scientific proofs could not at all convince the masses and win them over to a nut and fruit diet. Probably Densmore, too, originally came by his ideas through other ways than through science.

Nature and its laws are unchangeable from the beginning to eternity, and there never will be true successes in healing, and men can never become truly healthy, strong, and happy if they do not again take raw fruit, and above all nuts as their staple food.

The answer to this will most assuredly be, that diseases have indeed been cured without the fruit and nut diet, and that men have been well and strong. But men to-day have no longer the least conception of true health, strength and happiness, such as nature will award to him, who will again strictly obey all her laws, and of the healing successes that can be achieved.

I have already attempted, in the beginning of this book, to prove satisfactorily how incomprehensible and dangerous is the distrust which men have towards nature with respect to light and air. It is just as incomprehensible and injurious that they can have no confidence in the food which nature offers them. Is it not evident that all creatures are beautiful, well, strong and happy when feeding on their natural food; the deer on grass, the lion on flesh?

It is also well known that the orang-outang, whose intestines and organs of digestion are so like man's that they can be mistaken for them, lives entirely on raw fruit, and nevertheless possesses such enormous strength that he is the giant of the tropic forest. It is believed that man would not derive sufficient strength from a fruit diet. But with his artificial diet of meat, vegetables, leguminous seeds, bread and alcohol, he is to-day altogether infirm and weak in comparison with the orang-outang. He could, however, be much stronger than the orang-outang, if he ate truly natural food, and otherwise led a truly natural life, for as the highest creature, who is to rule over all the animals, who was the most highly developed, he ought greatly to surpass all animals in strength.

The myths of giants, Cyclops, and the Valkyries, also point to the original great strength of man.

Animals always prefer *unripe* and *half-ripe* plants and fruit. Every experience will confirm this. Children, too, who still have more instinct than adults, are generally fond of unripe fruit.

Even naturalists seem to note the fact that animals prefer unripe plants and fruit.

In Martin's new large natural history we find it stated that the orang-outang of the wilderness is especially fond of eating unripe fruit.

It is a well known fact that birds like the cherries best before they are quite ripe, but are just beginning to turn red. Birds will leave the ripe cherry-tree alone and turn to the tree with the unripe fruit.

It can be generally observed that animals like the tender, unripe grass and grain best.

They also like the dried grass and straw better when it has been cut sooner, and in a more unripe state than farmers usually cut it nowadays. The unripe fodder is also more wholesome and more advantageous for the animals.

Apples that are put by for use in winter are now generally picked half-ripe. They would have to stay on the tree much longer before they would be fully ripe.

That children get diarrhœa and skin trouble from eating unripe fruit proves most effectually that unripe fruit more than ripe fruit has an invigorating and stimulating effect upon the body, for diarrhœa and skin trouble are likewise only curative crises, purifying processes of the body.

One should therefore no longer fear *unripe* and *half-ripe* fruit, but should eat it. Our pampered tongue will also relish it more and more. Green vegetables are unripe herbs or unripe leguminous seeds, therefore green vegetables are more wholesome than ripe leguminous seeds and ripe grain, from which bread is baked.

Animals that are fed much on leguminous seeds and ripe grain, and especially when they do not work hard, always grow stiff in the joints and sometimes even die. On the other hand, horses that are fed on unripe fodder, even if it is in a dried state, do not get stiff. This proves that the leguminous seeds and the ripe grain are not according to nature, and cannot be recommended. For this reason the present-day vegetarians make a great mistake in recommending whole wheat made of full, ripe kernels with thick chaff, as the basis of human nourishment. This mistake has often enough been severely punished.

Many people think that dates and figs are not good for our teeth. The dates and figs that we eat are dried and, therefore, no longer pure nature. It may be that abundance of sugar in our *dried* tropical fruit is of a certain disadvantage to our teeth, but I doubt if this is so very bad. Moreover, tropical fruit is not absolutely necessary, I recommend it chiefly because it gives more variety to our table, especially in winter, which is very agreeable. Against fresh tropical fruit, like oranges, etc., such objections can, of course, not be raised.

To be sure, our fruit is artificially cultivated and no longer a spontaneous product of the earth, but it is still a product of nature that we relish in the raw state and can, therefore, be eaten just as well as berries.

Tropical fruits (dates, figs, oranges, almonds, etc.), do not thrive in the same climate with us and are properly intended only for the inhabitants of southern countries, but we can relish them raw, and they cannot therefore, be considered exactly as unnatural food.

We therefore act but very slightly contrary to nature when we eat tropical fruit in comparison to the very great departure from nature that man is guilty of when he eats leguminous seeds, potatoes, and the like.

Milk must always be taken *uncooked;* cooking only makes the milk indigestible. Sour milk can also be used.

Of course, fruit and berries ought in the first place to be eaten *raw* (uncooked). In the absence of fresh fruit, however, dried, stewed and cooked fruit can be eaten.

In the preparation of stewed fruit and fruit preserves no sugar or very little ought to be used. Artificially prepared *sugar* (not the sugar that is contained in the fruit) *is very injurious to the stomach.*

The unblued sugar, which can be found in the market, is, of course, better than the ordinary sugar.

Dates may be used for sweetening. Honey is permissible with bread.

It is necessary to eat slowly, and to masticate well. The stomach can digest food better that has been well mixed with saliva.

It is natural to eat raw fruit more slowly than cooked viands. If we only always stand by nature, the right thing will come of its own accord.

The transition from a meat diet to the present vegetarian diet (green vegetables, leguminous seeds, bread and some fruit) is very difficult, as a strong desire for fat, which the nut contains, will soon make itself felt. In the course of time there will also be other sensations of discomfort, although the symptoms caused by a meat diet and alcohol will disappear. That is why so many discontinue their vegetarian mode of life again. But with a diet of raw fruit, especially with nuts and raw fruit, the digestive organs are at once very much relieved, and the digestion very much improved. This clears the head also, and makes the entire being feel free and light-hearted, while a hitherto unknown sensation of well-being and joy pervades it. Since the body is now supplied with the substances it requires for its nutrition and development, an agreeable sensation of bodily warmth soon makes itself felt, and with a new sense of power and vigor there also comes new joy in life.

As for the pampered palate, that finally learns to relish the most tasteless things, even those that were exceedingly disagreeable at first, for instance alcohol and tobacco.

In truth, however, no culinary art can impart the fine taste to viands that nature gives to raw fruit which has grown and prospered in God's own sun.

If a person has only for a short time overcome his craving for unnatural food, he will learn to appreciate the real luxuries of a natural diet. He can always eat the raw fruit without craving any change, and will become more and more susceptible to the finest flavors, so that it would be very difficult for him to accustom himself again to the old mode of living.

This explains why people remain enthusiastic adherents to the fruit diet, even those who could be kept on the old vegetarian diet with the greatest difficulty only.

But in recommending this diet I must again call attention to the fact that the more strictly in accordance with nature we make this change in our food, the more and the stronger the so-called curative crises may appear. They may manifest themselves in various forms, by pains in the limbs, a temporary feeling of languor, and in other ways. They are always a good sign; they prove that the body is in full curative activity. The patient also distinctly feels the relief which the crises bring him, and will not be discouraged by them if he understands nature only to some extent.

Sometimes, too, with this thoroughly natural diet an excessively keen appetite sets in in the beginning, so that great quantities must frequently be eaten to satisfy it. This is also a good sign, as it proves that the body is now beginning energetically to build itself up.

An excessive appetite in the beginning need not alarm anyone, it will disappear again in time, and finally one will require a smaller quantity, in order to feel satiated than formerly with the unnatural food, and this lesser quantity will be eaten with greater relish.

Excepting the mother's milk, the food which nature provides for man is in *solid* form. The animals in nature that subsist on raw, juicy vegetable food, drink very little, the roe, for instance, does not drink at all. It is probable that man, too, was originally a non-drinker, since it is so difficult for him to drink without an artificial apparatus. But if one considers how much liquid food (soups) man eats nowadays, and what quantities he drinks (alcohol, spirits, coffee, tea, etc.), it is easy to see how greatly man sins against nature in this respect also.

Cures are achieved by Schroth's cure only through this circumstance that the patient must for a time avoid *all* liquids.

Whoever begins to derive his nourishment entirely from fruit will soon perceive that he is no longer thirsty and does not need to drink.

As for the rest, the only drink that nature offers, besides the mother's milk is water. Lemonade and fruit-juices may also be used.

An agreeable drink can be made in the following manner: One bottle of selters water or chalybeate spring water and add the juice of one lemon, and raspberry juice as flavor. This drink has been used at Jungborn on festive occasions, and has met with much approval. We always had a happy time over it.

If there must be drinking on festive occasions, therefore, it is not at all necessary to take alcoholic drinks. Glasses can be touched with fruit-juice, too, and toasts can be proposed to the Fatherland, to anyone's birthday, etc. High spirits, and cheerfulness need not necessarily be accompanied by intoxication.

Fruit-juices ought always to be simple, pure juices, such as our housewives prepare them.

To all the manufactured fruit-juice of to-day (that are advertised under high-sounding names, such as unfermented wines, etc.), there must always be attached some suspicion of adulterations, although some of these are often even prepared in good faith.

The unnatural thirst that is at present caused by meat, salt, and spices, calls for strong, exciting drinks. The flabby nervous system, too, wants sometimes stimulation; but when stimulated it finds itself more completely shattered In this way man came to be addicted to alcoholic drinks, spirits, coffee, tea, etc. I suppose it is no longer necessary to prove how alcohol is contrary to nature, and how much disaster in every form this monstrous demon has caused among mankind.

In small quantities, of course, alcohol is comparatively less harmful, than when taken in great quantities. Physicians who assume that beer and wine in small quantities are even strengthening, and therefore prescribe it to their patients, err most unfortunately. Even a slight artificial excitement through alcohol, which must always be followed by a much greater relaxation, is very harmful even to healthy persons; to the sick it must be still more harmful.

The harm that men cause to their health nowadays by the excessive use of alcohol, spirits, and tobacco, women try to achieve with coffee. Coffee is to-day a source of much sickness and misery among our women. As long as a woman does not wean herself from coffee she can never enter upon the road to true health. Coffee made from cereals is naturally not nearly as harmful as real coffee, but it is desirable that even the use of cereal coffee (malt coffee) should be more and more restricted and avoided, since much liquid food is always injurious.

The more fresh, juicy fruit man eats, however, the more does the craving for drinks and liquids subside.

Drunkenness can only be cured by a natural diet.

Opponents to the natural mode of living have all kinds of doubts and objections to offer. One immediately asks where all the nuts, apples, etc., are to come from if all people were again to live a natural life; another is full of anxiety about the many butchers, shoemakers, inn-keepers, apothecaries, etc., who will then be out of employment.

Everyone who to-day wishes to live on natural food can easily get what he needs for his nourishment.

As soon as the demand for fruit should become greater, however, great quantities of it could be raised on the surfaces now devoted to cattle-raising and to the cultivation of a great many things that are not only without value, but even injurious to man (tobacco, turnips, potatoes, grain, etc.).

To-day the space allowed to fruit is only along the public highway and other desolate and useless places and surfaces. The berries and nuts in our woods are actually looked upon as weeds and are exterminated.

Strictly speaking, the condition of man has deteriorated in the same degree in which he has deviated from nature in his mode of living, and in which civilization and science have advanced, and it will once more improve in exactly the same degree in which he will again approach nature. In the beginning there were no trades, men were happy then; if it could be that trades would again become superfluous, then *all* men would once more achieve earthly happiness, however unlikely that may seem to many.

I would implore every fruit-eater, even now, to do all in his power to foster fruit culture.

The human digestion in all its contrivances is arranged only for a fruit diet; fruit alone, therefore, can be easily and completely digested.

The process of developing foreign matter is, therefore, at once suspended where fruit is the only nourishment, and the digestive organs can devote themselves all the more to carrying away old, stored-up foreign matter; the fruit serves as a stimulus to this activity.

Considering the digestibility of raw fruit, and all the wonderful healing and vitalizing powers it possesses, it is obvious of what great importance a fruit diet must be in the curing of diseases.

The successes that have been achieved with a fruit diet are indeed wonderful. Through it health often returns in cases where all vital energy seems to have been extinguished, and nothing seems to remain but to despair. I have frequently convinced myself of this.

Why then must we still neglect fruit and have recourse to all sorts of unnatural foods and remedies?

Every animal when it gets sick instantly stops taking nourishment.

Man ought to eat as little as possible during sickness, at least he ought to eat only when the stomach demands food by means of a violent appetite.

Temporary fasting is of great advantage.

Jesus, too, thought highly of fasting: "Howbeit this kind goeth not out but by prayer and fasting."—Matt. 17:21.

Many believe that they must force themselves to eat when

they are sick and have no appetite, so that the body may not become too weak, but that is a fatal mistake.

When the stomach does not demand food, it is in no condition to digest it; it will then only be burdened with the food which it receives without appetite, which in sickness especially is very injurious, and may even become very dangerous. No well person ought ever to be urged to eat, but with a sick person this must be avoided all the more. Here, too, it would be very desirable that anxious mothers should not sin so much in this respect.

With artificial food there is always this danger, that men will eat too much, while with natural food (raw fruit) nature has so arranged it that it is not easy to eat too much. Therefore if a person eats fruit when he is sick, he need not be so afraid of eating too much.

In describing the natural mode of life my object, so far, has essentially been to point out the advantages that it brings to the physical part of man; I have tried to explain how those conditions that we call disease can be avoided and cured by a return to nature.

But in nature everything is in closest harmony, and in man, too, body, mind, and soul cannot be separated from each other. The body sustains mind and soul, and contrariwise, mind and soul always influence the body.

Man was originally created by God not only entirely healthy and beautiful, but also absolutely noble and good. He was the crowning glory of creation. The masterpiece of the all-wise and all-good God could not be full of imperfections of body, mind, and soul.

Men to-day possess sinful desires of all sorts, they struggle much against them with all the means in their power, but they again and again relapse into sin. If God had originally placed these evil tendencies into man, which he so often and so repeatedly tries to overcome with all the earnestness and all the strength that is in him, only to succumb every time, then God would not be a good God but an evil spirit, whose pleasure is not in goodness but in evil. But the sinfulness of man is the consequence of his own unnatural mode of life. The fall of man was through a forbidden food, a fall from nature, as I will show more fully.

In free nature, for instance, the animals indulge in the sexual act only for purposes of propagation. After the impregnation has taken place the animals do not only discontinue the sex act, they cannot even be forced to it by any means. Just so it is with man; the healthier he becomes, by leading a natural life, the more can he not only avoid immorality and other sins, but they become quite impossible to him. But only when he has arrived at this stage is man truly reformed. However, among all the various classes of animals there are even sub-divisions; for instance, the quadrumana are divided into apes proper and monkeys. The various races of men, likewise, have not all reached the same degree of development, some possess more imagination and reason than others. "Man," of whose blissful and god-like state, the myth of Paradise tells us, was meant to belong to the most highly developed race (i.e. the white race). Those men who were most highly gifted with reason, were also the men who were most exposed to the danger of achieving the highest culture and scientific development, and were thus destined to drift into the greatest misery.

We need not fear, however, that, by a complete return to nature, modern civilized man will finally return to the state of the savage races of distant countries, who are not much above the animals.

All the deviations from the original, healthy condition of the mind and soul have been caused by disturbances in the body. The foreign matter injures all the organs, even those that unite the mind and soul with the body. But no one thinks to-day that by caring for the body in accordance with nature, we can do away with such conditions as idiocy, insanity, absence of mind, ennui, ill-humor, melancholia, anxiety, sensuality, youthful excesses, vice, and crime, passion, hatred, envy, malevolence, etc.

At all events, all ethical culture, all the work expended on the mind and soul is in the main to no purpose, without the corresponding natural care of the body, and may even cause still worse conditions.

A Greek myth tells of the Danaids. These were the daughters of the King Danaos, who, upon the advice of their father, had killed their husbands on their wedding night. For punishment after their death, they were condemned to continually dip water into sieves in the underworld.

All those who are to-day working to make men better and happier without first leading them back to nature, are doing the work of the Danaids; they are forever dipping water into a sieve, which can never be filled.

Yes, all those lawgivers and philanthropists, who know nothing of the significance of a natural mode of life, often only increase the evil. Thus, for instance, we fight against public vice, prostitution, and thereby merely further what is much worse, and more dangerous, secret vice.

This reminds one of the struggle with the Hydra, of which the Greek myth likewise tells us. The Hydra was a monster with nine (or a hundred) heads, that devastated the region about the Argolian swamp Lerna. It was in vain to attempt to slay this monster, for two new heads grew for every one that was cut off.

The giant Hercules, however, subdued the monster and killed it.

All the evil in the world, the present dangerous monster among mankind, can also be destroyed, but only one thing avails: return to nature.

"So God created man in His own image, in the image of God created he him."—Gen. 1:27.

God is love, and in this respect man resembled God. Love of God and his fellows was originally the sole disposition of man.

When man fell from nature the consequent sufferings of the body were at once accompanied by taints of the soul. Sensual pleasure, in its manifold ugly shapes (especially sexual sensuality* the chief evil) was created, and man's love became tainted; hatred arose, from hatred grew envy, malevolence, and all the sins against God and our fellows. The image of God was more and more lost in man.

In nature we at once see that all creatures which live on flesh are vicious, while plant-eating animals are gentle and peaceable. As soon as the ape and the dog are fed on flesh they lose their docile disposition and become fierce and dangerous. Apes that are fed on meat only a short time, at once become unchaste in the worst degree.

The natural mode of living is not merely a stomach question, then; we wish thereby not merely to heal the sufferings of our body, but to reach higher ends, yea, the very highest end, of morality and virtue. Man's likeness to God will be restored more and more.

JESUS AND THE NATURAL MODE OF LIFE.

Jesus, the Saviour of the world, must be our staff and guide. Let us go to the Saviour for advice on all vital questions. Is the question of our nutrition of such small importance, then, that we need not be concerned about what Jesus prescribes in regard to it?

All religions give prescriptions with regard to food, the religion of the Jews, the Mohammedans, and above all the great society of Buddhists in India. It is a well-known fact that the Buddhists are not allowed to eat meat.

Can it be, then, that Jesus alone placed no value on food? Should the Saviour, who preached only love, and gentleness and

---

*The reproductive and digestive organs of man are closely connected. Animals in the lowest stage of development possess only reproductive and digestive organs. With man's unnatural mode of nourishment, sensuality is produced in the first place.

After the fall of man shame appeared. Man was ashamed, which was the first result of the forbidden fruit: therefore they had recourse to fig leaves. But shame is the sign of sexual impurity. The primeval, completely healthy and pure man was not ashamed.

peacefulness, not have known that this requires a natural mode of nutrition? Almost all mankind to-day are indifferent about their food, and do not see what great harm is done to body and soul by unnatural nourishment. But Jesus walked on divine heights, and should He not have known the great truth, the importance of obedience to the laws of nature with respect to food?

Oh, ye ignorant and fools, I should like to exclaim here! It is safe to assume off-hand that the Saviour did not walk in such dark error.

We see that although Jesus primarily preached the salvation of the soul, He was at the same time occupied, wherever He went, with healing the diseases of the body. Jesus well knew that the sufferings of the body could not be set aside.

In antiquity health culture was always a matter of religion. Priest and physician were always one and the same person. This was also the case with Jesus, He too, realized that body and soul could not be separated, if men were once more to be made sound, good, and pious.

By a natural mode of life we obey the laws of nature, which are God's commandments; conformity to nature must be a matter of religion.

I have often pointed out how Jesus always sought this union with nature. Jesus remained in the desert for forty days, He preached in the desert, on the seashore, and on the mountain.

Jesus always held up the mode of life of the animals in free nature as an example to men:

"Behold the fowls of the air: for they sow not, neither do they reap, nor gather into barns; yet your Heavenly Father feedeth them. Are ye not much better than they?"

When John sent word to Christ to ask, "Art thou he that should come?" the answer came back:

"The blind receive their sight, and the lame walk, the lepers are cleansed, and the deaf hear."—Matt. 11:5.

Jesus wished to be recognized by John by the healing of the diseases of the body.

When Jesus sent out His disciples, He bade them:
"Heal the sick, cleanse the lepers," etc.—Matt. 10:8.

People came to Jesus under the same circumstances under which to-day they come to the nature-cure method, after they have tried everything that science has to offer.

"And a woman having an issue of blood twelve years, which had spent all her living upon physicians, neither could be healed of any,

"Came behind him and touched the border of his garment; and immediately her issue of blood stanched."—Luke 8:43, 44.

And this word of the Saviour's also:

"I thank thee, O Father, Lord of heaven and earth, because thou hast hid these things from the wise and prudent, and hast revealed them unto babes" (Matt. 11:25), still holds with the nature-cure method to-day. They are only lay people, insignificant men, not great men of science, who have once more taught us what can really make men healthy and happy.

The Essenes thought much of the bath; they took one daily, and always thought it was a religious rite.

Jesus practised and taught bathing in the same way. Baptism in the Christendom of to-day is a remnant of this.

From the above we can see that Jesus not only healed a great many diseases, but also championed a natural method of curing.

But Jesus also preached a natural mode of life. The first Christians, the saints of old, as soon as they were converted to Christianity, withdrew from the world to nature; they always nourished themselves on vegetables, often from the abundant fruit alone that grew in the forests of the Orient. This is reported to us in the history of the Church. Saint Augustine is said to have eaten only fifteen figs a day. Surely the early followers of the Saviour knew better than the present misguided Christians what mode of life Jesus prescribed.

So, too, the old cloisters were in the beginning always built in the woods, in the midst of nature; vegetable food and other directions for a nature life were always among the rules of the cloister.

Nevertheless Christianity gradually fell away again from the natural mode of life.

Even behind the walls of those world-secluded cloisters, meat-eating, gluttony, and drunkenness soon held sway once more, and in consequence all sorts of sins and vices ran riot there. The monks well knew that this mode of living was not in accordance with the teachings of Jesus and the Bible. Therefore they hid the Bible and kept it from the people.

In this manner, only a few remnants were finally left in the Christian Church as reminders of the diet of Jesus: fasting in Lent, ember and vigil days, abstinence of meat on Fridays, Ash Wednesday and Holy Week, the Sacraments, etc.

John was the precursor of the Saviour. Of him it was said in the announcement:

"For he shall be great in the sight of the Lord, and shall drink neither wine nor strong drink."—Luke 1:15.

John lived in free nature: he dispensed with culture entirely, and wore only a mantle of camel's hair. And our Bible to-day tells us that John ate *"locusts and wild honey."*

But eminent theologians and Bible translators (for instance Bunsen), who are by no means vegetarians, and do not care to speak in its favor, are of the opinion that a mistake has here been made in the translation. They think that the words "locusts and wild honey" had better be translated as "sprouts of trees (fruit, like nuts) and sap or sugar of trees."

In the Orient many trees yielded a sort of sap or sugar, which was used as food. Or fruit especially rich in sugar may have been meant.

It is hardly credible that a pious man like John would have run after locusts to catch and eat them, without any preparation, when he became hungry.

There are, indeed, people who, besides other unnatural food, will eat locusts, but they first roast them and grind them to powder. But an artificial preparation of the locusts was impossible to John, this son of free nature, who had neither spider nor stew-pan. Even if there are some people who have been depraved to such an extent by unnatural food that they are again able to eat and swallow live locusts and beetles and the like, it is not at all probable that the great and holy John did it. But at all events it is impossible that John could have lived on live locusts all the time. In that case we should have to look upon him as a monster, not as the precursor of the Lord, whom the prophet announced with the words:

"Behold, I will send my messenger, and he shall prepare the way before me: and the Lord, whom ye seek, shall suddenly come to his temple, even the messenger of the covenant, whom ye delight in."—Mal. 3:1.

In consequence of the above error in the translation, we to-day have an indistinct and wrong impression of John the Baptist.

I now hope to show you John in a true light, so that we may be edified by him and appreciate his mission in every respect.

What is meant by wild honey is quite inconceivable. Is one to believe that John in the wilderness daily took the honey from the bees? I do not think that this would have been an easy task for him.

The translation according to which John nourished himself with the nut-like fruit of trees, is obviously the right one.

But John only wished to smooth the way for the great King that was to come: "Prepare ye the way of the Lord, make his paths straight." From John's mode of eating, therefore, we may infer that of the Saviour.

When the Saviour was born the wise men came from the Orient.

Now long before the time of Jesus there were the Buddhists in India who led a religious nature life.

It is safe to assume that these wise men of the Orient came from the Buddhists. Thus we see at once that there was a connection between the Buddhists and Jesus.

The theologians know that in the course of time passages of

the Bible have been expurgated and spurious passages have been inserted, and that in many ways falsifications and misrepresentations have taken place. Many philologists and theologians have exposed a number of false passages in the Bible.

I have already pointed out how the Christians have deviated more and more from the natural mode of life prescribed by Jesus, and how they have tried to conceal it. This probably explains how the first copyists of the New Testament, and later the translators, came to expurgate and falsify, at first consciously and finally unconsciously, the very passages relating to Jesus' directions for a natural mode of life. In this way we can explain how it came about that in the New Testament many passages, especially such relating to the natural mode of life, are wanting, and others that are still extant are so obscure and confused.*

Luther has given us the best Bible translation; it is pregnant with poetic beauty and very well adapted to the understanding of the German people. But in Luther's time the knowledge of a natural mode of life and its significance for body and soul, had become totally lost. This explains how Luther came to make many a bad blunder in his translation, which can mislead us in regard to the mode of life taught by the New Testament.

But there are still many passages in the New Testament which plainly show the Saviour's plan of nutrition, and other passages can easily be set right. This can be done especially if we no longer insist too rigidly on the meaning of single words, but have an eye to the spirit of the New Testament. I shall return to this later.

But whatever has been done to efface and obscure the teachings of Jesus with regard to a nature life, they cannot be obliterated from the soul of the people and from the customs

---

*The late Dr. med. Rich. Nagel, an old champion of vegetarianism, has given us some correct and good references and clews to innumerable, wonderfully forced Bible translations. Dr. Nagel's translations have for the most part not been brought before the public at all. But it is our highest duty not to overlook or forget any merits. Therefore I wish to mention Dr. Nagel in this place.

of the people, upon which the powerful holy institutions of the Saviour have made such a lasting impression.

On Christmas, the birthday of the Saviour, when the holy night descends, when the candles of the Christmas tree are lit, and holy Christmas joy and Christian love fill our hearts, we still eat nuts and apples. Nuts and apples belong to this consecrated feast of Christendom, and if we are not altogether thoughtless, we shall recognize in this old custom the food which the Saviour had once prescribed for us.

The great significance of the old custom of eating nuts and apples on Christmas is unfortunately not recognized at all.

Would that Christmas might become the perennial feast of Christendom, and that nuts and apples might again become men's daily food; then, too, the love that fills their hearts on that day would again prevail, and soon we should once more hear: "Peace on earth, good-will to man."

Jesus will but have gained in wisdom and holiness for us, when we have realized that He, too, preached the natural food, that the eternally inviolable laws of nature were not unknown to Him, and that He did not corrupt His body with all kinds of unnatural food. On the other hand, this knowledge will lead us to look upon the natural mode of life as something holy, something divinely appointed. Not until then shall we appreciate it fully.

But although Jesus did indeed prescribe a natural food, He was in this respect, too, considerate and gentle with His newly-won followers; in this respect, too, Jesus stroked the lost and misguided sheep gently and cautiously.

Jesus always thought very highly of John:

"Verily I say unto you, Among them that are born of women there hath not risen a greater than John the Baptist."—Matt. 11:11:

Jesus also valued and Himself adopted the diet of John.

But for the above reason, out of love and wisdom He was not so strict with regard to food as John. During the three years that Jesus taught, He did not, like John, live entirely on unprepared food, raw fruit, but ate also prepared food, cooked vegetables (also bread).

"For John came neither eating nor drinking (artificially prepared food and drink), and they say, He hath a devil.

"The Son of man came eating and drinking (cooked food, bread, etc.), and they say, Behold a man gluttonous, and a winebibber, a friend of publicans and sinners. But wisdom is justified of her children."—Matt. 11:18, 19.

These words of the Saviour show that He considered fruit as the only correct diet, and only deviated from it sometimes at the call of wisdom; and how He was misunderstood on that account on the part of His malicious opponents.

Jesus and the Bible would preach the true salvation of man, therefore they must especially preach the natural mode of life, for not until men practise this can they gain their salvation.

Jesus did indeed consider the soul higher than the body, and He did not wish that we should consider our nourishment too anxiously and painfully, and should thus be prevented from diverting our thoughts and senses toward a higher soul-life.

I think I have now considered every condition in the matter of diet. I have arranged the diet for the weak, who cannot at once break entirely with the old food, and for the strong, who desire to be led by the hand of nature to the sunny heights of health and happiness.

MEAT AND ALCOHOL.

Nature did not intend man to be a meat-eater, a beast of prey.

Man does not relish meat in the raw state without some sort of seasoning and preparation. He must at least have salt with his meat.

The beasts of prey are transported with voluptuous delight when they can kill an animal; they become intoxicated with the fresh blood.

But man, when he is not yet entirely brutalized, shrinks from killing; his conscience is always aroused when he raises the murderous steel against an animal, his fellow-creature. The death-rattle of an expiring animal still moves the most hardened man. Most people would not eat meat if they themselves had to kill the animal. The raw, unprepared flesh, the animal corpses in the butcher shops, are always a revolting sight. In some places, therefore, the law forbids meat being carried about openly.

And why will people, in this respect also, turn a deaf ear to nature, to instinct, to the sense of taste, smell, hearing, sight, to conscience? Is this, also, too simple? Why does man make laborious scientific investigations to ascertain whether he belongs to the class of carnivora, corpse eaters, or to the class of omnivora (pig, bear, etc.), to the classes, indeed, which always appear to us as vicious and cruel and which we despise?

It is only another proof of man's morbid desire for knowledge, if he does not investigate with the simple means nature has given him whether meat is suitable food for him, but rather studies the teeth and intestines for that purpose, and attempts to ascertain the ingredients of meat.

This latter way to truth is not in accordance with nature and must lead astray, especially since through man's unnatural life many organs have degenerated, and some have been similar in the various creatures from the beginning.

Several scholars, who certainly are themselves very much attached to their roast, have claimed that man was designed for a partial meat diet, according to the structure of his teeth, and there are many who thoughtlessly repeat this after them.

Nevertheless man is not equipped with claws or fangs, such as all beasts of prey possess, to seize and tear their prey. The digestive organs of carnivorous animals are likewise quite different from those of man.

Beasts of prey, for instance the dog, can eat the bones as well as the meat. Man cannot do that, which proves that his stomach must be arranged very differently from the stomach of these animals.

Let us but compare the eye-teeth of man with those of vegetable and fruit-eaters, and those of meat-eaters and omnivora, and we can plainly see that man belongs to the vegetable and fruit-eaters and not to the beasts of prey. The eye-teeth of men have no more similarity to the fangs of omnivorous and carnivorous animals, than the mouse has to the elephant. Just so the length of the intestines in man does not point to a meat diet.

But if meat has not been intended for man by nature, it is also injurious and harmful to him. Man does not become healthy and strong by eating it, but sick and weak.

It is claimed that man must eat meat on account of the fat it contains, which enables him to endure our cold climate. But why not acquire the requisite bodily warmth through the fat contained in the nut? The nut contains the fat that is natural to man and not the many other ingredients so injurious and poisonous to man.

The Eskimo of Greenland, whose country does not yield him nuts and vegetables, which could nourish him, also tries to endure the severe cold of the North by eating meat and animal fats. It may be that the animal fat does enable the Eskimo to live in the extreme north, but on the other hand, the Eskimo, on account of his unnatural food, is an ill-shaped, ugly specimen of humanity, and intellectually an idiot.

People are too apt to excuse their unnatural mode of life, their meat and alcohol habit, by reference to the *climate*. The climate is called in to quiet their conscience with regard to their great crimes against natural living. A fruit-diet, however, enables man more than unnatural food to endure heat and cold.

We cannot suppose that man, the most highly developed creature, was destined by nature to occupy only a small part of the earth. The Bible, too, says:

"Replenish the earth."—Gen. 1:28.

But it is not necessary that man should deviate from his natural food in order to spread over the earth.

Both the hottest part of the tropics and the coldest part of the north, are equally unfitted for the habitation of man. But if man should be designed by nature for the warmer parts of the earth, they need but begin a natural mode of life again. Their instinct would then reawaken more and more, and following this, they would gradually wander back to the warmer regions. In reality, however, the intermediate zones are best adapted for human beings, as I shall show further on.

Man, the image of God, who ought to be a gentle, merciful ruler upon earth, violates the divine impulses of his heart when he kills, or causes animals to be killed for his food. Man, at present, is continually soiling his hands with the blood of his fellow-creatures. This offence in obtaining his food must naturally be followed by most severe punishment.

Meat eating is therefore an offence against nature, an unnatural practice, which must have exceedingly bad and dangerous consequences. Unnatural meat and plant food is not digested by the stomach. Thus the meat that has been eaten is not digested, but rots in the stomach, and is continually fermenting in the body and blood, and causes, more than undigested, unnatural vegetable food many inflammatory and disgusting diseases, and also most ugly sins and vices.

Orestes, of Greek mythology fame, whose soul was oppressed by a horrible murder, was incessantly pursued and driven by the Erinnyes, the avenging furies. The conscience of humanity is at present also burdened with murder, and cannot find rest or peace upon earth.

The heating meat, with all the salt and spices that are required to make it palatable, always awakens the desire for strong drinks, for alcohol. Meat eating, therefore, opens wide the doors for that uncanny demon, alcohol. Meat has a foul, vicious brother that accompanies it. No one can fail to recognize the harmful, dangerous character of alcohol, even in the smallest quantities.

Alcohol excites the nerves, and transports man into a beautiful illusory world of dreams, which, however, is always followed by stale, empty reality, nausea and discontent. Man thinks he gets strength from alcohol, but this also is deceptive Artificial excitement is the most harmful thing for health. If we are not deceived by the momentary effect, we soon realize that the body is very much weakened by the alcohol, and that the nerves especially are shattered in the most alarming manner. Alcohol, therefore, works the greatest ruin to mind and soul; vice and crime are also among the horrible consequences.

The man who eats no meat finds himself continually in such a frame of mind that he is in no need of creating for himself a momentary, beautiful, but illusory dream life.

But if meat is so injurious to body and soul, the question presents itself to us whether the Bible and Jesus did not prohibit meat eating. Would that religion, the Bible and Jesus again played a greater part in our life in every respect!

Some especially grave mistakes have crept into the old translations of the Bible, whereby all its teachings with regard to meat-eating are mis-stated and unrecognizable.

The first law that God gave to man runs thus:

"Behold, I have given you every herb bearing seed, which is upon the face of all the earth, and every tree, in the which is the fruit of a tree yielding seed; to you it shall be for meat."—Gen. 1:29.

So we see that in this law man has not been charged to eat meat.

Besides this law, which was written into man's very soul, there was originally no other law given. God the omnipotent ruler could rule men by *one* law. If man had obeyed this first law, all the subsequent laws of God,* also the Mosaic law, and all the thousands and thousands of laws made by man up to the present day, would not have been necessary.

The first law of God is repeated Gen. 2:16 and 17, while a prohibitory law is added, and a punishment threatened:

"Of every tree of the garden thou mayest freely eat:

"But of the tree of the knowledge of good and evil, thou

---

*If man had not fallen from nature, had not lived a wrong life, the inclination to commit murder, to lie, to be immoral, to steal, etc., would never have arisen, and there would have been no need for those inner voices to awaken in man, which forbid all these sins against God and our fellow-men.

shalt not eat of it: for in the day that thou eatest thereof thou shalt surely die."

But what is meant by the tree of the knowledge of "good and evil"?

We can have no conception of a tree of the knowledge of good and evil; a tree cannot know.

However, the original language of the Bible was poor in words: there was but one and the same word for plants (trees) which were still rooted firmly to the ground, and plants that in consequence of a higher development were separated from the ground, i. e., animals. If a distinction was to be made between plant and animal some addition had to be made. The vegetable and animal kingdom are closely related. Science is at a loss to determine the boundary line between plants and the lower animals (microscopic animals, corals, polyps, etc.), But at present plants are still distinguished from animals in that we designate that as an animal which feels and perceives.

The Bible therefore adds the phrase, "the knowledge of good and evil," to designate the animal. In Gen. 2:9 the animal is also called "tree of life," i. e., a tree (being) which has life. It would, therefore, be more correct if the passage in the Bible would read: "being of the knowledge of good and evil," and by this being that can know what is the good and evil, harmful and useful, that has feeling like man, is meant the animal. *The fall of man, the first sin of man, therefore, consisted in the eating of the forbidden food, the flesh of animals.**

In a paradise myth of the Hindoos, the translation of which

---

*There is still another passage in the Old Testament from which it can be inferred with certainty that man first sinned solely by eating meat. In the beginning men still recognized their sin; they fought against it, but again and again became backsliders. Finally they tried to justify their sin; yes, they even made themselves believe that God had left it free to them to eat meat.

It would lead me too far to bring all the proofs for this here. Besides, I consider it useless.

is free from error, the eating of the flesh of animals is distinctly prohibited.

Only those creatures in free nature that eat meat, kill. Through a meat diet nature directly instills the desire to murder. Now when after the fall of man the first, and for the time being the only, bad deed was murder—fratricide; this proves that the fall of man consisted in the eating of meat, otherwise the deed would be inexplicable.

Moreover we hear of the skins of animals soon after the fall of man.

"Unto Adam also and to his wife did the Lord God make coats of skins, and clothed them."—Gen. 3:21.

Where were the skins to come from, if man had not already killed animals? The Bible shows how civilized mankind has gone astray. In the beginning men lived in a state of *paradise;* they lived on the fruit which nature yielded spontaneously. The first fall from nature was the beginning of the *chase,* and the fall of man was the chase. As a result of the chase men ate the flesh of animals and clothed themselves with their skins.

Now they fell sick, an inner restlessness made itself felt, just as the horse that is fed on ripe oat kernels, instead of on its natural food (grass), becomes restless, and must be put to hard work. Men likewise had to begin to work now, and cleared the forests; the age of agriculture began.

But in this way agriculture was but a punishment:

"Cursed is the ground for thy sake; in sorrow shalt thou eat of it all the days of thy life;

"Thorns also and thistles shall it bring forth to thee;

"In the sweat of thy face shalt thou eat bread."—Gen. 3: 17-19.

The curse of the Lord lay upon the soil.

While the earth produced fruit spontaneously, without trouble or labor on the part of man, the tiller of the soil to-day is suffering from bad harvests, weeds and the like, in spite of his hard labor. Care and anxiety are the lot of the farmer.

Instead of delicious fruit, man must now eat herbs (lettuce, cabbage, leguminous fruit, etc.) from the field. That is his punishment.

"And thou shalt eat the herb of the field."—Gen. 3:18.

All the products that man laboriously wins from the soil in agriculture are, moreover, injurious to his health; they destroy his earthly happiness.

After agriculture came grape-culture, and alcohol with its disgusting consequences made its appearance:

"And Noah began to be an husbandman, and he planted a vineyard:

"And he drank of the wine, and was drunken; and he was uncovered within his tent.

"And Ham, the father of Canaan, saw the nakedness of his father, and told his two brethren without," etc.—Gen. 9:20-24.

Then came the trades and the arts.

"And Zillah, she also bare Tubal-cain, an instructor of every artificer in brass and iron."—Gen. 4:22.

The art of building was also introduced. The tower of Babel was begun. And now arose the various languages. which resulted in the science of language.

But misery steadily increased, men were plunged more and more deeply into error, they continued to fall from nature and from God. Disease, sorrow and want, discontent and despair became greater. At last the Psalmist laments:

"The days of our years are threescore years and ten; and if by reason of strength they be fourscore years, yet is their strength labor and sorrow."—Ps. 90:10.

But ever and anon prophets and voices were heard that spoke against the falling away from nature, against meat-eating, while at the same time they alluded prophetically to the coming of the Saviour.

Then in darkest night a beautiful morning appeared: it was the world's Saviour.

Christ wanted to atone for the fall of Adam, He wanted to lead men back to nature and to God; He also wanted to banish that primeval sin, the eating of meat, from the world, for until this was done His glad tidings could not be received by men

But how could Jesus Himself have eaten meat then? The Saviour preached gentleness and mercy above all things, and could He have eaten the flesh of animals, which brutalized men, defying the voice of conscience and the voice of God within their breasts, had mercilessly killed? Jesus would in this case Himself have sinned against mercy, and would not have been free from guilt. Could Jesus have eaten meat that produces so much disgusting suffering of body and soul, sins and vices?

There is also a mistake in the translation of the New Testament, that corresponds to the mistake that has been mentioned from the Old Testament. In antiquity men tried to propitiate the gods for their sin of meat eating by offering an animal in sacrifice. Historians tell us that the Essenes, the sect to which Jesus belonged, had no animal sacrifices. For this reason we can safely assume that they ate no meat. This is also admitted by theologians.

Contrariwise those sects ate no meat who offered no animal sacrifices. Jesus and His disciples did not offer sacrifices; He even forbade animal sacrifices.

"I will have mercy and not sacrifice."—Matt. 9:13.

How then could Jesus eat of the Easter lamb,* the chief sacrifice of the Jews? The word in question, correctly translated from the text, is Easter meal. In the sense of the Jews, with whom the Easter meal always meant the sacrificial lamb, this could indeed be translated as Easter lamb, but with Jesus, who even forbade the sacrifice, it never could mean Easter lamb A good translation must not only be literally correct, it must preserve the sense.

C. Weizsaecker, who is no vegetarian, has made a translation of the New Testament in which many of the old mistakes

---

*The following argument turns on the word *Osterlamm* (Easter lamb) used in the German Bible for passover, and loses its force with readers of the English Bible.—(Translator.)

have been avoided. It has already received recognition, and has been introduced into our schools. In this translation of the New Testament the word passover is always substituted for Easter lamb in the passages in question.

"Where wilt thou that we prepare for thee to eat the passover?"—Matt. 26:17.

"Go and prepare us the passover, that we may eat."—Luke 22:8.

In contrast to the Jews, who ate the bloody lamb, the Saviour took bread for His Easter meal, gave thanks, broke it, and gave it to His disciples to eat.

There are still other passages in the Bible according to which the Saviour is said to have eaten meat. In various places in the New Testament we read that Jesus distributed fish among the multitude that followed Him, and that He Himself ate fish But it seems rather strange that in the Orient people should have taken fish with them upon a journey, when even we in our northern climate would not take fish with us on an excursion or journey, because fish decays much faster than other meat. It is said that the sect to which Jesus belonged had a sort of bread baked in the form of a fish. It was called fish, and was probably the fish which Jesus distributed and ate of Himself. This interpretation and translation is much more probable.

All the passages that can be found in the New Testament to-day approving or advocating the eating of meat are falsified. These passages are either spurious, wrongly translated, or wrongly interpreted. But it would lead me too far to furnish proof in the case of each separate passage. Whoever has grasped the spirit of the Bible, especially that of the New Testament, knows that Jesus expressly forbade the eating of meat, and above all things, that the Saviour did not eat meat. Yes, and if all the world had been eating meat until now, Jesus certainly did not eat it.

But I believe that the knowledge of this is of the greatest importance, and that it is the best means of salvation. The serpent was the tempter of man in Paradise. It said:

"Ye shall not surely die:

"For God doth know that in the day ye eat thereof, then your eyes shall be opened, and ye shall be as God, knowing good and evil."—Gen. 3:4, 5.

The wily serpent is the cunning of reason whence science was born. Science is still misleading men to-day, just as it did in Paradise. It is still teaching that great advantages can be gained for body and soul by leaving the paths of nature.

In most recent times a great scholar has even asserted that through our refined, artificial mode of life, men had developed into something higher and would finally become like gods.

But science is still deceiving and betraying us. Every sober, unbiased mind must recognize that men with their unnatural mode of life cannot become gods, but must become sick, wretched creatures, sinful, wicked, benighted beings, veritable devils.

We must be most careful, therefore, when the eating of meat is recommended to us by science, or on scientific grounds, with all sorts of sophistical reasoning and in the face of the law of God and of Jesus. In such an emergency we must listen to the voices of nature, which here utter an unmistakable warning.

But what stand did Jesus take with respect to alcohol? This is the next question that presents itself to us.

In the Old Testament we read:

"Who hath woe? who hath sorrow? who hath contentions? who hath babbling? who hath wounds without cause? who hath redness of eyes?

"They that tarry long at the wine; they that go to seek mixed wine."—Prov. 23:29, 30.

"Because he transgresseth by wine, he is a proud man."—Hab. 2:5.

"Thou shalt tread sweet wine, but shalt not drink wine."—Micah 6:15.

In Ephesians 5:18 we read:

"And be not drunk with wine, wherein is excess."

We know also that John did not drink wine or any strong drinks. At the last supper Jesus said:

"But I say unto you, I will not drink henceforth of this fruit of the vine, until that day when I drink it new with you in my Father's kingdom."—Matt. 26:29.

"New" means fresh, unfermented. New wine is fresh grape juice. From this passage we infer that Jesus, in order not to be too strict, and not to harm His cause thereby, may have made an exception for once, and have drunk wine (the Saviour was always mild and considerate) in order in this way to win people over to His side,* but that He always spoke in favor of grape *juice* and against alcohol.

Jesus wished to extend His career as a teacher of men only over several years. It is quite obvious that He did not mean the heavenly kingdom beyond when he spoke of His Father's kingdom where He would drink unfermented wine with His disciples, but He certainly must have meant the community of Essenes, who also called themselves God's community. At all events the beyond could not have been meant here. Jesus is known to have prepared wine at the wedding of Cana. But it is very probable that this wine was non-alcoholic, and for that reason was so greatly relished by the wedding guests. There are to-day still plenty of delicious fruit juices and the like, which are really more agreeable to the taste than real wine.

THE FIRE.

Solely through the discovery of fire has it been made possible for man to stray so far away from nature.

Only by the aid of fire could man artificially prepare all sorts of food, alcohol, medicines, etc. All the contrivances of civilized

---

*Herein particularly does the Saviour show the depth of His love and wisdom, that He did not proceed with too great severity in respect to food, but mildly. All those who are too strict and harsh in their opposition to an unnatural diet do wrong and harm their cause much. But it is also probable that in consequence of this very mildness of the Saviour, all His prescriptions in respect to a natural mode of life have been wiped out in the course of time.

life, that have brought in their wake diseases and all our present misery, have been made possible through fire only.

Man could not have turned away from nature if he had not had fire.

Fire, therefore, is the real beginning of man's misery. But to-day mankind no longer recognizes its enemies; it looks upon fire as a benefactor—a friend that has brought us many blessings and great welfare. But here, too, the consciousness of the truth has been kept alive in the soul of the nations. Many myths, especially Hindoo myths, regarded fire as a sinister, demoniacal element. The devil is represented as belching forth fire. The *Greek myth of Prometheus* tells us most impressively and beautifully how terribly the gods resented the discovery of fire by men, how severely man is punished for it, and how every evil has come into the world through fire.

Prometheus (i. e., He who reflects beforehand) stole the fire from heaven in order to make meat palatable to men. God Zeus was greatly enraged at this; he chained Prometheus to the Caucasus, where the vultures came and ate out his liver. But the liver grew again as soon as it was devoured, so that the vultures continually found new food, and Prometheus new tortures. Then also Zeus sent Pandora, a woman equipped with the most bewitching gifts by all the gods. Epimetheus, i. e., he who reflects afterwards, received Pandora. But she brought a box with her, which she opened, and out came all the evils, except deceptive hope, which remained behind in the box.

One can easily understand how fire to-day still works terrible mischief to man, such as the myth relates. If men had no fire with which to prepare meat by cooking and roasting, meat would soon not be eaten any more. Then we would no longer have all the instruments that are required to catch and kill the animals and prepare the meat. I have already mentioned that alcohol and medicine can be prepared only by the aid of fire. I have certainly proved sufficiently how all serious diseases are caused by meat eating, alcohol, and medicine. But it is also clear how diseases and suffering can be caused by cooking the rest of our food.

Animals always remain beautiful and well on raw vegetable food, if diseases are not caused in them in other ways, for instance by bad air. But if the grass, potatoes, turnips, etc., are cooked, the animals readily eat greater quantities of the cooked food, which, in its artificial preparation, slips down more easily, before it is well mixed with saliva, and this is very bad. Stuffing now begins, the animals grow stout and fat, ugly, languid and lazy; in a word, sick. The farmer always fattens his animals for half a year at the most, for although they eat still greater quantities after that, they no longer increase in weight, but even begin to fall off, while all sorts of diseases begin to show themselves. The stomach is now completely worn out by the long continued overfeeding; it derives much less benefit for the body from the greater quantities of food than formerly from the smaller quantities.

And yet these animals get their natural food, only in a cooked condition. If we now consider that the things which men eat nowadays are not only not intended for them by nature, but are made still more unfit, more indigestible and less nutritious, by the process of cooking, we can easily understand how injurious and disastrous food artificially prepared by means of fire must be.

The digestive organs are soon worn out, and foreign matter (undigested matter) is formed. This comes to light in various ways, in the shape of boils, skin disease, inflammations, fever, and all sorts of diseases. Physicians cut, cauterize, rub with salves, and prescribe medicines to suppress the symptoms of the disease, but the foreign matter continues to grow from the inner seat of the trouble, so that the painful labor must always be begun anew by the body. By his complete ignorance of the cause of the disease, man is chained fast like Prometheus, and must, therefore, quietly endure his tortures.

If we no longer employ fire in preparing our food, we shall be obliged to fall back upon our natural food, and physicians will then no longer find anything to cut and to cauterize.

Warm baths relax the skin and the nervous system, just so warm food relaxes the inner, digestive organs. It would be well, therefore, if *all* food and drink could be taken cold, at the most lukewarm, but not hot, as the latter must always be very injurious.

If man eats raw fruit he is in no danger of harming his body by hot food. He is also in no danger of eating too much, while, with the artificial, unnatural foods he must continually struggle against this, and is still always eating too much.*

Consequently, when men no longer cook, they gain the following advantages: women need no longer ruin their health before the cooking stove, the source of poisonous vapors, where they acquire their many troubles and diseases; they gain time for nobler occupations, can devote themselves more to their children and spend more time in God's beautiful, free nature; they need no longer prepare those viands, which for themselves as well as for their families are the cause of all diseases, and indeed of all unhappiness in the world. All members of the family will soon have a finer taste, be able to enjoy their food better, and will gain rare vigor and joy of life.

---

*This unnatural life of ours calls out in every way needs, desires, and cravings, the satisfaction of which, as man clearly perceives, result in great harm to him. He must therefore continually practise abstinence.

> Thou shalt abstain—renounce—refrain!
> Such is the everlasting song
> That in the ears of all men rings,—
> That unrelieved, our whole life long,
> Each hour, in passing, hoarsely sings.
> —Goethe, "Faust."

The school, the church, poetry and all the world are therefore continually preaching abstinence and renunciation, but we are nevertheless to-day pandering to all our desires. Body, mind and soul are again and again injured by the gratification of our morbid desires. For the healthy man, living a perfectly natural mode of life, the complete satisfaction of all his needs, which in this case are simply the voices of nature, is however of the greatest advantage to himself.

A diet of raw fruit (chiefly nuts) does very much to increase all the powers of the body, and still more all the original higher spiritual capacities and god-like faculties of man.

When several years ago, during the great strikes in English coal mines, horses that had been kept there, in dark, underground passages, for from ten to twenty years, were brought up from the mines into the daylight, they were frightened, acted as if they were insane, and ran back towards the dark, damp holes of the mines. Similar to these unhappy horses the woman appears to me, who also, apparently, is suddenly brought into too much light and sun when, the advantages which will accrue to her and hers if she will stop cooking, are presented to her. She, too, may quickly retreat into her dark kitchen, to stay there till thick soot settles down upon her perspiring face, and she no longer resembles that noblest of creatures, which it was God's intention to create in woman, but not a blackened stoker before a fiery stove.

Poor Cinderella, when will your prince come to lead you as queen to his throne of joy and happiness?

The drinker is chained to his cup, even if he realizes that he will end miserably. The scholar with shriveled body, yellow complexion, and bald head, cannot turn his back upon his laborious studies, although the true joys of life are receding from him more and more. Just so woman to-day cannot free herself from an unnatural occupation, from the cook-stove, even if true earthly happiness would begin for her and hers by so doing.

Man as originally created by nature, was absolutely beautiful. Greek art represents the perfectly beautiful woman by Venus (Aphrodite). Our women to-day are generally a great many degrees removed from this original beauty. But the only means of again becoming more beautiful is the natural mode of life, for this insures better health, and health is beauty. Do our women think they can gain the beauty they desire at the cook-stove?

> Love woman's being does encompass quite,
> Both prison 'tis and heaven to her soul.
> To humble love resigned, herself she gives,
> And serving, rules withal.

In free nature we do not find the difference between young and old as we do among men. The old animals are always the most beautiful, the strongest, and during mating time the happiest. Love is a tender flower, it suffers most of all by our unnatural mode of life, in the tempests of our present civilization, only now and then, in men's younger days, does it brighten up like a light that is about to go out. But no plan is more surely adapted to smother the soul's noblest impulses, than a smoky kitchen. A healthy woman, however, who always remains young and beautiful, can lead man—the whole world, by a tender chain. Would, therefore, that many women might free themselves from the kitchen, and find their way to true, continuous happiness in love.

Primeval man, before his fall from nature, before the fall of man, did not have to work to gain his livelihood, still less was he driven by inner restlessness and barrenness to fitful work: Not until the forbidden food was eaten did the curse fall upon man:

"In the sweat of thy face shalt thou eat bread."—Gen. 3:18.

If women only would take to the bath again, and have recourse to light and air, then a new joy of life would awaken in them again, too, and the desire to seek their conditions of life in other spheres than in the dark, smoky kitchen.

Pandora is our civilization. Civilization to-day also wears a brilliant, bewitching dress. Civilization has been made possible only through fire, and it still brings us all the evils, just like Pandora, although we celebrate it greatly.

We must once more become prejudiced, and unbiased in order to recognize the harmful and dangerous character of all our present civilized contrivances, all great discoveries and inventions, be it the art of printing or gunpowder, the railroad or the bicycle, the telegraph or the telephone. Men are completely dazzled to-day, they are looking through spectacles which make all the evils appear as blessings.

They quite overlook all the diseases, all the haste and unrest, all the nervousness, all the despair, which all these achievements of civilization have in their train. The blessings that are thought to have accrued from them are only shams.

Of course we cannot to-day at once dispense with fire once more, and cannot at once banish all unnatural practices from the world, we can only gradually return to nature.

WHEN SHALL WE EAT?

In all things nature gives her prescriptions accurately, she even tells us when to eat.

In nature everywhere we find that the animals feed chiefly in the evening. Every forester knows that game eats but little during the day, but towards sunset it begins to eat vigorously. To the fodder stations that are arranged for the game in the forest in Winter, when the ground is covered with snow, the animals come only in the evening, although they would be just as undisturbed there during the day.

Beasts of prey eat only in the evening or at night. In the menageries, too, the chief feeding time is in the evening.

Everyone knows, too, that beer and wine taken in the morning have a much worse effect than in the evening. The "eye-opener" is much more injurious than the "night-cap." The many banquets and drinking bouts that people indulge in at night could not be indulged in in the morning. After dinner one is generally tired, but this is not at all the case after supper. The body does not digest food readily in the morning, the stomach is more active in the evening and at night.

The members of Jesus' sect ate very little during the day, according to the intentions of nature, the most serious among them did not eat till after sunset (later the anchorites of the first Christian communities did likewise). In the evening they assembled for their chief meal, supper was at the same time a sort of religious service. Jesus also introduced the supper among His disciples, and a remnant of this is the holy communion of the present Christian Church, just as baptism is a small remnant of the regular bath, which Jesus prescribed, and which had the significance of a sacred rite to Him.*

Of course all sorts of subtle reasons are adduced with much show of wisdom against supper, although nature has designed it, but not one of these reasons is tenable.

Very little ought to be eaten in the morning. It would be best not to eat anything until noon. Fasting until noon, which is in accordance with nature, is not at all difficult. At noon it is also well to be careful not to eat too much (as little as possible). But in the evening one may unhesitatingly partake of a full meal.

My patients have always claimed that they never experienced such unmistakable good results from the treatment as when they fasted until noon. In taking a course of treatment, therefore, I emphatically recommend fasting until noon.

If one has not already eaten too much during the day, a hearty supper before sleeping causes no distress or disturbance. Regularity in one's habits, in diet, and the observance of meal times is of importance.

From such survivals as baptism and the holy communion, Christians ought soon to recognize the precepts of Jesus with regard to water and eating, then the salvation preached by the Saviour would also soon be theirs.

"Awake, O spirit of the first witnesses,
That stand as faithful watchers on the tower,
And ne'er in silence stand, nor night nor day."
—(v. Bogatzky.)

---

*Indeed, Christians ought not to be satisfied with being solemnly baptized once in their lives as children; they ought to bathe every day, if possible, and remember that they are thus fulfilling a holy commandment of the Saviour and God. Every bath ought in a certain sense to be a religious rite.

THE NATURAL MODE OF NOURISHMENT, CARE AND EDUCATION OF CHILDREN.

What a wealth of the sweetest and holiest sensations and joys does nature offer to man through his children! Children

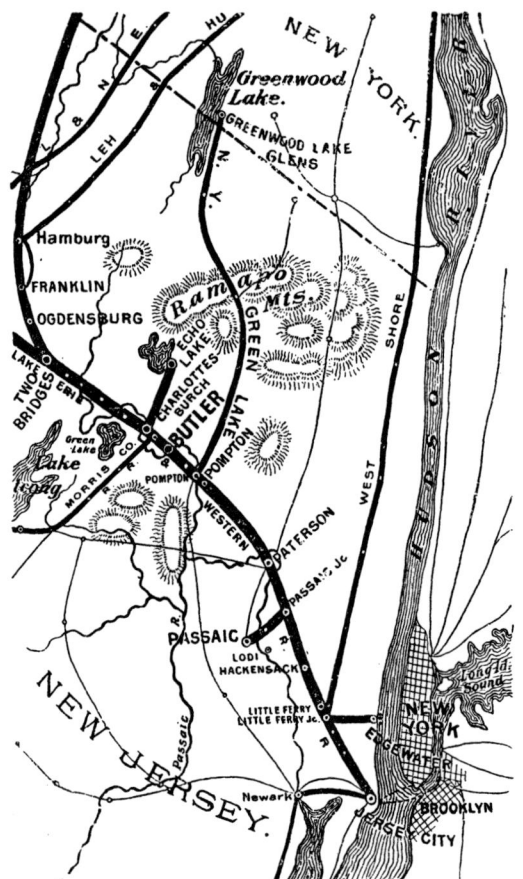

Map Showing Location of Butler, N. J.

are precious jewels that God has entrusted to man. But man assumes high duties and great responsibilities in having children, and he must devote especial care to their nourishment, rearing, and education. Here, too, nature ought to be our only guide, and her demands alone ought to be satisfied.

The human being is alive before it sees the light of day.

The woman who is to become a mother ought to realize at once that she has holy duties towards a new being, and that she has been chosen for a high purpose. During this time she ought to withdraw herself from the world of gossip, ill-will and envy, hatred and contention, she ought to avoid all excitement and restlessness, and abstain from all indulgences and pleasures that are exciting to the nerves and moreover disgusting. Instead of these she ought to contemplate the nature of God, with its calm and peace, and seek her enjoyment in nature. I have sufficiently described the mode of life, which is also the one a woman in this condition should follow. It is most important, too, that women should not be so unreasonable in their dress during that time. They do not know how heavily they can sin against their children even before they are born.

During the time when the germ of a new human being is developing, the slightest influence upon the mother and her mode of life is of the greatest importance, a fact which is too much overlooked to-day to the greatest misfortune of mankind. How many encumber the earth to-day who are weak-minded or complete idiots, who can find neither rest nor peace, and who end in vice and crime. Most of these unhappy people can trace their misfortune and misery to pre-natal influences.

Could this spectacle of so many wretched human beings but lead parents to realize what horrible sins they can commit!*

---

*I should like to call attention, in this place, to a little book: Dr. med. Rosch, "The Chief Cause of Most of the Chronic Diseases, Especially of the Permanent Troubles of the Female Sex," which certainly gives married people an opportunity to realize what grave offences they commit in regard to sexual intercourse. The idea seems to prevail to-day that within marriage there need be no restraint to sexual intercourse. This is a fatal mistake that must avenge itself upon the married couple themselves, and upon their posterity. Soci-

The woman, who in some measure lives a natural life, need not fear the hour of her danger, her confinement. She will be delivered with great ease. Should this not be the case, however, earth compresses on the abdomen will be of great advantage. Light and air are the first requisite in the lying-in chamber. Let the windows be open!

The new-born child should no longer be washed with warm water, it ought rather to be at once given a quick cold bath and cleansing, so that the tender life may be strengthened and assisted. At all events children ought to be bathed and washed only in cold water from the beginning, and at all seasons of the year; it would be the surest way of guarding against effeminacy

---

ety to-day pronounces sentence only on unchastity outside of marriage.

Sexual intercourse has but the one high purpose—the propagation of the race. Originally man, like every other creature, also followed exclusively the voice of nature in this respect. This voice spoke very distinctly to him, although only at long intervals. To-day man is here, unfortunately, the victim of a bad, morbid desire. The preservation of the race is not considered at all; on the contrary, people are very much annoyed by the fact that this intercourse does at the same time fulfil nature's purpose, which they even try to frustrate. How very much has man here placed himself into opposition with nature! Within very modern times the American people, too, have unfortunately sunk as deeply in this respect as other civilized nations, who have long been far in advance of the Americans on the road to decay. In all newspapers female "remedies" are openly advertised without reserve. But nothing is a surer sign that a nation is irretrievably on the decline than these universal, terrible offences against the highest laws of nature. Now there is no longer any limit to licentiousness, with all its disastrous consequences. It must soon become apparent how much harm is done in this way. But if people will once more begin to lead more natural lives, these offences against nature will stop of themselves, or can be successfully combated. Then also the demands that Dr. Rosch makes, in the little book just mentioned (an English translation can be had for 25c., postpaid, from B. Lust, 111 E. 59th Street, New York), can certainly be fulfilled. But unless they are, all struggle and all attempts in this respect will be in vain.

and sickness from the time of birth. In the very coldest season the water should at most be of the temperature of the room.

All swathing bands must, moreover, be dispensed with, light and air must from the beginning have every possible chance to penetrate the little body. The child must therefore often be left naked, the vital energy will thus be greatly stimulated in the young being.

When to-day a new human being is born, all the aunts and cousins are at hand, with teapots and the like, to receive the new citizen of the world, to bless him with their teas, and other unnatural contrivances, and this is actually kept up with man to the very grave.

But let us show these aunts the door, in order that all human unreason and all absurdities may from the start be cleared away from the path of our little pilgrim. This is the first great service we can do the child to-day.

When the human infant begins his worldly career, his first impulse is towards liberty, light, and air. Instead of these, he finds a dark room, with actually foul air, is put into bondage, so to speak, by swaddling clothes, and is packed away in thick feather-beds, so that he can hardly be expected to have the courage to live. If the child is ever taken into the open-air he is wrapped up in thick shawls, the baby carriage is so closely covered that the air and sun cannot penetrate at all.

To be sure, when people in the country, for instance, have little chickens or geese, they always take them out into the sunshine and are pleased to see how lively they are, and how they grow and flourish. The little infant, however, is always deprived of the strengthening air and the invigorating sun; it must not surprise us, therefore, if the children grow sickly and die.

The incessant crying of babies, which often quite exhausts them, and is such a trial to the parents, is the fault of the parents themselves. Give the babies more freedom, take away the pressing bands, place them in the light and air, and see how quiet and cheerful they will be and how they will prosper.

If, in consequence of all the mismanagement, the digestion of the child is very much disturbed, an abdominal compress ought to be applied. It may be the water compress of Priessnitz, but an earth compress is still more effective.

With all the inexplicable errors in the treatment of babies, which people commit nowadays, it is surprising that still more children do not sink into an early grave. This proves that man from the beginning is endowed with much more vitality than the animal, for the little animal could never stand all the unnatural treatment that the human infant must endure, but would surely always perish.

All this mismanagement of the children during the first years of their lives harms them, of course, for life. Let us have more nature, then, at all events!

The mother's milk is the natural food for children to begin with. By leading a natural life, as I have described it, during pregnancy and also during the time in which she must nurse her child, the mother can provide sufficient nourishment for the child. It is of course, entirely wrong to think that a woman can derive strength and nourishment for her child from eating meat and drinking beer and wine, during pregnancy and the time when she is nursing her child. On the contrary, her milk supply will in that case be less and wholly bad.

If in consequence of an unnatural mode of life, the mother has no nourishment for her child, the best substitute is a healthy wet-nurse. Otherwise UNCOOKED cow's milk must be given to the child, of course, only from the best and healthiest cows possible; from cows that go to pasture.

We are afraid to use uncooked milk on account of bacilli, and think we can kill and render them harmless by cooking.

Bacilli, like so many other microscopic animals, are only the products of fermentation. When there is foreign matter (disease germs) in the body that passes into a state of fermentation, bacilli will always form, just as the individual, who does not keep his external skin clean, will become the victim of vermin. If bacilli get into the body from without, they will not flourish there, unless they find a fertile soil, foreign matter. Therefore, if we but keep ourselves free from foreign matter, through a natural mode of living, we never need to fear bacilli; on the other hand, no precautions (cooking, disinfection, etc.) can protect us against them. Where disease matter is present, be it in the body or in the milk, the bacilli are even necessary. They are serving an important purpose.

If, by cooking the milk of sick cows, we kill the bacilli, the disease matter, which furnishes the soil of the bacilli, and which is the really dangerous matter, remains in the milk after all.

If the body of the child contains foreign matter in sufficient quantity, it can in no wise be protected from bacilli; if the contrary is the case, the bacilli can in no wise become dangerous. But uncooked milk with bacilli passes into fermentation more quickly than cooked milk, and is therefore more quickly digested by the stomach. The bacilli even aid digestion. By cooking the milk we only render it more indigestible, and therefore more injurious, so that the child will be retarded in his development.

The disease matter that may be in the uncooked milk is more quickly removed from the stomach again than the disease matter in the cooked milk. In cooked milk, moreover, as well as in all other cooked foods, all life has been killed. For this reason, too, it has no longer any real value for the body, it can no longer impart life and strength.

The "pasteurized" and "sterilized" milk is of course just as useless and injurious as cooked milk. For that matter, the cooking pasteurizes and sterilizes the milk also.

The infant, therefore, ought to be nourished with mother's milk or raw cow's milk, until it can eat raw fruit and nuts.

Oatmeal porridge and other baby foods so frequently recommended ought to be once for all discarded. It would be even preferable to give the children some cooked green vegetables and a little bread. They begin quite early to like fruit and nuts, which agree with them very well indeed. On a fruit diet children develop bodily, mentally, and with regard to their disposition and soul in such a manner that they are a heartfelt joy to the parents.

In all our artificial life to-day, in all the hopeless misery,

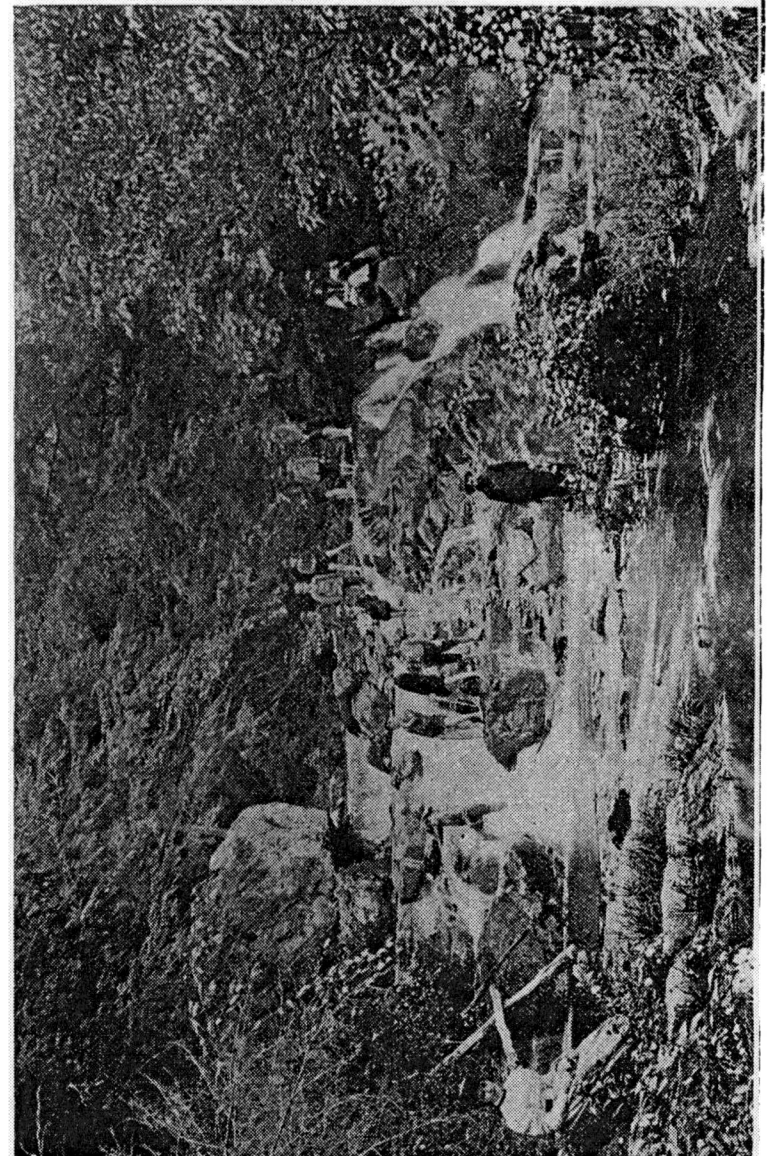

Waterfall in the Light, Air and Sun Bath Park, American "Jungborn," Butler, N. J.

there is still one paradise left, it is the paradise of childhood. But let the children keep the fruit, otherwise you will mar their paradise, and deprive them of much joy and pleasure. We can also let them eat HALF-RIPE AND UNRIPE fruit without misgivings. It is especially beneficial to them.

Jesus says:

"Suffer little children, and forbid them not, to come unto me."—Matt. 19:14.

The members of the sect to which Jesus belonged, lived in the country as mechanics and agriculturists. The strictest ones among them lived even entirely in the open-air, in the desert or on the mountains, and many of them again nourished themselves entirely from the spontaneous products of the earth. To those people, living strictly natural lives, children were often entrusted for education.

Thus John was sent into the desert by his parents, when still a child. It is said of him:

"And the child grew, and waxed strong in spirit, and was in the deserts till the day of his shewing unto Israel."—Luke 1:80.

The Saviour, too, especially wished to gain over the children to lead a strict natural life. Yes, if the children would begin to lead a truly natural life, it is obvious that they could attain to a degree of health and earthly happiness, such as adults cannot always hope to reach. I should, therefore, like to charge parents most urgently: let the children lead a natural life, guide them back to nature; you will reap the richest, most beautiful blessing for it here on earth, and God will reward you for it in heaven.

It is a well known fact that children who still have more of instinct, often rebel against cooked food, while they are very fond of fruit. Nevertheless they are often forced to the unnatural food by the parents, even with blows. In consequence of this the children naturally fall ill, and when they are to take medicine they again instinctively rebel against it, but the mother, whose heart beats in unbounded love for the sick child, must again force herself to severity, although her own heart aches under it. The child is made to take the medicine by force, and even in the days of sickness one does not always shrink from using the rod. But now the measure of unnatural treatment is full to overflowing, the little body of the child succumbs to it, and is soon resting in the cool ground. The mother stands at the grave with sore and broken heart, but her sadly benighted love can now no longer manifest itself for the child's ruin.

The chief desire of parents to-day is to have their children always fat. They are generally not satisfied until the children look like fatted pigs or trumpet-blowing cherubs.

Adults also frequently strive to be corpulent and fat, and to weigh much. Even if they don't exactly care to be pot-bellied they still seem to think the whole value of man depended on their avoirdupois, as that of fattened cattle.

But this is again altogether contrary to nature and completely wrong.

The animals in free nature (young as well as old) are always most beautifully proportioned, they are never bloated or thick and fat.

Man, too, is sound only as long as the body possesses agreeable proportions, has no bloated appearance, and is free from fat bolsters. A really beautiful form results only from a diet chiefly of raw fruit, which is also the only diet that insures a normal state of health. Children especially ought therefore to be nourished, and beautiful, and not fat and unsightly, Here, too, the Apollo of Belvedere may serve as an example, if one wishes to know how a body must look in order to be beautiful and sound.

One of the most dreadful, and fatal errors that mankind has ever made itself liable to in its ignorance of nature is vaccination.

It is proven scientifically and statistically that small-pox has been much less prevalent since vaccination has been made compulsory. But to him who again understands nature this only proves how injurious vaccination is. The young body that still possesses sufficient vitality to free itself from its inherited foreign matter, through the so-called children's diseases, to which small-pox belongs, is rendered powerless by the vaccine poison. Its entire development is thus interfered with, and instead of an acute disease, which under a natural treatment would have resulted in the greatest benefit to the body, a destructive, bad chronic disease commences.

Especially when the inoculation is repeated in the twelfth year of age it soon becomes plainly apparent that disease in various forms is beginning its work, as a direct consequence of vaccination.

Nobody knows when mankind will be redeemed from this horrible error, through which it legally imposes the greatest suffering, and misfortune upon its own children.

Scrofula, paralysis, epilepsy, various nervous troubles, and other chronic diseases, that are prevailing to-day, are frequently the result of vaccination, as I once more wish to emphasize.

After every inoculation the place ought to be treated with clay compresses, which must be frequently repeated for several days. The compresses ought to be large enough to extend beyond the place of vaccination. The child ought, moreover, to lead a strictly natural life during that time. In this way no harm whatever need be feared from vaccination.

If no pustules appear on the spot, after inoculation, the law requires that the child be vaccinated again, whereupon the above treatment must be repeated. The law does not call for more than three vaccinations, however.

I suppose it is not necessary to warn against anti-toxine in particular, which also is nothing but a dreadful inoculating poison. It may be that diphtheria may be subdued with it, but diseases that are a great deal worse—cancer, insanity and the like—may originate in consequence of this procedure.

Diphtheria, like every other acute disease, can also be cured easily and surely by the natural method, without ruining the child. Parents need no longer fear this present angel of death in the least, and need not in their anxiety have recourse to that horrible poison called anti-toxine.

All children's diseases are favorable healing crises, and there is no need of anxiety on account of them. In every disease (diphtheria, measles, scarlet fever, typhoid fever, etc.) the child must in the first place be made to lie or walk about naked in the room with open windows. The longer this can be done the better. The best thing, of course, would be for the child to walk about naked in the open air, if that were possible. The water-bath must also be taken, and earth compresses on the abdomen; in the case of diphtheria around the throat. Moreover the sick child ought not to be allowed to eat anything, or only very little, and only nuts and fruit. As soon as it is at all possible the child is to be allowed to go out of doors again (if possible barefooted). It will be surprising to see how quickly children's diseases can be cured, and how bright and lively the children are after it. By the acute diseases the young body frees itself from much foreign matter and refuse.

By our many anti-natural practices to-day (wrong nourishment, living in unhealthy, stuffy rooms, absurd clothing, etc.) children are made exceedingly delicate. Even from the demon alcohol they are not always protected. The boys in the high schools early try to imitate the vices of the adults. They even try to boast of their beer drinking, cigar smoking, etc. A better example on the part of adults, especially teachers, could do an infinite amount of good here.

In consequence of effemination and all sorts of unnatural habits, and through the unreasonable demands of our present school education, from which all good is expected to come, the nerves of our children are at an early age overstrained and weakened. Thus all sorts of sensual desires are early aroused in the children, which they have not the power to resist. The most dangerous enemy of youth, self-abuse, shows itself. Watchful parents can soon discover from the shy demeanor of the poor child, who often struggles against his vice with bitter self-reproach and great suffering that he has fallen a prey to this worst enemy of youth. Parents ought never to punish in such a case. The mental and spiritual development and perfection of the children must be brought about in quite a different way than by all sorts of force and punishments. Punishment, especially corporal punishment, ought never to be resorted to. But it is an especially mistaken policy to attempt to cure a child of youthful vice by severe punishment. At such a time the child is in especial need of love. Let the parents lovingly and gently treat the child with the remedies of nature, water, light, air, diet, exercise, etc., and soon he will be rescued from the clutches of the dangerous enemy, and be once more bright and cheerful.

If this is not the case, the children grow up deprived of all the joy and pleasure of youth; life itself becomes a burden, and the otherwise so cheerful boys and girls become weakened, enervated, cross and pessimistic youths and men, maidens and women, whose dull eyes look sadly into a world of torture and pain.

The habit of wetting the bed, so frequently found among children, may also easily be overcome by a natural treatment. Here, too, punishment is actually a crime.

Once more I wish to recommend *going barefooted,* especially for children, and once more would I call attention to their clothing, which must be as simple and natural as possible. Boys (also men) ought, among other things, to dispense with the *vest,* this intermediate article of clothing intended to give extra warmth to the chest. The chest especially ought to be very accessible to the air, and ought to be left as free as possible. In children's clothing this may be easily arranged.

I have had the opportunity to convince myself repeatedly how young people, who permanently led a natural life, became mentally capable to a remarkable degree. Such boys, who had been considered backward pupils, soon began to learn with ease, and to outstrip their companions without taking any pains to do so.

Also physical strains and hardships, such as our present military service demands, could be borne by these young people with remarkable ease. In this respect, too, they greatly distinguished themselves.

I have repeatedly called attention to the fact that the natural mode of life has a very great ennobling influence upon the soul: this, too, may be observed in children. Yes, the natural mode of life is the foundation upon which alone we can build up a true morality and nobility of soul. Therefore in leading a natural life we should strive with all our power towards soul perfection, and make this an object in the education of our children.

What, then, is a natural education of children?

Man is originally the image of God, the highest essence of love. Education, therefore, if it is to proceed in the spirit of nature, must strive to restore this image of God as much as possible.

Jesus says:

"Thou shalt love the Lord thy God with all thy heart, and with all thy soul, and with all thy mind.

"Thou shalt love thy neighbor as thyself."—Matt. 22:37, 39.

These words alone contain the true, natural education of man. All the innumerable volumes that have ever been written on pedagogy, all the endless lectures that have been delivered on this important subject, do not come near saying what the above short words of Jesus contain. One is determined to-day to educate youth through science, but it is as the apostle says:

"Knowledge puffeth up, but charity edifieth."—1 Cor. 8:1.

The boy, who has with great difficulty learned his first Latin vocabulary, already looks with pride upon his playfellow, who goes to a lower grade school, and soon drops him. Thus the more the boy advances in knowledge, the more is he led by conceit and pride, which is most disastrous. But we must always discriminate between the external hollow sham, which our present artificial education mostly produces, and the inner worth of man. Our youth of to-day is drilled, they are taught all kinds of external fine forms and manners, but the heart and disposition are not developed. The soul, instead of being ennobled, retrogrades. The vulgar, uneducated children, whose life is an unnatural one, by no means deport themselves in an exemplary way, but their unrefined, coarse demeanor is nevertheless better than politeness and friendliness that are not heartfelt. The latter is fraud and deception. Therefore children ought to lead natural lives; it will again teach them the love of God and of man, and love alone makes us better. We ought to train them to truly love their fellows, for conversely we may say: Who loves his neighbor as himself loves also God. Young people must learn to love God, and bear only goodwill and friendliness in their hearts towards their fellow-men, and manifest it to all alike, irrespective of rank. Parents in whose heart this divine spark is not yet quite extinguished, or where it has been revived, will themselves find ways and means to call out and cultivate love in their children. In this way alone can true education and true virtue be achieved that will result in blessings to the child and be his only salvation throughout life. Only by a natural mode of life and true love of his fellows is the child brought to the threshold of a life full of joy and happiness, which will stay by him under all circumstances.

Sorrow and want can never reach such a child throughout life.

Many parents to-day think that happiness for their children is to be found only in a higher school education. This is a source of great anxiety to them: all considerations of health are pushed into the background, and thus they provide only for the misery of their children. But they would so much like to see their children occupy high positions and draw large salaries, surrounded by splendor and dignity.

Do not allow yourselves to be deceived by the splendor which often but surrounds inner discontent and wretchedness. Only he is happy who, in the full possession of health, lives in great simplicity, and with few wants, close to nature—a free man with love of man and trust in God in his heart.

The child that is continually overburdened with mental strain and work, and is enervated thereby, looks forward to a life of sickness and satiety, hard struggles and bitter disappointments, even if there are prospects of high positions, honor, fame and riches. Our present mental overburdening of girls is still less comprehensible and more useless than that of boys. Girls' and women's nature is least fitted to bear up against mental work.

Parents who have realized that happiness is not enthroned upon the heights of human society, but that it is to be found in the first place in the breast of every individual, and then especially in the lower, peaceful circles, will take this into consideration in choosing a calling for their children.

It may indeed be a difficult task to-day for many to choose the real joys and true treasures of nature for their children, in place of the deceptive pleasures, and blessings of civilization, of science and of riches.

But parents who have penetrated to correct conceptions, and are not led by pride, but are independent of the general mistaken views, and can think for themselves, will be sure to limit the school education of their children to that which is most necessary under present conditions. Let them but think, in matters of school education: The less the better, and they will surely find the right calling for the child.

Fruit culture, and many a little trade and business will in future afford opportunity for the most beautiful, most independent, and most wholesome lives. One need then no longer hope to find salvation in a scientific school education, but in the undisturbed health of body and soul resulting from a natural mode of life, and the love of God and his fellow-men.

This is the true philosophy of life ; let us begin to practise it on ourselves, and especially on our children, then our present nervousness, the disease of the century, will soon disappear, and make room for a new happiness of mankind.

In consequence of various hereditary weaknesses children to-day are different from birth in body, mind and soul. If parents should attempt to train them by force to that which they desire to make of them, the result would chiefly be disastrous and bad.

Let parents take their children as they are given them by nature, care for and educate them in the natural way I have described, and gratefully accept the result.

Let nature have her way, therefore, even in the education of children. This is a very important principle in education.

CASES AND CURES.

Reports of cures, letters of thanks, etc., have no value in themselves.

We know that sham cures can be achieved by unnatural means. A disease is apparently cured; that is, it disappears, and another much worse disease is produced. The second disease need, of course, not show itself at once, and it may even not seem to be as bad, according to our present conceptions, as the first; in fact, however, it is always much more dangerous and destructive. Many invalids, especially of the nervous type, re-experience an improvement, and think themselves cured, and write letters of thanks, and reports of their happy cure, until in the course of time comes disillusion and bitter, painful disappointment.

If we consider, moreover, how frauds are often practised in order to obtain favorable reports of cures, we can easily understand how the greatest swindlers in secret and patent remedies may produce a great many brilliant reports of cures.

The people must, therefore, acquire sufficient penetration to judge in how far any system or method of curing coincides with the requirements and laws of nature; for any system or method of curing the sick that in its applications follows nature in every detail, must *always and in every case* lead to health. This holds true whatever symptoms may appear in the course of the cure, and however inexplicable they may seem to misguided men of to-day.

I should like to see my method receive the confidence of the people because it satisfies, in every respect, the requirements of nature. For no other reason do I bespeak confidence in my cause. I shall therefore not communicate many of the letters of thanks that I am daily receiving, nor report many brilliant cures. I shall only relate a few successes that have been achieved through my method, especially at the Jungborn, by way of practical elucidation of my theories. In doing so I shall add some reflections that may still seem necessary.

INFLAMMATORY RHEUMATISM.

J. R. at B. was suffering from inflammatory rheumatism. The case was a difficult one, since R. had had an attack of inflammatory rheumatism only half a year previous to this one (this, therefore, being a relapse), and was badly poisoned with nicotine. The patient was suffering excruciating pains; the limbs, especially the hands, were twisted and bent. The parish physician was of the opinion that the case would be of long duration, and was about to send the patient to the hospital. The physician had warned especially against exposure to the air. R. was now taken to a light-and-air cottage. It was in the month of May, and a medium temperature prevailed. The patient was at once stripped entirely, and placed for a time on the bare ground. He was thus taking a light-and-air bath. He also received the natural bath in the open-air. The light-and-air baths and sun baths were frequently repeated during the day, and a water bath in the open air was taken daily. After each of these procedures comfortable warmth was restored by a warm bed, consisting of soft woollen blankets, which soon resulted in copious sweat. The diet consisted of nuts, almonds, fruit, tropical fruit, raw milk, butter, a little bread.

With this treatment R.'s pains subsided during the first day, on the second day his limbs straightened out, on the fifth day he could already take a walk, and on the ninth day he could again go about his vocation.

After a fortnight R. took the reckless and inexcusable step of returning to his old habits of life, to meat eating, alcohol drinking, and tobacco smoking. But nevertheless his sickness did not return.

SERIOUS NERVOUS DISEASES.

A. S. at B. suffered greatly from nervous disorders for nine years. Finally he became entirely incapacitated for work, and became subject to spasms, during which he would fall to the ground. The disease drove the patient to despair. He had received some relief at a nature-cure institution, which, however, was not permanent. After a few weeks of my treatment, a most decided improvement was already apparent. Remedies: Light-and-air baths (going naked), often all day long in warm weather, the bath, earth power. Diet: Nuts, fruit, tropical fruit, milk, butter, a little bread. Until noon S. ate nothing at all. The patient became especially enthusiastic about sleeping on the bare ground. After just ten weeks of treatment S. was remarkably fresh, and full of energy for work. But it was his opinion that this great result, after his long, vain search for relief, was due to his utilizing the power of the earth during sleep. S. declared that he had never in his life felt so strong and fresh as since he had taken the natural treatment under my care. With great enthusiasm and devotion he continued the treatment at home, as far as possible: the bath, fruit diet, fasting until noon, sleeping with open windows, light-and-air baths in the room. He was inconsolable because he no longer had an opportunity for sleeping on the bare ground.

SERIOUS TROUBLE IN THE HEAD AND DEAFNESS.

W. P. at H. The patient had fallen from a scaffolding, striking on the head. It was evident that W. P. was well charged with foreign matter, which now found its way to the injured head, causing a serious diseased condition there. P. was entirely incapacitated from work. He had already been deaf upon one ear since his childhood. The ear had been operated on, and P. was under the impression that the drum had been cut out. Moreover P. could not distinguish anything with one eye, although he could see; everything was indistinct and double. P.'s head trouble had been pronounced incurable by the medical faculty in G. A course of treatment lasting eight weeks, in one of the best nature-cure institutions, had also been without result. He came to me and remained under treatment for eight weeks. After a fortnight a most decided improvement began to set in, and P. was overjoyed in marking his continued progress. The fear of taking cold, of which the patient was greatly possessed, was soon overcome.

P. had only hoped to cure his head trouble, and was greatly surprised when, during the last two weeks of his cure, he could again hear with the ear that had been deaf. He had not expected to have his hearing restored; indeed, he had thought it quite impossible. P. continued the treatment at home, took the bath, observed the diet, and part of the time also slept in a summerhouse in a garden, situated outside of the city.

He wrote to me: "I need hardly describe to you how much my health has improved during the last six months. I have been made happy—more than happy—by this new method of healing." Later on I heard that even his eye was better.

The remedies in P.'s case were likewise: the bath, going bare-footed, the light-and-air bath (in warm weather and sunshine often all day long). The patient was very enthusiastic about sleeping outside of the light-and-air cottage under the sky (in good weather).

Diet: Nuts, fruit, tropical fruit, milk, a little bread and butter.

P. had already been a vegetarian for about a year before coming to me, living on leguminous seeds, potatoes, bread, and only some raw fruit. But it was with the greatest difficulty that his family could keep him to this diet.

But it can easily be explained why patients do not like to adhere to this form of nourishment, for after the first relief experienced from the change, the general health is apt to become even worse in the course of time.

After P. had lived for a short time on the natural diet which I recommended to him, he became so enthusiastic about it that he energetically set to work to win his family over to it, and successfully.

With almost all my patients I have made the experience that they willingly and enthusiastically adhered to the natural diet, which is so very simple and requires so little work of preparation.

In the beginning of the treatment P.'s appetite increased enormously so that it could hardly be satisfied, but this soon subsided.

BAD STOMACH TROUBLE AND CONSUMPTION OF THE SPINAL CORD.

S. von N, at St. P., aged forty-two years, suffered for several years from a very bad stomach trouble and consumption of the spinal cord. Several professors had diagnosed cancer of the stomach, and consumption of the spinal cord could be recognized from the way he threw his legs in walking. When the patient came to the Jungborn he was almost unable to eat anything.

He vomited some forty times during the night. He was placed in a light-and-air cottage at the Jungborn. A compress of wet earth on the abdomen at once put a stop to the vomiting; when the compress was taken away the vomiting began anew. This plainly showed the effectivenesss of the earth. Sometimes the patient took the natural bath; as soon as he was able he frequently took a light-and-air bath.

When v. N. had been the Jungborn for ten days he had no more vomiting spells, even after the earth compress was discontinued. From that time on the patient began to improve remarkably. His appetite was excellent, and he could satisfy it on the fruit diet without hesitation. There was not the least distress after eating. The consumption of the spinal cord also began to get well.

RETENTION OF THE URINE, INCIPIENT DROPSY.

L. G., at M., thirty-three years of age. The patient had been seriously ill for two years, so that he was obliged to give up his occupation on account of his condition. He suffered with retention of the urine (incipient dropsy), accompanied with complete derangement of his digestive functions. He could no longer urinate except by artificial means, his legs already began to swell. The patient claims to have consulted seventy(!) medical men during the two years of his sickness, among them some twenty (!) distinguished professors. Besides this he had used many other cures, the Warner Safe Cure, the Gluenicke Cure, sea baths and the like, and also had experienced the illusive successes of such unnatural cures, but in reality his illness increased continually. He was dangerously ill and almost paralized with fear of death, when he came to the Jungborn in the middle of September. The urine was already seeking new outlets through canals that could be recognized externally. In several places on the legs below the knees it was flowing as a malodorous liquid from open wounds. The great danger of this condition was at once clear to me. G. was immediately taken to a light-and-air cottage at the Jungborn, so that the purest air could have free access to him. Then compresses of moist earth were put on the abdomen and the region of the kidneys. These compresses were frequently renewed. Sometimes the patient had to come out of his light-and-air cottage to take a light-and-air bath (go naked) outside, especially since he could soon again walk alone without aid. He allowed the earth-power to act upon him as much as possible.. The water bath was not employed so much in this case. In the beginning the patient received only raw fruit (nuts, fruit, berries), later on raw milk, butter and bread was added.

With this treatment nearly two quarts of urine passed off in the natural way as early as the second day, and there was a normal movement of the bowels at the same time. On the third day G. could walk again, on the fourth he could run. In the second week the wounds on the legs were healed, and G. could then already make rapid walking tours into the mountains, lasting from three to four hours.

This rapid, incredible success caused great excitement at the Jungborn. G. left us after two weeks without a trace of his former severe suffering about him.

I must here call attention to the fact that this brilliant success was achieved at the end of September in the *cooler* season, otherwise the result would have not been so rapid.

A HIGH DEGREE OF NERVOUSNESS.

R. in W. suffered from nervousness in such a high degree that he had completely given up his occupation since six months. At night, especially, R. was entirely without sleep and restless, almost raving. He took chiefly light-and-air baths. On the fifth day, after a light-and-air bath, on a very cold, rainy day in April, he became quiet. He continued to improve rapidly, and was soon restored to his profession. For the rest R's treatments followed the usual regime. But the rapid result was achieved by the *cold* light-and-air baths.

In nervous troubles especially cold light-and-air baths are most effective.

PNEUMONIA.

L. in B. was ill with pneumonia, and had for six weeks, during which he was treated with medicines, been suffering great pain. Of course, L. had been anxiously confined in a room until his arrival at the Jungborn. After I had talked his fear of catching a deadly cold out of him, he at once, after his arrival, went about naked for hours. On the evening of the first day L. was already quite happy. In his opinion he had gained more in one afternoon, by the simplest means, than six weeks of vain endeavor had done for him. L. continued the treatments only for a few days, and was then cured and very happy.

Here we see how easily and rapidly success is achieved in acute diseases.

DISTURBANCE OF THE DIGESTIVE FUNCTIONS.

Miss L. in B. suffered for years from severe disturbances of the digestive functions. A movement of the bowels could only be brought about by artificial means. On a diet of raw fruit and the rest of the treatments (light-and-air baths, going barefooted, etc.) regular movements of the bowels set in on the fifth day. This, of course, brought great relief and a feeling of great comfort.

This stubborn and dangerous trouble that afflicts so many women to-day, and brings so much intense suffering and misery in its train, can be cured so easily and surely.

DROPSY.

A. Z. in B. was afflicted with dropsy and had been pronounced incurable by the physician. At the Jungborn Z. at once began to take light-and-air baths diligently. The swollen places, especially the abdomen and legs, were treated with earth compresses. Of course Z. also lived in a light-and-air cottage at the Jungborn, in which as many windows, etc., as possible had to remain open at night. Z. was also obliged to keep a very strict natural diet. In this way a striking result was already achieved in the first week.

O. at H. took treatment for dropsy at the Jungborn during only twelve days. The success, however, was so great that upon his return home his physician was greatly surprised.

But in such severe diseases, we ought never to rest satisfied with a course of treatment of such short duration. O. scarcely paid any more attention to his dangerous disease after his return home, for which, of course, he soon had to suffer severely.

THROAT TROUBLE.

K., teacher in R., was afflicted with throat trouble for years, and had been treated without result until he came to the Jungborn. Earth compresses around the throat in connection with the rest of the treatments soon effected a cure.

SCAB ON THE HEAD.

Paula P. at E., a child, suffered from a thick scab on her head. By a fruit diet, light-and-air baths, etc., care was taken to cleanse the body within from foreign matter. The head was covered with moist earth, directly on the scab, which seemed to be very agreeable to the child. After four weeks the scab had disappeared.

CONSUMPTION OF THE SPINAL CORD.

R. K. at B. had consumption of the spinal cord and spent fourteen weeks in vain at a large and celebrated nature-cure institution. At the Jungborn K. was very much strengthened by light-and-air baths. The legs were treated with earth compresses. Already after a few days a marked improvement could be observed. After fourteen days K. could again walk for hours. The throwing of the legs in walking disappeared more and more, so that after this time the disease could hardly be recognized any more externally.

We have seen repeatedly that even the diseases, which are generally considered incurable by science, have lost all their terrors before a truly natural treatment.

TOOTHACHE.

O. P. in I., suffered from the most excruciating toothache for weeks. P. was actually writhing in pain. Various dentists could not help him by filling the teeth and applying their dangerous pain-killing remedies. Then P. applied earth compresses to the place on the cheek where the pain was most severe. After continuing these for several days the pains disappeared entirely and P. was very much surprised to be delivered from his tortures in so simple a way, and regretted that he had formerly, in similar cases, allowed dentists to ruin his teeth still more. Several years have passed since this time. Although P. had formerly often suffered from toothache, he has never been troubled since that time. Earth, therefore, does not quiet pain temporarily, it does not deceive, it cures thoroughly, it takes away the cause of the pain.

TUBERCULOSIS OF THE BONES.

G. R. in B. suffered from tuberculosis of the bones of the foot. He had been in the hospital for half a year. The foot had already been operated on twice and a bone had been removed from the instep. But the foot could not be healed, and before long R. would have lost his foot or leg by amputation. At the Jungborn the loam compress, in connection with air, fruit diet, etc., here again did excellent service.

I particularly regretted the operation in the case of this strong, young man. All the pains and anxieties that it caused were unnecessary, and the foot would have healed much better and quicker without it. The bone that had been taken from the foot could, of course, not be replaced: but the foot was healed, nevertheless, and once more was fit for use, although R. limped somewhat.

TYPHOID FEVER.

Anna G., a child in K., aged ten years, was taken with typhoid fever. The mother asked my advice by letter. I wrote her that she must in the first place let the child go about naked in the room by open windows, as often and as long as possible; moreover, that she must give the child nothing to eat, or but very little, and that she must let it take the natural bath perhaps once a day. In this way the child was completely cured from typhoid fever in from two to three days. Naturally the mother undertook this simple treatment without the knowledge of the physician. The latter was therefore very much surprised to find the child cured in a very few days, from this dreaded and dangerous fever. He then tried to gloss over his surprise by saying that he must have been mistaken, and that the sickness could not have been typhoid fever, while before he had made the statement that the spots that appeared on the skin of the child, plainly indicated typhoid fever.

With our simple, natural method we may indeed often surprise and embarrass physicians.

The mother and little Anna then came to see me at the Jungborn and told me how much brighter and healthier the child was since she had had the fever. Of this we all had the opportunity to convince ourselves at the Jungborn, for we were all greatly pleased with the bright, cheerful child. But if the mother had been completely self-possessed and clear from the beginning, and could have treated the child correctly when the very first signs of the disease appeared, the typhoid fever would not have developed at all, and the child would have been cured in several hours. The disease matter would then have been thrown off in another and easier way.

Would that mothers could but realize that they need not, in cases of sickness, live in dread anxiety for their children, their precious jewels. I can confidently assure all mothers that it is always an easy matter to avoid a serious illness for their children, or, indeed, death. The best thing for mothers to do is of course to protect their darlings from disease by a natural mode of life.

GENERAL DEBILITY.

Miss A. O. at E. was very weak in consequence of nervous disorders, and was especially afflicted with a sense of fullness in the head. She could walk but little. After Miss O. had taken treatment at the Jungborn for a fortnight she could already take a walking tour of eleven hours' duration in one day, without being even tired. This certainly proves that a fruit diet, light-and-air baths, etc., produce great strength. It is the common belief to-day that men grow strong on a meat diet, but here we see again that Miss O. had become very weak and sick on a so-called nourishing meat diet, and on a fruit diet became well rapidly and physically capable.

CONVULSIONS.

Mrs. G. at B. was taken with convulsions; when a clay compress was placed on her neck she at once regained consciousness. Here we see how the clay compress can always be of the greatest use in daily life.

FISTULA OF THE RECTUM.

J. Z. at J. was afflicted with a fistula of the rectum and had already been operated on when he came to the Jungborn. Z.'s condition seemed to me critical. He always was obliged to carry a rubber pillow with him in order to be able to sit at all. I had myself given up hope in this case, since I could not reach the sick part directly with the clay compress, or bring any external influence to bear on it. But Z. was cured after all. I will here cite some passages from a happy letter that I received from him. May the high praise that Z. gives to the Jungborn be placed to the credit of the cause.

"To-day I can say that I am entirely well. I can go about my work again as usual, and whom must I thank for this? Only the Jungborn with its beautiful divine nature. The baths, the earth compresses, everything agreed so well with me. I could only remain at the Jungborn for a short time, but want to advise every sufferer to go to the Jungborn, one can be sure to attain what one wishes there, namely health; I am thoroughly convinced of it. The Jungborn is the very best health resort, this mode of living and this eating was a princely repast for me. The Jungborn will never be forgotten by me. I wish I could have stayed there only a little while longer, it would have given me the greatest pleasure."

From Z's lines one can see that a nature-cure, diet, etc., as it is most thoroughly practised at the Jungborn, can by no means be called ascetecism, coupled with deprivations, denials, etc. On the contrary, the true joy of life is to be found only in a natural life.

The case of Z. has again taught me that one ought not to despair even in the most serious cases of sickness, but ought always to try a nature cure. In the most desperate cases brilliant cures are often still achieved.

BLINDNESS.

W. S., brewer at F., had been entirely blind in one eye for

some time. Medical art had tried all its skill in vain. At the Jungborn S. could already see a little after a few days; after several weeks the eye was perfectly well. "The blind receive their sight, and the lame walk." The clay compress worked wonders with the eye also, as so often before. When S. came home his physician was much embarrassed by this success. But S. was so enthusiastic about the matter that he at once had every arrangement made in his garden so as to be able to continue the mode of life and the treatments as much as possible.

CHOLERA INFANTUM.

Willy K. in L., aged two and a half years, was taken with cholera infantum. The fever rose to 91 degrees F. The mother, who was acquainted with the old method of nature-cure, gave the child two baths in the course of the day. This reduced the fever somewhat, but it soon rose again. The next day the father of the child, who knew of my simpler and surer method, came home. He held the child naked in his arms at the open window for an hour and a half, whereby the fever was reduced 5½ degrees F., Next day the temperature again rose 1 degree F., but sank as soon as the child had another light-and-air bath. Now the fever did not return any more, and the child was entirely well, that is, cured.

Mothers have been sorely alarmed, time and time again, as their children were taken with cholera infantum. How much excitement and anxiety was caused by sending post haste to the doctor and to the apothecary, how much harm was done to the little body by the medicines, and how often did the little being find an early grave! What a bother are the packs, steam baths, etc., of the old nature-cure method, where the cure is not achieved till after several weeks, often weeks full of pain, and often with all manner of painful consequences. With my method we can calmly look the enemy in the face, and know no fear, because we are led by the hand of nature who will never desert us. A few light-and-air baths, which require no apparatus, no blankets, etc., and which cost nothing, and in a few days our child is well again, and skips about with more than usual cheerfulness and spirit. May this example help us to realize how easily we can get the better of acute children's diseases, and avoid all anxiety. Why should we then still fear acute diseases? But we must again learn to understand simple nature, then we will also take the proper precautions to make our children well and keep them so.

DISEASE OF THE SEXUAL ORGANS.

H. F., student at N., suffered for years from nervous weakness. A sense of fullness in the head almost incapacitated him for work, so that he became tired of life, and often thought of committing suicide. Physicians had diagnosed the case in most contradictory ways, and all found different causes for the trouble. For about three months F. had taken Kneipp treatments, which improved his condition somewhat, but did not result in a cure. When he began to try my method there soon was a change. After a fortnight of treatment, gonorrhœa set in. F. now told me that he had had sexual intercourse with a girl some years ago, shortly afterwards he had experienced pains in the sexual organs, for which he had used a salve that a professor prescribed for him.

At the Jungborn the gonorrhœa was soon cured, and with it disappeared the nervous trouble, while his ability to work and his interest in life returned.

H., a student at H., was likewise taken with gonorrhœa after eight days' treatment at the Jungborn. He had had this malady once before, but it had disappeared again, although he had not used any remedies for it. Neither had it reappeared during two long courses of Schroth treatments, which he took in the meantime.

I have already called attention to the fact that the sexual well-being of man is most disadvantageously influenced by an unnatural mode of life, and that all sorts of uncleanly and disastrous vices are caused by it.

The sexual well-being of man is connected with the love of the sexes, this great and holy power, that stirs the body and soul of man to its very depths, and with which nature combines the great purpose of propagating the race. Now, if this mysterious and holy sphere is disturbed and desecrated by all sorts of vices, it is evident that some special disaster must follow; instead of sweet joy we then have disgust, sickness, satiety of life, even pestilential diseases.

Sexual immorality defiles and corrupts man more than anything else, and it is most necessary to call attention to the matter, however unwillingly I touch upon this sad, dark side of our present human life. There exists to-day unspeakable corruption from this source, and an enormous amount of disease; it is therefore a duty to enlighten men on this subject, especially our youth.

In consequence of unnatural practices in the intercourse of the sexes, a very dangerous poison is developed. Naturally sexual diseases first arise in the sexual organs. The first stage of sexual disease is gonorrhœa. This may in a certain sense be considered an acute sexual disease. The urethra, is, so to speak, in a catarrhal condition, as it is endeavoring to throw off the poison, and the pus therefore issues in drops from the tube.

From the two cases mentioned above we see that with a wrong mode of life gonorrhœa cannot be sufficiently eliminated, and with medicines the dangerous poison can be fixed and permanently lodged in the body. The first case also shows how dangerous wrong treatment can be. I can therefore not sufficiently warn against all unnatural procedures in sexual diseases, since the consequences can be very serious indeed, such as severe nervous troubles, blindness, consumption, cancer, etc. The only safeguards are correct nature-cure treatments undertaken at an early stage. We also see from the above that the old nature-cure methods are not sufficiently effective in sexual diseases. The first case furthermore teaches us how meaningless and valueless diagnoses are. With purely natural treatments we can rob gonorrhœa of all its dangers.

Chancre and syphilis are still more dangerous stages of

sexual disease than gonorrhœa. These, too, can in the first place be recognized by the formation of ulcers on the sexual organs. If chancre or syphilis do not receive the right kind of attention, the poisoning of the body proceeds apace, which manifests itself from time to time in various symptoms; by all sorts of skin diseases, ulcers all over the body (even in the mouth), so that the afflicted person is often obliged to shun human society on that account. The poisoning can, moreover, manifest itself in the most dreadful, most horrible diseases that we know of: epilepsy, insanity, consumption of the spinal cord, St. Vitus' dance, etc.

Unfortunately, for these pestilential diseases the word holds good: "I will visit the iniquity of the fathers upon the children unto the third and the fourth generation."

But all this mischief is chiefly caused by the lavish use of mercury preparations. They not only render the body incapable of throwing off the poison of the disease, but they introduce still another horrible poison into the body. The treatment with mercury is a dreadful crime against humanity and against all laws of nature.

Syphilis, too, this scourge of mankind, can be cured by natural treatment and the more recent the case the quicker the cure. In old cases patience and perseverance will be necessary. But the cure ought to be undertaken in any stage of the disease, there is always a chance to improve and help.

All friends of humanity ought to help here, and show men the only sure way to put a stop to this dreadful disease, which has to-day spread among all classes.

DIABETES.

This disease, too, is greatly feared. Medical science prescribes an almost exclusive meat diet for it, but it is well known that in this way diabetes has never been cured. This disease is like all the rest, a consequence of an unnatural mode of life, and can therefore only be cured by a strictly natural life. On account of the widespread erroneous view that a meat diet is necessary in diabetes, it is often very difficult to induce the patient to accept a fruit diet. But this unfortunate prejudice must be overcome, and the perception must take root that the name of a disease is always a matter of indifference, that, moreover, we can no longer make any distinction between the separate diseases, but that all diseases must be treated in the same way, strictly according to the prescriptions of nature. When men have once recognized this only correct method of treatment, they will no longer fear diabetes.

BOILS.

Mr. A. at L., twenty-seven years of age, had been suffering with furuncles all over the body for two years. Hitherto the patient had healed them with so-called Hamburg and similar plasters, or, more correctly, had driven the matter back into the body with salves and similar allopathic remedies. In consequence of this unnatural treatment, the entire left leg began to swell up in such a way, that he could walk only with the greatest difficulty, and was quite exhausted when he arrived at the Jungborn. The entire upper part of the thigh was already so much affected that it was quite black. The case was exceedingly critical, and many a physician would have considered it necessary to amputate it. The universal remedy loam, the only effective remedy for boils and swellings, there too did its duty completely. By compresses of moist earth, which were placed upon the most inflamed part, in this case the upper thigh, the matter gathered and as early as the fourth day of the patient's stay at the Jungborn, a veritable stream of pus and blood issued from the affected spot. This made a hole the size of a dollar into the flesh, from which a mass of foreign matter was brought to the surface daily.

By continued treatment of the wound with a clay plaster the wound gradually healed.

Besides the clay, which was the chief factor in this cure, the aromatic air prevailing at the Jungborn, the nut diet, as well as the sun, and also the rain, did much to eliminate the foreign matter. The urine of the patient, in the days when the boil was discharging abundantly, was bloody, and it is to be assumed, therefore, that the elimination of foreign matter went on by this channel also.

Boils very frequently occur in the beginning of the treatment according to my method. This is easily explained and a very favorable symptom, for it is a sign that the eliminatory function of the body has been greatly stimulated by the treatments. As long as it is at all possible nothing whatever ought to be done in case of boils, but nature ought to be left to take its own course. If the pain gets too severe it can be alleviated by clay compresses. But boils must always be treated with cold clay compresses only. They must not be cut or pricked open. When they are ripe they will open of themselves, clay compresses will then greatly aid the discharge of the pus.

The boil is exceedingly beneficial for the body, it is often accompanied even by fever, which proves most of all that the body is in the state of curative activity, during the process of the boil.

I have often observed that patients with boils would not be persuaded to discard warm water compresses (or also warm hayseed compresses), and have then always convinced myself that this treatment was wrong and contrary to nature. With the warm compresses the boil often ripens before its time, and we are thus working against nature, the body does then not nearly get the advantage from the boil that it does with col l clay compresses, and every unnatural treatment always has its disadvantages. Only after cold clay compresses does the body experience a really grateful relief, and the wound, too, heals most quickly in that way.

If one takes thin, soft linen, wets it and spreads it with clay, it will generally adhere like a plaster, and no further bandage is needed to keep it in place. One generally soon finds out what is the easiest way to treat a boil with clay. I must here remark once more that in the case of open boils the clay or the earth must be placed directly on the wound.

The elimination of foreign matter from the body through

a boil is very great. It is not only the disease matter that flows from the boil in the form of pus that is expelled. I have often observed that the greatest quantity of foreign matter is discharged through the urine while a boil is running its course. I have often found big heaps like sponges in the urine. Boils are therefore not to be feared but welcomed.

CHRONIC HEADACHE.

M. in M., suffering from chronic headache for years. M. was relieved of his protracted headaches by a clay compress on the neck during the night.

TETTER.

N. N. in O. was suffering for years from corrosive tetter. All remedies had been tried without avail. After applying six compresses with moist earth the tetter dried up and disappeared. What a simple and rapid cure of a very disagreeable trouble! I know of some brilliant cures by my method in cases of long standing.

SNAKE-BITE POISONING.

Recently the following report made the round of the papers: "In the village of Recale near Caserta a young girl of twenty, while making hay, was bitten in the foot by a snake a few days ago. Her foot and leg soon began to swell, and the girl suffered great agony. Her father placed her on a pushcart and took her to Caserta. When they arrived there the whole right leg and arm of the poor sufferer had swollen to enormous dimensions. The physicians declared that the girl was past cure. The patient, moreover, lost consciousness, and her father brought her back to Recale more dead than alive. Here he made a last desperate effort to save his child by resorting to a remedy which tradition said had saved a girl of the village bitten by a snake centuries ago from certain death. He dug a hole in the garden, put his daughter naked into it, and then covered her up, leaving only her head free. The Mayor attempted to force the father by calling in the police to take his daughter out of the hole, but the entire village took the part of the father, the men armed themselves, and there would have been a bloody collision if the Mayor had insisted on the execution of his order. The girl was "dug up" again only twenty-four hours later, completely cured. This strange occurrence has been confirmed in the 'Corriere di Napoli' by the prefect of Caserta."

In our part of the country, the common adder is perhaps the only one of all the dreaded poisonous snakes. From the above well authenticated report we see how easily blood-poisoning by snake bite can still be healed, even after, in consequence of wrong treatment, a most dangerous stage has been reached, and the poison has already penetrated through the whole body. We can therefore feel all the more convinced that a poisonous snake bite is without any danger whatever, if moist earth is at once applied. If ever anyone should be bitten by an adder, therefore, let him at once apply moist earth to the affected place, and renew it in the beginning every hour or two. He will then have nothing to fear, especially not if he also leads a natural life.

The same as snake bites the bites of mad dogs can be rendered harmless by the prompt application of moist earth. The skill of Professor Pasteur is entirely uncertain and unreliable, but the skill of the great master, nature, never fails us. If indeed there ever has been a case where rabies have been avoided through Pasteur's method, we may confidently assume that the health of the person in question has thereby been impaired to such a degree that he is doomed to disease, in a way that is still more tormenting and more dangerous than rabies.

From this we again see what a very important place earth occupies as a healing application, that it is indeed an invaluable and cheap *universal and household remedy.*

DISEASE OF THE SPINAL CORD AND OBESITY.

H. at F. suffered from diseased nerves and spinal cord, was *entirely paralyzed,* and weighed two hundred and fifteen pounds.

It was with great difficulty that he could be transported to the Jungborn at all. On the journey it always took at least four men to carry H. into another car when a change had to be made. There seemed to be no longer the least hope for H. He remained at the Jungborn for four weeks, and soon wrote me from his home:

"To-day I can joyfully exclaim: your method of curing has truly done wonders in my case of severe nervous and spinal disease, coupled with complete paralysis of both legs! During my stay at your institution there was already a substantial improvement, as you will remember, and this did not only endure, but kept on increasing, although I have been actively engaged in my business, from morning till evening, since the day of my return.

"Of course I have strictly observed all your directions with respect to diet, earth compresses, baths, etc. My general health has improved exceedingly, and I have lost fifty-five pounds in weight, as a result of the treatments. I thank Providence for enabling me to find your institution."

At the Jungborn H. was often buried in the earth with his legs, and sometimes up to his chest, which proved to be very effective. For the rest the treatments, in this case also, were as usual.

CHRONIC INFLAMMATORY RHEUMATISM.

Ph. at F. (fifty-nine years old), suffered from chronic inflammatory rheumatism for years and was finally quite paralyzed. A course of treatments according to the old nature-cure method had not had any special result. Ph.'s condition became more and more serious, finally one leg was to be amputated. In his greatest need my book fell into his hands. By taking the bath, the fruit diet, light-and-air baths, etc., a cure was effected in an astonishingly short time, to the greatest astonishment of his friends. The leg was saved.

Gout, rheumatism, lumbago, sciatica, and all diseases of this kind come from bad humors in the blood. They can all be healed by a true nature-cure (but not by packing the body in warm wool, by warm baths, etc.), and all the pains and tortures that they cause ought not to be endured any longer.

MISCELLANEOUS.

Mrs. S. of H. "It is with great pleasure that I write you once more in my mother's behalf, to thank you with all my heart for all your goodness and kind endeavors. During her four weeks' treatment at the Jungborn my mother has so fully recovered, and is so refreshed in body and mind, that she is quite rejuvenated in spite of her sixty-three years of age, and everybody who sees her is perfectly amazed! She must then always give a thorough report of the Jungborn, and of all the good things that suffering mankind experience there. My husband and I are true champions of your cause, and we, too, often think with pleasure and gratitude of the hours spent with you.—M. G."

"I am happy to tell you that I have passed my examination satisfactorily. I am chiefly indebted to the diet that I observed during the last weeks before the examination for keeping up so well during the ordeal. I was always full of life and never lost courage. I am quite a different person now, and am taking a new interest in life.—E. St."

It would lead me too far to add more testimonials of the remarkably favorable results that have already been achieved by a truly natural mode of life and by the treatments, even in cases where the old nature-cure method had been entirely barren of results. I shall only mention a few more cases, that are of especial interest.

LARGE WOUND FROM THE BITE OF A DOG.

A. N. in E. was bitten by a large dog that was universally feared for his viciousness. There were two wounds; the one was so large that it seemed incredible that a dog could inflict such a wound with his tusks. It was about an inch and three fifths in length, about three fifths of an inch deep and two fifths of an inch wide, the dog had actually torn out the flesh. It was therefore, much worse than a cut of the same length and depth. The friends of the wounded man were, therefore, in great anxiety, since dog bites are generally very dangerous. I cooled the wound with cold water, then put *moist earth* upon it, and bandaged it with a wet linen cloth. This application was renewed every morning. The patient led a natural life according to my method. In this manner the patient did not suffer *the least pains* from the start, and was not for a moment hindered in walking, running, climbing mountains, etc. The lesser wound was already healed on the second day, and the larger wound showed not the slightest alarming inflammation, or gave any other discomfort or annoyance to the patient. In three weeks the deep, large wound was healed. Whenever the bandage was taken off a great quantity of very malodorous liquid matter came away. Earth is peculiarly adapted to draw disease matter from the body and from the wound. For this reason it is so very healing in cases of insect, snake, and mad dog bites, and in *vaccine* and other blood-poisoning, as I must once more repeat.

The use of alcohol, tobacco, etc., is especially dangerous in case of wounds.

I have already mentioned that we find all creatures of nature that eat meat to be bloodthirsty. But beasts of prey are seized by this passion only when they must satisfy their hunger. In meat-eating men, however, this murderous poison manifests itself in a most disgusting and abhorrent manner. For man meat-eating is not natural, it must therefore necessarily cause morbid desires and passions. There is, moreover, an uncanny demon that plays havoc with man, called alcohol; at present it is penetrating old and young and makes fearful monsters of people. Man does not kill only for the sake of food, he even lays hands on his brother.

In order to regulate this savage murderous passion of man, and to let it appear a little less gruesome, the art of war has developed. In war, then, mankind satisfies its innate uncanny desire to murder, to be sure according to the rules of civilized warfare. Floods of human blood are shed, and in the uncanny jubilation of victory are mingled the dying groans of human beings, and the sad lament of innumerable broken hearts of brides, mothers, and fathers. Through his unnatural mode of life man has reached the greatest monstrosity, war. Jesus said:

"Put up again thy sword into his place: for all they that take the sword shall perish with the sword."—Matt. 26:52.

In case this wildest passion of men should once more be let loose, in case peaceable governments should no longer withstand the people's greed for war, for this eventuality I wish to call especial attention to the bandage with moist earth.

The wounded warrior always has earth at his disposal, he can even moisten it with his own saliva. If he cannot make a bandage, he need only fill the wound with earth. If a bullet cannot easily be removed with the hand, he can calmly allow it to remain in the body. Extracting the bullet by cutting is injurious, even dangerous. As soon as the warrior has filled or covered his wound with the earth, his pain will cease, and the way will have been prepared for the most favorable healing process. If the bandage with moist earth has once been introduced, the danger from wounds in hospitals will no longer be so exceedingly great in time of war, and there will be a stop to the many operations and amputations. And after the war there will no longer be so many cripples walking the earth without arms or legs, as witnesses to the extremest human misguidance and degeneration.

M. A. at B. took treatments according to my method for about three-fourths of a year, for a *very severe,* old, and longstanding nervous trouble, after all other remedies had failed. The old nature-cure method had brought him relief and a little improvement. As a child he had never had any of the children's diseases (small-pox, measles, scarlet fever, etc.), and in later years, too, he had never had an acute disease or cold. A. had considered this as a good sign of health; in truth, however, it was just because his body did not possess sufficient vitality to purge itself of foreign matter, through acute diseases, and colds, that his severe nervous trouble had taken possession of him, and would surely soon have brought him to the insane asylum, or to an early grave, had he not taken the natural treatments. Soon after the treatments A. became subject to many, often very large boils and carbuncles, which with the natural treatment, always brought him great relief. In the course of time light acute diseases set in, even severe diarrhœa, accompanied by cholera symptoms. After these crises, too, A. always felt very much refreshed and well. At last a very severe influenza made its appearance. The patient looked very pale and miserable, and felt very weak. He took to his bed in the light-and-air cottage depicted on page 66. The cottage remained open on all sides, although it happened to be very cold, rainy weather in March, and a very cold, piercing wind blew through the place. Sometimes the patient took a light-and-air bath for twenty or thirty minutes, in the cold weather, that is, he walked about naked (without any clothes whatever) outside of the light-and-air cottage, in the open air, and sometimes he took the natural bath. He hardly ate anything at all. After A. had been lying in the light-and-air cottage in the midst of pine and birch trees, for several hours, he felt great relief. The foreign matter began to loosen, there was copious discharge from mouth and nose, and soon perspiration set in. In three days A. was cured of the influenza. After this severe crisis he felt that he had made an immense stride towards health. He was very happy and thought he had not, during the whole course of treatment, made anywhere near as much progress. A. is still continuing the cure with continued great results and is still sleeping in a light-and-air cottage.

Was not this a simple, cheap, and happy cure?

With the unnatural treatment of to-day, how long do men still suffer from the consequences of influenza? For many even the sequel is death. But those who die of it are often better off than those who survive the wrong treatment, and are "cured," but in whom, in truth, the light acute disease has been changed into a chronic disease (consumption, cancer, asthma, etc.), and who are thus given over to protracted invalidism, great tortures, and terrible misery, unless, indeed, they happen to find the right cure later on.

It is entirely erroneous to think that only especially hardened, and strong natures may venture to make use of air in the above manner. Air is always helpful and harms no one in any case. The delicate and weak experience the greatest strengthening effect and the greatest relief from light-and-air baths at the lowest temperature.

But angels might come down from heaven and bring this message to men, and still they would not believe it.

Whoever has no summer house, or light-and-air hut at his disposal, ought at least in every case of sickness, (acute or chronic) leave the windows of his bed room open in summer and winter, and then too expose his bare body to light and air again.

If the healthy man needs air, above all things, for the preservation of his strength and vigor, how much more necessary must it be for the sick organism. That air is actually feared in sickness is a dangerous and fatal delusion, for which men must suffer bitterly.

The opinion also prevails, for instance, that in measles, scarlet fever, etc., children must not go out into the air too soon, and even the windows are darkened in the sick room, that no light can penetrate.

But in this manner many children are made unhappy for life, (blindness, deafness, weak-mindedness, etc., are the consequences) or the little earth mounds in the cemeteries increase in number, at the sight of which everyone's heart is moved, because one involuntarily feels that these tender buds were broken, before the blossom could unfold, against God's intention and will.

I know a child that had light-and-air baths during an attack of measles, and that went out walking in the fresh, cool air on the third day, while the windows of the sick room were always kept open. All the cousins and aunts of the neighborhood were indignant at this unprecedented recklessness of the parents, and a physician made the statement that such foolhardiness would avenge itself severely even if the consequences did not appear till half a year had elapsed.

But the child, who has since been kept on a natural mode of life, is prospering wonderfully, although several years have passed since that attack of measles, and is the joy of its parents' hearts. Yes, children above all are such wonderfully appreciative patients in a natural cure.

With holy awe people to-day send to the apothecary for remedies, that have been invented and brewed by men who themselves are groaning under their load of disease and pain, and the people who attempt to cure themselves in this manner are considered sensible. But the remedies of nature have always been ridiculed and derided, as well as those who, in order to free themselves from their disease, have resorted to nature in order to regain their health and happiness—a happiness of which men in their present sad state of existence can have no conception— because they again observe the laws of nature and the commandments of God. Is this not the same as deriding God Himself?

In the above reports of cures we have seen that all patients were treated in the same manner.

Only the earth compresses, by which a local effect was to be produced, varied according to the disease.

I now observe that almost all patients took compresses on the abdomen, even if this was not especially stated in the report.

Likewise in all cases great importance was placed on going barefooted (without sandals) on the bare ground.

Often, too, the body or parts of the body were rubbed and stroked by proper persons. This was chiefly done after the natural bath, and contributed much to the surprising results.

The true healing method must be simple, and must possess the unity which nature itself has. Whoever attempts to individualize in the healing of diseases, only shows a morbid desire for knowledge, for science, whose chief mission it is to reduce, individualize, specify, classify, numerate, etc.

Of course the cure progresses more rapidly in one case than

in another; that depends on how much the vitality can still be stimulated.

The return to nature, the natural mode of life and curative process, must soon become a joy and a pleasure, it must not be a torture and a burden.

A gentleman once wrote to me: "It is a pleasure to be sick at the Jungborn."

The more rapidly and the more fully we return to a completely natural mode of life, the better the result will be in all cases, but not all people can again return to nature with the same dispatch without experiencing hardships and discomforts on account of it. This depends greatly on how far the diseased condition has progressed, and how much the internal organs, especially the digestive organs, have been ruined. Everyone can best judge for himself in this matter. Everyone must, therefore, have complete *liberty* in taking the treatments; there must be *no compulsion.*

All the practices may be suspended, especially the water and air baths, if at any particular time the patient feels very much disinclined to them. Let there always be freedom in the treatment of the sick, no compulsion.

I have intentionally never attempted to describe and treat the various diseases, with their manifold phases and symptoms, in detail. I have considered it my task only to point out the remedies of nature that are at any time the best and surest in *all* diseases, and in *every stage* of a disease.

Let no time be lost in: *skin diseases, kidney trouble, liver complaint, consumption, feminine diseases, epilepsy, obesity, eye and ear troubles, diseases of the throat and nose, bladder trouble, sexual diseases, head trouble, sciatica, gout, stomach trouble, heart disease, paralysis, spinal disease, influenza, children's diseases, diphtheria, measles, etc., etc.,* but begin at once, as soon as the first symptoms of a disease appear, to undertake a cure as nearly as possible according to the directions of nature.

Why should one, in case of sickness, first await an examination and other useless and mistaken stuff before acting? While the examinations that are at present customary to determine a disease, and the other preparations for all sorts of difficult and unnatural treatment are pending, a patient may often even become well again.

After all that I have said so far everybody ought to be perfectly clear as to what to do in any case of sickness. I certainly have sufficiently dwelt upon the importance of avoiding diseases by a correct, natural mode of life. But if this has not been done and anyone is taken with pain and distress, or if any acute or chronic disease whatever sets in, then keep calm, and be assured that in a truly natural cure, with the means that I have pointed out, all diseases, even the most dreaded (diphtheria, typhoid fever, cholera, etc.), are entirely without danger.

At all events see to it that there is pure, fresh air, apply earth compresses, take light-and-air baths, the water bath, have the body rubbed, leave off eating, until the appetite becomes very urgent, and then restrict the diet to raw fruit as much as possible, live chiefly in the open air, go barefooted, use the earth-power as much as possible.

About the spiritual influences that are of the most curative significance in days of sickness, I shall speak more fully later on.

Whoever has so far followed my expositions intelligently, will know that the same mode of procedure holds for *all* cases, and will not ask for particular directions and a special course of treatments for every individual case.

I cannot prescribe special treatments for all the different diseases, as is done in other health treatises; for a truly natural cure is, in the main, the same in all cases.

If, for instance, the case is one of typhoid fever, then let, first of all, all the windows in the sick room be opened, even in the colder seasons. Then the water bath is to be administered, and after it a light-and-air bath, whereupon warmth must be restored by rapid walking, if this is possible, or by wrapping in warm woollen blankets. The light-and-air bath can be taken frequently in every season of the year, in the open air is best, otherwise in the room; one soon becomes convinced of its effect. The duration of the light-and-air bath is from fifteen minutes to several hours; the longer the better.

An earth compress on the abdomen is most advisable.

The moist earth draws the heat from the abdomen and dissolves the foreign matter there.

In respect to diet, the rules repeatedly laid down by me must be observed.

The friends of the patient often wish to show him special attentions and love. Even if they are convinced of the correctness of the fruit diet, they will bring the patient all sorts of drinks and foods, for instance, fruit juices, non-alcoholic wines, fruit soup, honey, all sorts of fine tropical fruit, and the like. But this is entirely wrong. Even if I have said that such things are permissible, it is nevertheless better for the sick to use such dainties sparingly if at all. They are apt to deceive the tongue, to lead one away from a simple natural diet, and especially to beguile one into eating and drinking too much, which is always very injurious.

To remain in the open air as much as possible is greatly to be recommended.

The treatment of cholera is the same as for typhoid fever. In cholera as well as in *all acute and chronic diseases an earth compress on the abdomen, the chief center of every fever, as well as of every disease, is always very beneficial.*

The treatment for measles, influenza, pneumonia, etc., is likewise the same.

If a chronic disease (nervous disease, consumption, dropsy, and the like), has made its appearance, the same remedies of nature are again applied. But the manner of treatment must be so arranged that it can be continued for months, even years. The best thing, of course, is to keep on with the cure indefinitely.

In consumption, as well as all lung troubles, it is of great benefit to apply an earth compress to the chest, in dropsy to the swollen parts, in abdominal troubles and sexual diseases on the abdomen or on the sexual parts.

In the case of wounds, ulcers, (cancer), and in all skin diseases, the earth compress is, of course, the main thing. But even in these cases the general treatment of the whole body must not be neglected.

I wish once more to call attention to the circumstance that in all diseases and for all conditions, *fasting until noon* is of the greatest hygienic advantage. If anyone finds these too difficult, let him eat but *very little* in the morning.

If a cure in this manner is not undertaken altogether too late improvement and convalescence will be sure to follow. Nature never fails.

Let every sick person begin his cure with this implicit confidence, and with the serenity that comes of such confidence, and he will soon regain complete health.

All sorts of remedies and applications, which are not in accordance with nature, are always recommended to every sick person from all sides, but these are always useless, and always carry even harm in their train. We should, therefore, at all events, adhere to the simple nature-cure.

If, perchance, the result should not come as rapidly as we expected it to come, we must still remain tranquil; we must be patient and not allow ourselves to be misled into unnatural practices. By unnatural practices a true success cannot be achieved, we always do ourselves much harm by them, without knowing it.

Medical science to-day fears so many contagious diseases, and spreads much terror abroad in this way.

But if we can still heal all these dreaded diseases, we ought to be able to deprive them of all danger of contagion. Whoever, therefore, takes up our cause *may entirely lose all fear of incurable as well as contagious diseases.* This fear does a great deal of mischief.

Only through this simple, natural, uniform method can men once more become free and independent with regard to the care of their health and their sick from a special healing class. They will then once more exercise sovereignty over their health, their most precious, earthly possession, and will be free from the present unworthy, and oppressive slavery to all sorts of doctors. In this field, too, people ought to begin to aspire to *golden freedom*.

Mankind has fought and struggled so much for freedom, this precious boon. Will they never care to gain the freedom over their own bodies, over their health?

SEA AND MINERAL BATHS, HIGH ALTITUDE SANITARIA.

Doctors nowadays are very fond of sending their patients to the sea-shore, to get the benefit of the sea air. But it is my opinion that man is not a water fowl, but that his original home was the forest. Primitive man did not live by the sea, paradise was a forest that extended all over the earth.

All this craze for baths with mineral springs, as well as salt baths, sulphur baths, and the like, is also entirely wrong. If we want to find health we must not look for it among those who make yearly pilgrimages to the various baths, for here, especially, we find disease and invalidism in every possible form. But in these circles sickness is more a matter of fashion, and many a one returns from the bath sicker than he went.

Therefore I must also admonish those of higher society, who really have the desire and the wish to get well: "Return to Nature!" The invalid and the man in need of recuperation must not go to the sea-shore, not to the mineral and salt baths, no, let him avoid all trouble and everything unnatural and go into the forest! O, how beautiful is the forest with all its magic, the rustling and whisperings of its trees, its cheery birds in the branches, its quiet and peace, its delicious air! In the forest the fetters of the disease loosen most quickly. In the forest the patient is most easily diverted from everything conventional, from everything low and vulgar, and therefore soon regains his health both of body and soul.

In the protected localities, in the protected valleys with their springs and babbling brooks, not on the inclement windy heights, but in the protected valleys do we find a luxuriant vegetation, here flourish flowers and fruits. Man, too, can therefore not flourish and grow well upon inclement windy heights, but only in the mild valleys, where the sun-rays gather.

The cold air applications can, of course, be made just as well in the valleys and protected places. But the roughness and inclemency of a cold climate is less perceptible here. The cold, however, which is very important remains here, too.

On the heights, to be sure, the bacilli, so greatly feared today, are said not to prevail, and it is for this reason that elevations are so often recommended by physicians. To go to high altitude sanitaria has also become an actual fad in our time. It is well known that this theory of bacilli has already produced many absurdities and done much harm, and that the opinions of scientific physicians are subject to continual change. It is not bacilli, but a wrong mode of life that cause diseases, let us therefore return to nature and fear neither diseases nor bacilli.

WHEN OUGHT ONE TO UNDERTAKE A NATURE-CURE?

It is often believed that summer is the only season adapted to nature-cure, and the greatest value is placed upon sun-baths.

Animals may indeed come out of the thicket for a few hours of the day, while the sun is shining, to lie down in the sun, but then they again withdraw into the cool shade. The Germans who emigrate to foreign countries, for instance to Brazil, etc., generally do not live long. In the intermediate north (not exactly in the coldest regions) men always attain to greater age than in the southern, warmer countries. It is well known, too, how many kinds of fever and skin diseases, to which innumerable people fall victims, occur in the hot zones.

To be sure the sun loosens disease matter and promotes all growth and development on earth. But whoever takes too many sun-baths is very much weakened. Every sick person always suffers from too great inner heat, which weakens, and often completely consumes him. Therefore cold air applications strengthen men above all things, and restore their health. Through cold light-and-air baths man gains strong nerves and strength, which is of chief importance.

In the cold seasons, when the air and water applications can probably be of only short duration, the nature-cure treatments are of wonderful efficacy. Alone through a fruit diet and earth compresses, through rubbing and stroking the body, which I here wish to emphasize once more, through breathing the air, which is purest in cold weather, very much can be gained during the cold seasons, but I once more lay stress on the great efficacy of cold light-and-air baths, even if they are of but short duration. The spring and autumn of the year ought to be valued most highly as a time for curing. In spring when all nature is born anew, man too ought to gather fresh strength for a new life, and also in autumn an invigorating breath passes through nature.

In the summer the cool mornings and evenings and the cool days should be especially chosen for light-and-air baths. Also rainy seasons have an especially curative effect. The curative effect of going barefooted is greatly enhanced on wet ground, in wet grass, etc. Wet ground is the very best conductor to lead off disease matter. Those who always avoid the cold, who perhaps go to warmer countries in winter, never get well. their animal heat especially grows continually less.

The want of animal heat in our present anæmic, nervous generation is actually alarming, but only through cold light-and-air baths, together with a natural diet (nut diet), can animal heat be once more restored. In taking a nature-cure you can also make yourself warm and comfortable in clothes, beds and rooms, after the cold applications, but you cannot regain animal heat by the warmth, cold air must accomplish that. In the course of time warm clothes, beds, rooms, etc., will become less and less necessary. The cold light-and-air baths can never be taken too long, they never do harm, but each one may be led, as regards time, by his own supply of animal heat, for everyone must be able to get thoroughly warm again afterward, in order to feel quite comfortable. Cold air is better adapted to restore animal heat than cold water. Anæmics can take the water bath very short or omit it entirely.

We know, too, that the nations in our temperate northern regions (it need not be the far north) have always been the strongest and most enduring. Let us recall, for instance, the ancient Germans, who in their primitive strength crowded out the refined and effeminate civilized nations of antiquity, the Greeks and Romans. The Germans were once the strongest people that the world has seen. Now, too, it seems as if the Germanic people, after they have passed through all the defects of civilization, were destined to lead the way back to nature. Out of its midst, apparently the new race will come that will permanently attain to the high aims of true health, and true happiness, and will thus enter upon the truly higher development of mankind.

Those who cannot take air baths in the open, must, of course, take them in every season of the year, in an unheated room in which all the windows are open. In taking this bath one must always be entirely naked.

It is also very desirable that the water bath, if any way possible, be taken in an entirely cold room. (The bath may be very short, according to circumstances). Only with beginners an exception may perhaps be made, and the room be warmed somewhat.

Let us therefore no longer fear the cold, but let us again expose ourselves to it more and more; in that way we shall soon acquire more strength and health. This more intimate relationship with cold air can also be arranged in such a way that no harshness or great discomfort need to be experienced thereby.

MY RELATION TOWARDS THE OLD NATURE-CURE METHOD.

I am unfortunately having the experience that many of the adherents of the old nature-cure method are unwilling to follow me in my progress, there are even some among them who are violently opposed to my cause. But I share this fate with many who before me have had new ideas with respect to the nature-cure method.

When Schroth in his time attempted to perfect the Priessnitzian water-cure method by a dry diet, he encountered his chief opponents among the followers of Priessnitz.

The attacks that have been made on Father Kneipp by the adherents of the old nature-cure method were much worse and more malicious than the warfare that was waged against him by the physicians and laity who stood outside of the nature-cure method. And yet the venerable, worthy Kneipp rendered very great services to nature-cure. He popularized going barefooted, he introduced douches, which correspond to the rain in nature, and has at least shortened the time of full and half baths (to several seconds) while he denounced warm baths altogether, which is of great importance.

It can readily be explained, how it is that the adherents of the old nature-cure method should make a hostile attack upon everyone who would introduce some progressive innovation into their cause, who would add a new stone to the edifice that it may grow more and more into a magnificent temple of God. The reasons for this lie deep down in the nature of the sick being known as civilized man.

Man is happy and proud in the possession of an acquired knowledge, the more so if he has reached it by special training, and through a special course of instruction. Now if another person comes along who goes a step further in this knowledge, the former involuntarily feels uncomfortable.

In such a case it is customary among nature-curists to accuse the innovator of going to extremes. They forget that what they believe to be the correct thing had also been denounced as extreme by their predecessors.

Let me now test my system with regard to extremism. The transition from the present general mode of nutrition to my diet is much easier than to the present vegetarian diet. On my diet patients quickly regain their health and grow strong. It corresponds more fully to the directions of nature, which must always be of great advantage. The manner in which I advise my patients to again enter into relationship with light and air fulfils but a small part of the complete relationship that nature prescribes, but this latter is of the very greatest advantage and blessing to the sick and entirely without hardship.

And what of the remedies of the present nature-cure method? I do not wish to say anything against compresses, abdominal bandages and packs, they correspond somewhat to the bandages, and compresses with moist earth. But even the packs may be injurious in their effects, weak patients, for instance, cannot stand them. But a truly natural water application ought indeed to agree better with the weak than with the strong. With the natural bath and the earth compresses, this is the case. Full baths, however, and warm baths, which are doing much harm again of late, and especially steam baths, enemas, etc., are entirely against the design of nature, and therefore do the very greatest harm. All the artificial apparatus and contrivances that are necessary for this kind of curing, prove that they are not at all in conformity to nature.

The applications of electricity, which must be produced by the aid of an apparatus, and electric light baths are unnatural. Also the light-and-air baths, and sun baths in glass halls, in a sort of hot-house, for which provisions are made in many institutions, are bad, they do harm in that they always lead away from nature again.

Nature designed fruit to be the food of man. All chemical investigations and determination of the ingredients of food lead astray. We have had enough of the theories, so often put forward by medical science, about albumen, nitrogen and the like, which man must take into his system through food. All these theories have always caused no end of harm. Those who have nourished themselves according to these scientific doctrines always suffered for it severely.

But nature-curists also frequently drop into the same error as medical men. Of late years much is said about the necessity of food containing nutritive salts, and this is having a bad effect on the nature-cure method. I have also called attention to the fact that green vegetables are less injurious than leguminous seeds and cereals, and know well enough that we cannot as yet quite exclude green vegetables from human food-stuffs. Nevertheless cooked vegetables are an unnatural food. In consequence of the nutritive salts theory, however, many consider green vegetables as especially wholesome, and place great value upon them as a factor in nutrition. This, of course, is entirely wrong. But even chocolate and cocoa with the addition of nutritive salts are greatly in vogue, and are used in the belief that they are very conducive to health, because they have been prepared and recommended by nature-curists. But chocolate and cocoa, with the addition of nutritive salts, spoil the stomach just as much as they do without this addition, and this is where the greatest danger lies in human nutrition.

All those who often and regularly drink nutritive-salt chocolate and cocoa, in the belief that they are wholesome foods, will soon have occasion to experience an impairment of their digestion. Therefore, so long as science has a hand in the nature-cure method, mischief will still be done.

Oat-cocoa is, of course, just as unsafe and injurious as nutritive-salt cocoa.

The old nature-cure method entirely overlooks the close connection between body and soul. The human body is not like a machine, and it is on account of a more highly developed soul that man stands high above the animal. The chief thing for man is his soul life. We must take this into consideration especially, if we want to heal diseases.

The old nature-cure method knows nothing of the wonderful curative effects achieved through soul influences, especially by fellow-feeling and love, that is cherished in the heart, and by true trust in God; they do not consider a true, natural soul life and its great significance for curative purposes. For this reason it is entirely powerless in many diseases. (especially nervous diseases.)

I have often been obliged to test the truth of the words:

"We are used to see, that man despises
What he never comprehends,

And the Good and the Beautiful vilifies,
Finding them often hard to measure."
—Goethe "Faust."

And many a time during the last years, while making bitter, sad experiences, have I learned to understand the words:

"Yes of the kind which men attain!
Who dares the child's true name in public mention?
The few, who thereof something really learned,
Unwisely frank, with hearts that spurned concealing,
And to the mob laid bare each thought and feeling,
Have evermore been crucified and burned."
—Goethe, "Faust."

I am ready to sacrifice everything for my cause, even my life. But whatever I shall suffer through my cause and whatever I shall lose, I shall never deny one word of it, and I shall never beg for human favors.

Men would in vain try to shake the mighty mountains, and the lofty rocks that surround my home, but it would seem still more useless for men to attack the eternal truths upon which I take my stand, and for which I at any time am ready to sacrifice all my strength, and my whole life. But still I would like to offer the hand of friendship to the champions and adherents to the old nature-cure method, who have until now been more or less unfriendly to me.

I owe the old nature-cure method infinitely much, I have through it found the way to nature. But if, driven by necessity, I investigated and obeyed the laws of nature still more than has hitherto been done, and if I regained my own health after severest sickness, and true joy in life, and if a great many others have through me found the way to the fountain of all life, to true piety and happiness, can I then be silent concerning that which I learned in painful struggle, and what I have achieved, and only because a few people don't like it? It is very difficult too to stop up this silver spring. It will, after all work its way through all obstructions.

All my opponents, if they could not be convinced by my book, should have come to the Jungborn; it is always open to them. Here they might have convinced themselves of the results.

If a truly natural method of curing should come into vogue, who would be injured thereby? Can there be any greater gain for the nature-cure method than to achieve more and ever more brilliant successes? Only by successful results can the attacks upon the nature-cure method be silenced.

Many more and better results can still be achieved than in the past, we can heal more quickly and more thoroughly, and can help in many, many cases where the nature-cure method has failed hitherto. In a word, quite a different state of health can be achieved than has hitherto been known, if for our bath we will only observe the form which nature prescribes, place more value upon light and air, and, also in this respect, consider the demands of nature; if we will not overlook the earth, and remember, in respect to our nutrition, that in making our choice of food, even from the vegetable kingdom, we must regard the designs of nature, and choose the fruits.

The time of eating, too, must correspond to the conditions prevailing in nature.

The manner in which I have so far spoken of the successes of a truly natural cure, of the healing of the body that can be accomplished, of the wonderful influence of a truly sound body upon mind and soul, and of the happiness of man that will result therefrom, the manner in which I have done this may indeed seem like exaggeration, like frenzy and fanaticism. Since the nature-cure method has so far not adhered closely enough to nature, *it was not sufficiently harmonious and especially not simple enough.* In this way no true health could be achieved so far, no true vigor and strength and ennobling of the soul. I mention this with no intention of blaming the adherents of the present nature-cure method and of our present vegetarianism.

In calling their attention to these mistakes, I would at the same time direct their attention to the precepts of nature, for the sake of suffering mankind that entrusts itself to them, and for whom it would result in the greatest blessing, and for their own sake, that they may take still more pleasure in their work than hitherto.

Meanwhile no one should permit himself to waver, but should look into and try the matter himself, and whoever will subject himself to a process of the natural cure according to my directions will soon experience in his own person the good results that were promised and accept the lesson. It costs nothing to make the experiment, and it may be made everywhere. Whoever makes it will soon feel that he is once more in harmony with nature, and that he once more shares in the original pleasure and happiness which nature has in store for those who tread her paths.

When in wood and glen young flowers put forth fresh shoots and all things renew themselves, when in love's sweet joy the nightingale sings her song, and gentle zephyrs fill the evening air, the sick heart of man, too, trembles with a vague inkling of all the wonder and magic bliss within the realm of nature pure and undefiled. Then we feel how health and happiness may still be had.

Once again I extend my hand to the champions of the old nature-cure method and plead for peace. While the nature-cure method is making its way by virtue of its profound truths, it is not right that its champions and adherents should waste their time in angry controversy. Let us not ourselves stem the tide which is powerfully pushing on.

EVERYONE HIS OWN DOCTOR.

Nature offers her prescriptions to all men in the same way. One man does not get more from nature than another in regard to what is best for his health and happiness. Therefore it is incomprehensible why one should not wish to be his own doctor. We need only to listen to nature and to follow her lead. Everyone must indeed once again become his own doctor, or rather once more select nature as his sole doctor, before we can look for true health. But this is the very lesson that modern man is so slow in learning.

Modern nature doctors indeed preach, "Everyone his own doctor," but in case of sickness they insist on an examination of the patient and begin to "particularize."

All this proves that they are ignorant of the true nature method, nor can everyone be his own doctor along such lines.

After one has again come to a true understanding of nature, he knows instantly what to do in case of sickness. What need of an examination, and what is the use of the name of the sickness? If it were of advantage to be informed concerning interior conditions, and processes in the human body during health and illness, nature would have constructed it so that we could readily look into it, she could have made it transparent or provided it with openings. But if the examinations are not desired by nature, they are always useless, and even very harmful. However, people nowadays are possessed by a perfectly morbid craze to let someone ascertain their particular disease and give it a name. But no exact and definite conclusions concerning the nature and course of disease are ever to be drawn from all the examinations by means of percussion, auscultation, or by studying the face, the nails, the hair, the handwriting, etc. In this regard nature is too mysterious for us. We come to see this especially when we observe the divergencies of various examinations. The more examinations, the more diagnoses.

To rely on and base a line of procedure on the result of a given examination, whether conducted by means of physiognomy, phrenology, or graphology, will also teach us that in most cases we have made a mistake.

Examinations are consequently entirely useless, yes, they are even always very injurious.

I know of a case where a physician, who is regarded as an authority, told a man after he had examined him that he was very ill and would surely die, within a few weeks. The man was stricken with fright, and immediately began to waste away until after a few weeks he died. Now granting that he was severely ill, it is evident that the positively expressed opinion of the physician, aroused such a firm conviction in the man that it aggravated the disease and hastened his death. Other physicians who had known and examined the man were indignant and amazed at this tragic end.

I have myself often observed, that patients who are frequently examined are always in a state of unrest and excitement. The state of their disease always depends on the result of the examination by a physician, or a nature-curist, or any man whatever who is subject to all sorts of errors. Patients have to suffer much in this way, and I pity them all the more, because it is so much harder for them to get well under such conditions.

Many diseases that did not exist before have been caused by such examinations, light diseases have become serious and portentous; more difficult to cure or even incurable, only by being ascertained through the examination of some medical authority. The powerful spiritual influences should be taken into consideration here.

We must always try to divert a patient, skillfully and quietly, (but without compulsion) from his disease. There is nothing that will more surely call a patient's attention to his disease than an examination.

Everyone knows himself well enough that he is sick, and everyone feels his local troubles better himself, than they can be ascertained by any other person by way of an examination.

But whoever has a particular nack for examining patients, can earn much money, by taking advantage of the present craze of men to always want to know the name of their disease. The success of the celebrated shepherd, Ast, proves this, who could diagnose diseases from the hair of the patient, but was nevertheless unable to cure anybody.

I have often been told by nature physicians that they well knew that there was no sense in examinations. But, they say, men to-day want to be examined, listened at, and felt over, and want special directions for every disease,—a harmonious, strictly natural mode of procedure is too simple for the patient. For this reason they (the nature physicians) made it appear as if they themselves considered the examination and individualization important and necessary. With this same intention patients are also often given all sorts of remedies (homœopathic remedies, herb juices, etc.).

It is true that it is often most difficult for men to-day to grasp what is simplest. But if a physician, against his conviction and knowledge, treats a man with all sorts of make-believes and remedies, is not that deception and fraud? But whoever has fully grasped the sacred significance of the nature-cure method, to him such deception and untruth will no longer be possible. Let us make a clean sweep, therefore, let there be nothing but truth and honesty in the nature-cure method. We shall some day have to give an account of ourselves to God. In this way alone can mankind once more be saved. Truth and honesty are the only right things after all. Away, then, with all examinations, all individualization, and all other hocus-pocus nonsense, with all charlatanism and swindle!

Whenever we wish to arrive at some knowledge of the interior of a sick body by an examination, there is always an inner voice to protest against it, and this, too, is the voice of nature which we must heed.

Unfortunately there are still many nature-curists who want to know all sorts of things about the inner diseased conditions, about the course of a disease, about the curability or incurability of a patient. Yes, men always want to be wise, wiser even than God, and therein lies all the misery of the world. Some nature-curists even deliberately try to show how very learned they are, and use all sorts of Latin, scientific, incomprehensible and high-sounding names and expressions, in order thus to make an impression on their patients, and to gain in their eyes. But, poor patients, do not allow yourselves to be dazzled by this! If we look closely we shall soon discover that all this knowledge is of no use, and is nothing but error. Indeed, errors are the rule with such nature-curists!

"For we know in part, and we prophesy in part."—1 Cor. 13:9.

Here, too, I should like to request nature-curists to set a noble and good example and to acknowledge and confess humbly and honestly, that they also know nothing. This, indeed, is the right kind of knowledge in this case also, to know that we don't know.

In this way suffering mankind would be most greatly benefited. It would be the surest way to again teach men to become their own doctors.

We need only to lead the sick to a purely natural mode of treatment and of life, which should be the same in all cases of sickness, and for which we need not to know or understand anything, when we can follow the voices of nature in good faith without sophistries and subtleties. All the rest we can then leave to nature and to God.

To these arguments of mine, many nature-curists have retorted that in this way all physicians and all nature physicians would become superfluous, and that they would thus undermine their own chances of making a living. But nature-curists ought to remember above all things that mankind to-day is being devoured by its selfishness, and that the world cannot grow any better either for the individual or the masses until unselfishness once more holds sway, and that it is to be wished, therefore, that nature-curists above all others should no longer think of their own advantage, their own living, in pursuing their holy calling! Nature-curists ought only to think of the blessing that is to come to all mankind from our cause.

The sick who are forever seeking for advice from one book or another, from one physician or another, can never acquire peace or health. Did primitive men have any advisers or physicians to assist them in the care of their health? Therefore I again exclaim: "Return to Nature!"

General and all-round health and happiness can return to the world only when everyone again understands nature, and when everyone becomes in truth his own doctor. Not until then will people no longer be helpless and perplexed in any condition of life, or at any moment, not until then will they be free and independent in the care of their health, and can thus soon become sound. In this way alone they are also proof against all great disappointments, and other great dangers in regard to their health.

It is indeed very difficult nowadays to lead men back to nature in this respect also, and teach them to be their own physicians. But when we once thoroughly understand and accomplish it, it is a source of much joy to us. We often observe to our own greatest surprise, how quickly people will feel and do the right thing in the minutest detail. For them there is now no longer any lack of insight or any doubt. Everything that they now do for their health they do gladly, with firm conviction and great enthusiasm, which calls forth great and important curative forces in the body. The consciousness of no longer being subjected to another in unworthy slavery, produces a rare sense of gladness and happiness, and the sufferings and diseases of the body drop off more and more like loosened scales; the heaviest, most oppressive fetters which sickness had placed upon the body get loosened more and more.

Men will then also have regained their complete *liberty* in the care of their health, a highly to be appreciated earthly possession, whose influence should be a special blessing.

God in His wise providence has given man liberty in the choice of his mode of life, which the animal has not (the animal cannot prepare its food artificially or make clothes). Unfortunately man's liberty has led him to desert nature, and has brought all his misery upon him. But if through his liberty he finds the right way again, and once more returns to nature and God, not from compulsion like the animal, but in consequence of a true understanding, and in obedience to his own free will, he enters upon the highest phase of his development.

Man now approaches more and more the ideal being from whom all the animal attributes have been sloughed off, while the Godlike attributes are taking their places, and are developing more and more. At all events Providence was working towards the highest end when from the start it gave man liberty.

For this reason man must always be allowed his freedom, no compulsion must ever be brought to bear upon him, especially not in the matter of his health. Only in perfect liberty can man really get well.

Yes, it is not so difficult to cure diseases, but we must again understand the voices of nature, everyone must indeed become his own physician.

I have always considered it as an especially high mission to teach men to become really their own doctors, and I shall continue to work in this direction, for I realize more and more how important this is for man.

I have also been told that many patients have been cured by the mere faith they have had in their physician. But how often, on the other hand, have men been deceived in their faith in men and human skill, and how difficult is it, therefore, to place one's faith and trust in a man!

Can men no longer place their trust in the great Physician in the heavens above? God always can help and does help if we only trust in Him again.

> "Oh trust in God who takes his stand,
> He surely has not built on sand."

If even the faith in a poor, erring man can sometimes cure and help, what great help must come to us if we give our faith to the Almighty, all-good God, who created and sustains the world, who guides heaven and earth, and who has the fate of every man in His hand, who includes all beings in the great universe in His infinite love!

But to-day we leave God entirely out of consideration; we think God is no longer necessary to us. There are so many professional healers at present, and there is so much science that we think God is superfluous.

I want to cry out to all sufferers and all invalids who are

groaning and lamenting: Place your faith not on the skill and knowledge of men; look aloft, rather, to the Almighty and all-good God; obey again the laws of nature, which are God's laws, and if you have the right kind of trust in God, He will always help you, and all your troubles and ills will soon disappear.

To be sure, the way in which to-day theology and the Church practise the various religions and observe the worship of God, and cultivation of the soul, is not the way in which we can be won and led to higher earthly blessedness. But him who will follow me still further, I can perhaps also lead on to trust in God and to the holiest and best fountain of life.

I have already frequently indicated how the sick particularly need the love and help of their fellow-men.

If well-meaning and otherwise suitable persons only place their hand on the sick portions of the body of invalids, they frequently experience instant relief. Think of the cures that Jesus achieved merely by the laying on of His hands!

Rubbing, stroking, and kneading can very often be practised on the sick by suitable, healthy and worthy persons in the simplest, most unskilled manner with the greatest curative effect. I repeat this again and again.*

By the touch of a healthy person health is not only transferred to the sick person, but the cure can also be explained in such a case by the disease being conducted away. But the healthy person does not suffer thereby, he even gains if it was a deed of love.

When limbs are fractured, dislocated, etc., they must first be placed in the right position by others, before earth packs, etc., can be applied. In many other ways, assistance, attention, and

---

*In this place I would once more like to call attention to a good remedy against cold feet, from which so many people suffer to-day. Besides the general remedies (especially going barefooted, etc.), it is very good to have cold feet thoroughly rubbed by strong persons with very warm hands. Such rubbing will in time restore more and more warmth to the feet, just as the rubbing of the whole body will always raise the animal heat of a person.

favors bestowed on the sick are advantageous or necessary. Yes, there must be a continuous flow of love towards the invalid, serving him and acting for him in the right spirit. When this love is genuine and true and acts in the spirit of nature, it can often achieve marvelous cures.

But for all this, no one need thoughtlessly and without a will of his own entrust his health to another, as is so frequently the case to-day. This does not at all imply that each one cannot always be his own physician.

The nature-cure method is of late gaining unprecedented popularity. The effect of this is, of course, that the champions of the nature-cure method, especially those that actually practise it, are violently attacked and persecuted by scientific physicians, and, unfortunately, often in a very hateful and unjust manner. The physicians, of course, frankly admit that they are defending the "interests of the medical profession"—yes, there is not so much fighting done to-day for the general welfare, for the welfare of unhappy, suffering mankind. But one must not really blame the medical profession for this; it is the general state of affairs at present.

Is there any other class that does not energetically stand up for its own interests, without being in the least concerned whether others, especially the common welfare, gains or loses thereby?

Physicians to-day do indeed leave no stone unturned to destroy the nature-cure methods; they are continually appealing to the aid of the police and the law for this purpose. It certainly does not speak well for medical science that it must ask protection in this manner. The nature-cure method will not lose by the oppression and persecution that is directed against it by physicians; its great power and truth will only be tested and strengthened thereby. It will now be forced to react against this oppression, and will thus only gain ground all the faster, and in the struggle that is forced upon it, it will achieve a splendid victory.

The medical doctors will then be driven by their own interests to draw more and more largely from the nature-cure method,

Of course in this struggle between nature-curists and scientific physicians many low and ugly practices are resorted to. But this whole war, the whole question of doctors, can only be finally decided and solved in that all doctors at last become superfluous, and everyone again becomes his own physician.

At first, of course, single individuals, possessing the right spirit, must direct men to nature and her voices, and to the right way of finding their souls' salvation. But all preachers of nature ought in the first place to strive to teach men to be their own doctors, for in this way they will give them freedom, health and happiness.

From what I have been teaching everyone can at any time undertake quite independently a purely natural cure, and lead a natural life *either for a time, in order to free himself from some sickness, or for his whole life, for the attainment of the highest earthly happiness.*

But whoever undertakes such a cure and leads such a life, faithfully and in accordance with nature, must under all circumstances remain steadfast, and be his own physician, and must not be led astray by any objections, advice and subtleties on the part of others, either medical or nature doctors, and also lay persons.*

AGRICULTURE AND FRUIT CULTURE, VETERINARY SCIENCE AND VIVISECTION.

I have already shown that nature originally voluntarily offered food to man, just as to every other creature, and I have

---

*Here I must once more observe that no one in taking the treatment must be deterred by crises, which may manifest themselves either as pains, discomforts, or a feeling of weakness, etc., and which in some cases may set in early, in others later.

The crises are always favorable symptoms; they prove that nature is engaged in curative activity. But if man is always disconcerted whenever nature is trying to help and cure, and will even work against it, with all sorts of unnatural remedies, how can he ever become healthy?

also shown the reason why man still disregards the gifts of nature.

Agriculture, which always comprised cattle raising, has from the start been a punishment, a curse for man's falling away from nature. Hard labor, sorrow, and care were always to go hand in hand with it.

"Cursed is the ground for thy sake; in sorrow shalt thou eat of it all the days of thy life."—Gen. 3:17.

The tiller of the soil could therefore never expect joy and happiness.

Within the last fifty years, moreover, a great and disastrous change has taken place in agriculture by the so-called "separation." Single tracts in the field mark, belonging to individual holders have been thrown together into large joint fields. The reason for this was an attempt to utilize the field mark far more than has hitherto been done; for every corner and every strip of land that has been lying fallow, or had been planted with hedges and trees, is now put to use. And the tendency is no longer to plant bushes and trees, because they give shelter to birds and cause them to multiply. And the birds, of course, also derive their sustenance from the fields, which one begrudges the little songsters.

This has at the same time been the opportunity for transforming the great pasture lands, the large green meadows, that formerly beautified the field marks, into tillage. The pasturing of the herds, especially of the cows, was discontinued because it was known that cows would yield more milk on stable fodder. Since that time cows generally stand, from the time of their birth till the day of their death or slaughter, tied to their crib in dark, stuffy stables, and always on their own dung. They are thus forever deprived of every free movement and of all pure, fresh air, which is an appalling cruelty.

The field mark formerly appeared like a garden—yes, even like a carpet, with its interspersed hedges and trees, and green meadows; but to-day it makes a most uninspiring and dreary impression. The sight of a field mark to-day is no longer pleasing and refreshing.

All this, even the cruelty against the animals, has come about because the land owners wished to make more money out of agriculture and stock-raising. For this reason, too, all sorts of artificial, chemical fertilizers, and innumerable machines have been invented and introduced. The feeding of the animals in the stables is also made more and more artificial, and in fact is horrible.

But rarely can it be shown more clearly than here that all striving and struggling for earthly mammon strictly speaking leads but to misery and poverty.

The countryman labors on his land in the sweat of his brow, from early morning till late in the evening, and if he ever for a moment looks up to refresh himself, the old fields and meadows, variously adorned with bush and tree, no longer delight his eye. No longer do flocks of birds sing their glad, cheering tunes to him in his hard labor. Yes, the rich farmer of to-day is in truth very poor.

In consequence of the unnatural fertilization, the products of the soil indeed become more abundant, but they are also much more harmful to health since then.

By a sort of prostitution he can draw more milk from the cows, that are bloated and distended by their artificial stall-fodder, but the milk is by far less wholesome. The farmers at present live not only on milk that is less wholesome than formerly, they also eat the flesh of those fattened animals that have been reared on their own dung, which must naturally result in still more sickness and suffering for them.

The greater abundance of money among the farmers, moreover, makes it possible for them to acquire many other unnatural habits. There is more unnatural clothing worn in the country now, and going bare-footed, for instance, has become almost a thing of the past. Indulgences and pleasures of all kinds that are detrimental to health have been introduced. The sons and daughters are more frequently sent to high-schools and boarding-schools for a scientific education. Everywhere there are now agricultural schools, dairy schools, domestic-science schools for country girls, etc. The country population everywhere aspires towards enlightenment and education.

But one can soon perceive that all this has not brought the country people happiness. All kinds of sickness and diseases, that were unknown to the old country people, and sin, vice and corruption have made their appearance in the country. The old peace and contentment, the old piety, have disappeared.

In the manner above indicated the country people intended to achieve more gain and to improve their condition, but instead of the good fortune they expected we now have "the destitution of the agricultural districts," which is incessantly proclaimed and deplored. Discontent and misery now put in an appearance everywhere, which was never the case formerly.

And the farmers likewise do not see that they themselves are to blame for all these evils. They look for the causes elsewhere. They are now incessantly combating all sorts of institutions and laws; here, too, the State is to bear all the blame.

And yet here, too, all endeavors will be in vain; only one thing can help:

"Return to Nature!"

In the first place farmers ought no longer to strive for treasures and delights and all sorts of apparent advantages through education, luxuries, etc., which never make happy but only have an external glitter which always deceives. They ought to begin a natural mode of life and return to the old simplicity and few wants, then they would indeed be able to live happily and without care.

It is, however, not to be expected that farmers will soon come to see things in the right light and will turn back. But the single individual can nevertheless begin to lay the foundation for greater happiness, for health and contentment.

I should especially like to urge farmers to turn their attention once more to fruit culture. It will certainly give them greater pleasure than agriculture.

Yes, when farmers shall seriously begin to devote themselves to fruit culture, they will have taken the first step toward a real improvement of their condition.

With the cultivation of turnips, hops and tobacco, with that horrible fattening of cattle, and the like, the farmers of to-day are engaged in an enterprise out of which nothing but disease and disaster can come to mankind.

The money which they receive for their products is in a certain sense the wages of sin, and there must also be a curse on it.

But with fruit culture farmers will promote a cause which will regain for mankind true salvation and happiness. God will reward the fruit-farmer for his work, and he will have more pleasure and satisfaction, more rest and peace, than the agriculturist.

Every labor is also "worthy of its reward," and farmers will be more and more able to live on fruit culture. Everyone knows that fruit is very much sought after of late years, and is ever gaining in value. Even people who have as yet no comprehension of a natural mode of life and of healing still begin to eat much fruit. This proves that the masses are now unconsciously being led back to nature.

I cherish the firm conviction that this movement will in future be much more rapid and much stronger. For this reason many can now turn to fruit culture; they all have the very best prospects, if they at the same time restrict their own wants. In the future enough money can be earned by fruit-culture.

It is sufficiently taught to-day that fruit culture can be so arranged as to yield good returns almost from the beginning. More attention must be paid to the cultivation of berries, strawberries, gooseberries, raspberries, etc., and must be planted beside dwarf fruit and half-stem fruit. In this manner fruit plantations can yield returns from the very first year, and can soon become very lucrative.

In fruit culture, too, we must avoid many unnatural practices; do everything in the simplest manner, and conform as closely as possible to nature; then we shall soon find the right way.*

I would also strongly urge the cultivation of *nuts* (hazelnuts as well as walnuts).

Foresters are to-day regarding the *hazelnut* as a nuisance, and are actually trying in every way to exterminate it. The hazelnut will put up with and grow in the most stony soil, on the most barren mountain, where hardly anything else can grow. But even these places are no longer given up to it. The nut shrub is never cultivated in woods and forests like other trees, and yet by rights it deserves the very first attention. Thus we see that man even eagerly seeks to destroy the hazelnut bush, which nature spontaneously produces without the labor of man, and which gives him the food which he absolutely needs in order to get true strength and health; while on the other hand, with great labor and at great expense, he cultivates the food that is of little use to him, and even injures his health. But if man always acts in such an unreasonable manner, is it then difficult to explain how all this sorrow and want, all this infinite misery and disease have come into the world?

Let us therefore again make room for the hazelnut bush in our woods, and let us plant it in the gardens; it will soon yield a rich harvest, and if we again live on nuts, an even stronger, healthier, nobler and happier race of men will arise. The nut bush will then also become the most beautiful ornament of our gardens and fields. Yes, entire forests of nut bushes must, in the course of time, again adorn our German Fatherland.

---

*Although I am 'here speaking in favor of fruit culture and fruit plantations, and would like to win people over to it, I cannot give any special directions as to how fruit culture can be pursued in the simplest and most natural manner. But everybody can get full instructions from the book "Joh. Bottner. Praktisches Lehrbuch des Obstbaues." (Verlag der Kgl. Hofbuchdruckerei Trowitsch & Sohn in Frankfurt a. d. O., geb. $2.00) or to the Naturopath Publishing Co., 111 E. 59th St., New York. The book contains a great many illustrations, which will make fruit culture clear in every respect to any lay person.

Only in the Hartz there are still solitary places, in the midst of stony debris, where not even the pine, which is certainly very modest, will grow, where one still finds the hazel-bush; everywhere else it has been exterminated. But in making excavations in the Hartz (even on the Brocken) nuts have frequently still been found and traces of former rich nut forests. In the same way we have proofs that the hazel-bush originally grew all over Germany in greater abundance than any other species of shrub or tree, and that there have been great nut forests.

The old Germans, as I have already mentioned, in the beginning allowed nature to provide for them entirely with her nuts and other fruit. When the Germans began the CHASE (the FALL OF MAN), which was soon followed by the use of alcohol and other unnatural practices, they deteriorated and became more and more brutalized, and finally developed into an enervated and miserable race just like the rest of the civilized nations, even if the inner corruption manifests itself to-day in a refined form and is surrounded by an illusive glitter.

One actually becomes deeply moved by observing how nature, in spite of all the opposition of unreasonable, foolish man, is determined to let the nut grow, in order to offer it to man as food. If he would now extend a helping hand to nature and, for the first at least, again give fallow places and mountains over to the nut, or even devote fertile land to it, upon which so much that is worthless and even injurious to health is now cultivated, the nut would soon again grow among us of so fine a quality and in such abundance that it could hardly be all consumed, and could finally be had almost for the asking.

But the nut is indeed the chief food of man; he can live upon it for the greatest part of the year almost exclusively, and in this way alone be truly strong and healthy. The old Germans have demonstrated this to us.

But if now the nut were again to be grown so easily and so abundantly that man could have it for the gathering, cannot mankind see that it could then easily free itself from all want and material care?

Let everyone, then, who has come to recognize the truth, do his share to again encourage the culture of the nut, on private lands as well as on public domains.

In the same way as against the nut, mankind to-day sins against the berries of the forest (huckleberries, raspberries, strawberries, etc.), and what I have said with regard to the nut holds equally for the berries also.

Just the most necessary and most important shrubs and bushes man does not cherish, but even destroys them.

Would that it might soon be different in this respect.

The countryman who is only concerned about his own and his family's maintenance, who does not care to gather false riches, who wants to be and remain healthy and happy, who knows wherein true riches consist, can easily achieve his ends with fruit culture.

In this manner the farmer needs to till much less land; he can let out or sell superfluous land, needs much less hired help, and domestic animals especially become more and more unnecessary. He need, therefore, no longer take advantage of his fellow-men or of animals.

It seems to me that a farmer, with only a rudimentary knowledge of the right kind, who desires to be healthy and happy in a natural mode of life, and for this purpose turns to fruit culture, must be better able than anyone else to create for himself a paradise on earth.

Man has sacred duties also towards *animals*. Animals, too, are God's creatures, and man ought to take pity on them when they are sick, and ought to lend them a helping hand. But nowadays man sins against his domestic animals, his faithful helpers, in that he exposes them in every way to an unnatural life, as I have already shown above. May I succeed to show men the right way in this respect also!

I have already shown how the many diseases to which our domestic animals are liable arise from the bad mistakes of our present agricultural system, from artificial stable feeding.

If man were to be tied like that, deprived of every free

movement, and forced to breathe in continually the fumes of his own excrements, would we not soon see that we were robbing him of his health in the most cruel manner? Men are continually sinning like this against the animals. This wrong cries to heaven and calls down severe punishment upon the head of man.

Also the feeding of animals with decayed turnip leaves, slops, etc., produces bad results.

Therefore domestic animals must again be let out of their dark, stuffy stalls, away from their dung, into the fresh air, into the pastures.

If the common pasturage for cattle cannot at once be reintroduced, every farmer ought to have a pasture of his own to which he can drive his cattle at least sometimes. It is absolutely necessary to have such pastures to keep the animals in health, and for cases of sickness among them. If the farmer has such a pasture, it will be an easy matter for him to cure his animals of disease. In most cases they need only be taken to the pasture night and day and kept there till they are well again. The animals like to lie on the ground, and are especially invigorated when it rains. In many cases, especially in skin and leg diseases, in lung trouble, etc., it is well to make clay compresses, or to bury the animal in the ground, for instance, mangy dogs. Short douches with water may also do good service. When the animals are returned to the stable we must take care that there is plenty of light and air, and the dung must at least be removed daily.

One need pay no attention to the animals after they are driven into the open air, into the pasture. They can be left alone to follow their instinct.

When horses are sick their shoes ought to be taken off, and they ought to be driven to pasture.

For animals, too, we need not fear colds. They may be left outside in cold days and in bad weather. In Winter, when there is ice and snow, they ought at least to be driven into the open air at intervals.

I think that whoever has understood me in my treatment of

men must know how to treat the diseases of animals correctly.

The hoof and mouth disease, so common to-day, is the direct consequence of stable feeding, Pasturing the animals in the open air generally suffices to cure them in a few days of this disease, about which veterinary doctors, and even the government, are so greatly troubled.

Besides providing pastures, green fodder ought also again to be fed more freely. For the Winter good hay must be provided, and a liberal supply of turnips and the like.

The grass that is to be made into hay is always mown too late at present; it is always allowed to get too ripe. If the grass were mown earlier the hay would be more wholesome for the animals, and the meadows could be mown oftener, and in that way made to yield more.

To-day a certain artificial strength is produced in horses by the excessive feeding of oats. For this reason the horse is much more liable to all sorts of diseases than those animals that are fed with green fodder and hay, as the ox, for instance. Horses can only become healthy and strong if they, too, are again driven to pasture, and are again fed on green fodder, hay, turnips (carrots), etc. Consider the horses of the Steppes, that eat only grass; how healthy, strong, enduring and beautiful they are!

In some parts of Germany the horses are likewise fed only on grass (in Winter on hay, carrots, etc.), and they are healthy and very sturdy. Of course, if animals are again put on green fodder, on a natural diet, we must not be disconcerted if in the beginning crises should set in. The crises will be the more violent the longer the animal has been fed in an unnatural way.

I have shown how much people have already harmed themselves by wearing clothes. But we have even begun to spoil our animals, especially the horses, by covering them with blankets. It is entirely wrong to cover horses on every occasion, when they have become warm, or when they must stand in the rain, with blankets. Horses ought never to be covered. Horses, too, can never be harmed by the air. When the time comes that men are no longer afraid of the cold air, and will even in a heated condition calmly expose themselves to air and draughts, they will perhaps also lose their anxiety with regard to horses.

Plenty of stories are of course told of horses catching dangerous colds. But these have only come about because, in animals, too, men no longer understand nature, and have subjected them to wrong treatment during colds. If animals have taken cold that is all the better reason for taking them out into the fresh, free air, then nothing whatever need to be feared; we shall only see them become all the healthier and fresher. Away with all blankets for animals, therefore.

In the treatment of animals, therefore, we need also only to adhere strictly to nature.

The castration of animals is also a brutal wrong on the part of man.

And in this place I would like to say a few words on vivisection.

In our times scientific researches are made on *living* animals, by cutting open their bodies and observing the workings of the inner organs. Furthermore living animals are sometimes deprived of their eyes, they are even burned out, their tongue is cut off, in others the stomach, liver, or some other organ is taken out of the body in order to be replaced later on. Science in this way practises the most atrocious cruelties and horrors that actually cry to heaven.

If science had the least ennobling influence on man, such brutalities would be utterly impossible to professors. It seems to me that vivisection more than anything else tramples under foot all the nobler impulses of man.

Researches and studies against which all the admonitions of conscience, all the voices of nature and God must at first powerfully rebel, and which can only be continued after all these divine impulses of the human breast have been smothered, can in no wise result in good. No. Such acquisitions are laden with curses and carry unspeakable harm in their train. At the sight of such scientific proceedings one must needs exclaim: "Woe to you, scholars, you degenerate men!" I have frequently shown how all vaccine poisons, anti-toxins, operations, these achievements of cruel, scientific research, destroy more and more all health among men, and are largely the cause of the misery that is abroad in the world, in a thousand different shapes. Yes, this whole misery of mankind is largely caused by the wrong medical treatment of men in times of sickness.

But this curse can be taken from us again only when men will listen to the voices of nature alone, and will recognize how simply nature offers us the necessary rules of hygiene, and how all those studies and scientific labors, with all their cruelties, lead only to disaster.

MENTAL AND PHYSICAL WORK, FRUIT CULTURE AND SPORT.

I have already said that the chief requisite for a sick person was physical and mental rest. We must adhere to this in all cases.

The animal, when it is sick, always seeks rest.

But mental workers to-day have gradually been brought into such a restless, excited condition that one must needs advise them to do physical work in order to induce mental rest. Physical work must therefore often be resorted to in order to gain mental rest, which is first of all necessary.

In the beginning men worked neither physically nor mentally in the way they do to-day.

In their higher soul-life, in their unclouded love for one another and for God, their life found its true contents, and true joy and gladness, it was surrounded with a wonderfully poetic glory. The life of the more highly developed men, such as originally lived in pure nature, as it is described to us in the myth of paradise, was without labor and trouble; it was pure joy and blessedness.

Our present intellectual and scientific pursuits and achievements have not been able to compensate us for those pure joys, and the unclouded happiness, which man lost by his fall from nature. They have only been still more the cause of all our present life-weariness, all our satiety and despair.

Men have not developed any more highly through their unnatural mode of life, their present intellectual and artificial education. They have, on the contrary, sunk very low in all their sinful lusts and vices, through the corruption of their organs of sense, their instincts and conscience; in all their intellectual and spiritual darkness, yes, they have indeed sunk far below the animal.

If men could only begin to realize this thoroughly, they would then no longer place so much value on their present intellectual work and education.

After the fall from nature began our physical and intellectual work and all these so-called "delights" and "blessings" of civilization.

But with the present intellectual labor, and all the beneficent contrivances, which especially the great inventions of modern times have brought us, such as railroads, the telegraph, the telephone, etc., with all the rest of the institutions, of big cities especially, and with all our present social amusements and entertainments, we find only those delights and pleasures that are in keeping with our unnatural mode of life, alcohol drinking, tobacco smoking, etc. In reality they are not pleasures and comforts, but only ordeals and tortures, delights that result in disgust, satiety, shattered nerves, and disease. The intellectual pleasures, like all the other pleasures of civilized man, are only a momentarily agreeable, artificial excitement, a transitory intoxication which is always followed by a feeling of dissatisfied, discontented, and painful satiety. Everything injurious to health can never be a benefit or a blessing in any other way.

In spite of all intellectual labor and industry, how barren and empty, how tedious and unsatisfactory is our present life!

The emaciated scholar, with pale face and bald head, often sighs:

"O full and splendid moon, whom I
Have, from this desk, seen climb the sky

> So many a midnight,—Would thy glow
> For the last time behold my woe!
> Ever thine eye, most mournful friend,
> O'er books and papers saw me bend;
> But would that I, on mountains grand,
> Amid thy blessed light could stand,
> With spirits through mountain-caverns hover,
> Float in thy twilight the meadows over,
> And, freed from the fumes of lore that swathe me,
> To health in thy dewy fountains bathe me!"
>
> —Goethe, "Faust,"

How has true wisdom been lost more and more, in spite of all scientific education, how have men grown worse and more corrupt with it! At the most we find much hollow show among men to-day, much external glitter, without heart culture, and without inner worth, no humility but much pride, and haughtiness, but—no happiness.

Of course we cannot to-day all at once avoid all intellectual labor and all schools; only gradually can we return to nature. But we ought to begin to realize that excessive mental work and mental unrest, more than anything else, undermine health and destroy the peace of our soul, and our earthly happiness.

We are superior to the animal by virtue of our intellect and reason, but in attempting artificially to increase and improve upon what we have received from nature we in reality only destroy. Is not the end of excessive mental work frequently mental darkness and insanity?

Let men c   ·· +o live in the right way in accordance with natu   ~~te the faculties and powers of

The way and their hap· to be altogetl mals.

Let us

and in the lecture-room, at the desk of the official and in the office of the merchant to the most necessary transactions Our reading, especially the reading of newspapers, ought to be restricted or entirely stopped. But above all things I would like to implore every philanthropist to strive to relieve the children, the growing up generation, of the heavy burdens which the schools at present impose upon them.

Much of our completely useless talking, disputing, writing, studying, meditating, investigating, etc., ought to be discontinued. Instead, we ought to approach nature, devote ourselves to the pleasures she offers, practise brotherly love, and in this way gain joys and rich blessedness which will always promote health and elevate mind and soul.

I should like to advise all scholars, whose minds have reached a torturing degree of restlessness in consequence of continual artificial development and incessant exertion, to try and associate for some time with good, worthy, uneducated workingmen as with their brothers, without pride. They will then soon experience how quieting and agreeable the society and conversation of these workingmen is, in which all great intellectual stimulation and excitement is wanting. They could thus also best realize wherein lies the chief cause of the nervousness and general ailments of our present society.

Scientific education has in reality made men neither wiser nor better. The educated classes therefore have no reason to feel themselves superior to the uneducated. This is pride that always avenges itself. Let men once more practise humility, let them again *descend* to their poorer, uneducated fellow-men, here they can again find and regain health.

The pleasures of civilization are vices that never satisfy, but always arouse more vehement desires, and although man suffers from them, he cannot get along without them. People also often find it very difficult to restrict, or leave off intellectual work, although they themselves realize that they are injuring body and soul by it, and are destroying their happiness. Their mind can find no rest, it is forever morbidly occupied with useless reflec-

Sorry:

The defect on the previous page is that way in the original book we reproduced.

tions and inquiries, with cold calculations and useless researches. But if men will only begin to live a natural life they will also find more rest again. Physical work will materially aid them in this endeavor.

In our time gymnastics and other sports are a part of the daily program.

I for my part cannot see anything natural in all this artificial bending, winding, straining, stretching—in these gymnastic feats indoors, either with or without apparatus.

There is particularly much sickness and nervousness among gymnasts. Great strength, artificially acquired, is by no means health. Athletes, circus riders, gymnasts, etc., are known to die young.

To the physical culturists, therefore, I would say: "Return to Nature!" Come forth from your musty, dusty rooms and halls, out into free nature! Even games in the open air are much better than gymnastics.

As for the rest of our modern sport of every description, there is nothing natural about it, even if it is practised in the open air.

In our present time of haste and worry people have enthusiastically welcomed and adopted cycling, in order to do homage also in this way to the spirit of unrest that has to-day reached its height. But if nature had intended man to hasten or fly across the earth she would have given him ostrich legs, or wings, that he, too, could fly along high in the air like a bird. Man distinguishes himself from animals by his erect position, but on the wheel he sits huddled up like an ape.

Men at first enthusiastically welcomed the bicycle, like all other great achievements of civilization. To-day, however, they are already beginning to realize how much sickness and how much mischief cycling bears in its train. Many, also, are already getting tired of cycling; it does not seem to be rapid enough for them. Now they would like to have flying machines, in order to fly with furious rapidity like a bird, across countries and continents in a short time.

Beautiful, quiet walks, in beautiful surroundings, in woods and mountains, during which the heart and the spirit expand, are better and healthier than all sports and all cycling.

Let us again turn to physical labor. But is physical labor according to nature if it was not included in the original scheme of nature? some one will ask me. Man has destroyed paradise; he must restore it. Now, if physical labor were injurious man would have to continue to do harm to himself, and for this reason alone the restoration of paradise would be an impossibility.

Of course, the labor of our laborers, from early to late, year in and year out, is unworthy of any man.

Fruit culture affords an opportunity for the most agreeable and best physical work. With fruit culture we promote the cause upon which depend the rescue and redemption of mankind, and through which men will again be led to health and happiness. In future every one ought to raise his own fruit as much as possible; it must become less and less a matter of business. Whoever raises more fruit than he needs for himself can, if he is able, give it away, make presents of it to his friends, and thus cause much pleasure, while in making presents of other things (money, etc.) he frequently causes no pleasure, and does no real good, often even mischief. The labor involved in fruit culture is so fascinating, so agreeable, it gives so much pleasure and joy that it is for this reason very conducive to health. If we only begin to see things in their true light, and realize that the most natural is always the best and noblest, then the labor of fruit culture will soon be considered much more advantageous, and much finer than all gymnastics, cycling, and all other sport, and all our present so-called noble pastimes.

Men will then also everywhere find an opportunity for physical labor at fruit culture. If he cannot engage in it himself he can always assist friends and acquaintances.

Here, too, it is particularly necessary that individuals of superior insight and independence should arise to set an example in spite of the erroneous opinions of the masses.

Could not professional and business men, and even laborers,

acquire a piece of land, and in connection with their calling arrange on it for themselves and families, and perhaps for some friends, a life as nearly as possible in accordance with nature? Fruit-culture, as I said before, holds out the promise of profit for such an enterprise, while at the same time it will produce much happiness. Such a place would afford an opportunity not only for physical labor, but for going bare-footed, for light-and-air bathing, etc. It could soon produce the entire food for the family, and satisfy the greater part of the continually lessening needs of people that have again turned to nature, so that calling and business would become less and less necessary for procuring a livelihood. Such people would gladly forego all the expensive pleasures and indulgences of our present civilization and society, the many costly dresses, etc. Many could, by such investments, again create the most beautiful, the happiest, independent and free careers for their children. Acquaintances and friends could in this way also be helped.

The return to nature can in this way be made possible to people with scanty or no means at all, since capitalists are always willing to advance money at a low rate of interest on land that is to be devoted to fruit-culture, and is thus sure to rise in value from year to year.

The chief need to-day is that people should again withdraw from the great cities, the hot-beds of everything unnatural, of all disease and corruption. If one were in a condition to avoid even the vicinity of great cities, and live entirely in the country, that, of course, would be best. In the country true human happiness, in complete simplicity and frugality, is again attainable. But if possible the spot for such a blessed retreat ought to be chosen near some woods, in the midst of beautiful nature. In the woods man again finds his home; here alone many a hunger and longing of man can again be satisfied.

It is important that there should always be several friends and comrades, to co-operate in creating for themselves a pure, noble nature-life, in the manner described. For in the first place men must be in a position to cultivate friendship and love, for without this they can never gain anything for themselves, and never be happy and blest.

In this way the return of humanity to nature must proceed gradually, in perfect quiet, without violent changes, without destruction and revolution.

Goethe's Doctor Faust sought all his happiness and well-being in science. He did not find it there, however. Lamenting and despairing he breaks out into the words:

> "I've studied now Philosophy
> And Jurisprudence, Medicine—
> And even, alas! Theology,—
> From end to end, with labor keen,
> And here, poor fool! with all my lore
> I stand, no wiser than before,
>
> *   *   *   *   *
>
> And see that nothing can be known!
> *That* knowledge cuts me to the bone."

The learned Faust is only thirty years of age, still young, therefore, but thoroughly sick in body and soul.*

Faust now surrenders himself to the devil, who appears to him in the person of Mephistopheles. He introduces Faust to

---

*On the first Easter day Faust takes a walk with his Famulus Wagner. Here we have the man of science striving for something higher, who is in vain looking for happiness, and the dry, case-hardened scholar.

> "That brain, alone, not loses hope, whose device is
> To stick in shallow trash for evermore,—
> Which digs with eager hand for buried ore,
> And, when it finds an angle-worm, rejoices!"

Round about the two scholars the populace makes merry and shouts in excessive glee. Even the people, with their unnatural mode of life, are strangers to the quiet, noble joys of the purely natural man. But still this boisterously merry populace comes closer to our hearts than the two enervated, obtuse, speculating and disputing scholars.

all the sensual pleasures of civilized man, and at times causes illusive visions to appear before him.

But neither in this way does Faust find rest and contentment; ever new desires only are aroused in him. Soon Faust sighs:

> "Thus in desire I hasten to enjoyment,
> And in enjoyment pine to feel desire."

Mephistopheles also offers Faust a magic potion, in order to imbue him again with pleasure in life, similar to the way in which man tries to put himself into a brief intoxication by the use of alcohol. When, for the purpose Mephistopheles leads Faust to the witches in the witches' kitchen, the latter asks:

> "I shall recover, dost thou tell me,
>   Through this insane, chaotic play?
> From this old hag shall I demand assistance?
>   And will her foul mess take away
> Full thirty years from my existence?
>   Woe's me, canst thou naught better find!
> Another baffled hope must be lamented;
>   Has Nature, then, and has a noble mind
> Not any potent balsam yet invented?"

Mephistopheles replies scornfully:

"Once more, my friend, thou talkest sensibly.
   There is, to make thee young, a simpler mode and apter;
But in another book 'tis writ for thee,
   And is a most eccentric chapter.

   * * * * * * * * *

   Good! the method is revealed
   Without or gold or magic or physician.
Betake thyself to yonder field,
   There hoe and dig as thy condition;

Restrain thyself, thy sense and will
   Within a narrow sphere to flourish;
   With unmixed food thy body nourish;
Live with the ox as ox, and think it not a theft
   That thou manur'st the acre which thou reapest;
That, trust me, is the best mode left,
   Whereby for eighty years thy youth thou keepest!"

Faust answers:

   "I am not used to that; I cannot stop to try it—
   To take the spade in hand and ply it;
   The narrow being suits me not at all."

This remedy which is here given as issuing scornfully from the mouth of the devil, Goethe has also proclaimed ironically to all mankind; that is, Goethe himself considered this as the correct remedy, but did not wish to state it as an alluring one. Otherwise he would have described the life in nature, that can rejuvenate man, and alone lead him again to happiness, in a different way.

The great genius sought for truth and light in the error and night of civilized humanity as only mortal man can seek for it. His Faust proves this. Nevertheless in this labyrinth in which he, too, was wandering, he did not find the thread of Ariadne, which alone could show him the way out. In his time he could not attain the knowledge of the true return to nature, through which alone salvation and happiness can come to mankind.

Goethe would otherwise not have referred so contemptuously to the union with nature, through a natural mode of life, through retirement and physical labor with unmixed food (raw fruit). Man is not to become a hermit; he needs at least the society of several people. But this offers enough opportunity to practise brotherly love, which gives life its proper contents and true happiness.

When man shall again live a natural life he will no longer stand below the animal; he will not live "with the ox as ox," for he will then have risen above the animal, and will again have become a true man, the image of God.

Raw fruit, this noblest result, which nature produces in the vegetable kingdom, this *living* food, is, as I have repeatedly said, the very foundation upon which the ennobling of man, his elevation to something higher, can take place. Yes, if the great Goethe were living to-day, when the time for the redemption of man is about to fulfil itself, he would put his wonderful muse into the service of the great, holy cause, and would preach and sing of a natural mode of life. Goethe would then not have led his Faust, who despaired of science, along the path of destruction with the devil; he would, on the contrary, have rescued him from despair by leading him back to nature. Goethe, too, was seeking for the true salvation of the soul, but he did not recognize and find it upon earth.

When sweet Gretchen, Faust's beloved, asked him how he stood with God and religion, he answered:

"Leave that, my child! Thou knowest my love is tender;
For love, my blood and life would I surrender,
And as for Faith and Church, I grant to each his own."

* * * * * * * * *

"My darling, who shall dare
 'I believe in God!' to say?
Ask priest or sage the answer to declare,
 And it will seem a mocking play,
 A sarcasm on the asker.

* * * * * * * * *

"Hear me not falsely, sweetest countenance!
  Who dare express Him?
  And who profess Him,
  Saying, I believe in Him?
  Who, feeling, seeing,

Deny His being,
Saying: I believe Him not!

* * * * *

"Vast as it is, fill with that force thy heart,
And when thou in the feeling wholly blessed art,
  Call it, then, what thou wilt,—
Call it Bliss, Heart! Love! God!
I have no name to give it!
Feeling is all in all."

This is an evasive, entirely obscure answer of Faust, which does not satisfy the reader either.

In the same way, however, Goethe himself went his earthly pilgrimage in error and in the dark, with respect to his God, and the salvation of his soul, until he ended it with the words: "More Light!"

But who of all the great celebrated scholars, poets, musicians, painters, etc., has been happy? None of them found the way to salvation.

Still I should like to pray to-day that the spirit of the great Goethe may help us to lead all men from error and all night to truth and light.

I wish once more to caution sick people to do physical work only when it is suited to their case, and then to practise it always according to their strength and within reason. In all cases one must begin to work with moderation, and must never force oneself to it.

Men to-day, from the laborer to the rich man, are forever multiplying their desires and wants; the more they have, the more they wish to gain. They continually demand more luxuries of every kind; they wish to rise higher and higher, to increase their business, to earn more and more money, in order to be able to give their children a still more scientific education, and to start them out in life with still greater riches. But all this for which people are incessantly striving, and for which they are forever laboring and working, are treasures which moth and rust corrupt, possessions which in reality burden us and our children with ever more worries, with disease and disaster. In this way man must continually work and worry, and it would be of course entirely wrong, if he would demand of his fellow-men, or even the State, to take his work and cares from him, or if he would suddenly want to stop working.

But if man returns to nature, if his demands and wants are continually lessening, he need no longer work so much, either mentally or physically. He can then enter into closer communion with nature, devote himself in love to his fellow-men and to God, and find his happiness in higher spheres. Neither does he then need to work all the time to fill his empty, barren life, and to forget for a time his dissatisfaction and despair.

In that way, too, no one can find anything suspicious or wrong in the greater leisure of another one. To-day labor is a necessity.

I mention this in order not to be misunderstood in regard to my conception of labor.

In many cases where men cannot at once wholly or even partially lay aside the unnatural features of their work, as well as many other unnatural things in life, much is gained if they only again recognize the worthlessness and harmfulness of these infringements of nature, mental work, mental overburdening, all institutions of civilized life, honor, fame, riches, etc. They can then more easily renounce all these things, and will no longer strive after them with so much unrest and haste, and especially not worry about them. They will then also not be sad and sorrowful when they lose them.

This will suffice to free many a spirit, and many a glance will be cheerfully directed towards higher, true joys and possessions, and here, too, whoever seeks will find.

THE FAMILY, HOME AND COUNTRY.

The family is the smallest circle into which men unite. Marriage is the bond by which Church and State keep the family together to-day. But is this bond always a safe one? is it always also the true bond which nature ties? Sensuality and money, and other ignoble, sordid motives (high position, rank, etc.) very often bring couples together to-day; true love is generally wanting. Very often love is a violent passion, reared in sensuality and founded on selfishness. Passionate love wants wholly to possess another individual of the opposite sex. But passion is transitory. The Church and State bond avails nothing here.

Thus we often have in marriage the external fair appearance with much hidden misery.

In spite of the firmest ties that are externally drawn about marriage, the real bond between the couple is frequently a very loose one, and generally they are entirely unfaithful to each other.

Not only he breaks the marriage vow who openly separates himself from his wife and who openly commits adultery.

Jesus says:

"Ye have heard that it was said by them of old time, Thou shalt not commit adultery:

"But I say unto you, That whoso looketh on a woman to lust after her hath committed adultery with her already in his heart."—Matt. 5:27, 28.

Yes, if we could always examine the hearts of married people we would very often find underneath the external bond, inner void and desolation, unhappiness and unfaithfulness.

The more men will again wander on the paths of nature, the more will they be bound only by true, serene, blissful love, which does not care to conquer, to possess, but only to give, and in this way will gain all. True love wants to be free, and may and should be free; it cares nothing for rules; it will not tolerate limitations and fetters; it is pure and faithful, and requires no legal compulsion. Only in union with nature will men again find real, serene, pure, beautiful happiness in love, which is also of such great importance in the matter of health. Thus alone can the right bond be tied by God and for all eternity.

> "To yield one wholly, and to feel a rapture
> In yielding, that must be eternal!

> Eternal!—for the end would be despair.
> No, no,—no ending! no ending!"
> —Goethe, "Faust."

When children again lead a natural life, then love of their fellows can again be successfully cultivated in their hearts. But, above all things, the relationship between parents and children, the entire happiness of the family, can in this way become much more beautiful. Yes, many a sorrow, and distress, will then be spared the parents, and the children will experience great blessedness and joy in purest love for each other, and for their parents. All the members of the family will then be closely united by a most beautiful tie; instead of the external appearance we shall find true, quiet, inner happiness, which all sorts of sickness and suffering can no longer undermine and destroy.

Family ties are being destroyed more and more nowadays. Scientific education, the struggle for existence and a livelihood, for which the requirements are becoming greater all the time, continue to demand greater sacrifices. And for this the tenderest ties of heart and soul are rent asunder.

Children are often separated from their home, from the loving hearts of father and mother, at a very early age. Far countries and seas often divide parents and children, brothers and sisters. But in the distance often a great longing arises, an ardent desire for home, for father and mother, for brother and sister. All the treasures that have been found in the distance cannot quiet this longing, this desire.

But why has nature created all these tender ties between the members of a family, only that men should tear them asunder and cause themselves much suffering and woe thereby? No, these, too, are voices of nature that demand obedience!

The more that men again return to nature, the smaller will become their needs and demands, and all their conditions will improve. Then they no longer need to leave their homes and their beloved ones. Many a tear will remain unwept by the eyes of father and mother.

Man is no bird of passage and no Norway rat; nature chains him to the place where he was born—to his home. Why are men continually changing their abode? Cannot every one remain where nature has placed him? When men again build dwelling-places for themselves in the midst of nature, when they again lead nature lives of greatest simplicity, then again will they be drawn more and more to their home, for it will then be easier for them to find their livelihood there and true happiness.

The individual families constitute the community, and these again form the nation; they all have a fatherland. Every animal keeps to his pack, and you, too, dear reader, I would fain admonish:

"Ans Vaterland, ans teure, schliess dich an,
Das halte fest mit deinem ganzen Herzen."
—Schiller.

"To the land, so dear, of thy fathers, hold fast,
Adhere to it with all thy heart, my son."

But natural men are the most willing and the most inclined to stand by the fatherland.

The Germans have attained their object of long striving and struggling; they again have a united German fatherland. But the German people are not happy for all that. Not the warlike equipments, not the great armies can in truth secure the fatherland; only the contentment and the strength of the people can do it.

But the contentment, and the strength of the people, are being lost more and more, and they can be regained only by a return, on the part of the people, to simplicity and to nature.

To-day the people mostly turn their inner discontent against the State and its institutions.* The people choose their own

---

*Men always look for the cause of their misery outside of themselves, although they are always themselves to blame.

In the first place, diseases are ascribed to wrong conditions in nature. There seems to be a sort of belief that nature is forever on the watch for a chance to harm and even to kill us with air and cold, and by making us take cold.

representatives, who make the laws, and officials are appointed to guard these laws and see that they are obeyed. But still the people are always dissatisfied with the laws and the officials.

On the one hand all sorts of demands are always made of the State nowadays; every one is trying to derive more and more benefit from the State or expects some beneficent institution from it. On the other hand every one is always dissatisfied and refractory when the State demands the taxes which it needs to satisfy all the demands of the people.

The whole life of civilized mankind to-day consists of contradictions.

All the contentions and strife of political parties are a result of the inner discontent and selfishness caused by an unnatural mode of life. Every one thinks only of his own advantage and that of his party. Everywhere every one is anxious to take, but never to give.

Politics are the science of patriotism; they destroy patriotism.

Only the nation that once more enters into close relationship with nature, contains within itself the secure power to protect itself against warlike neighbors, greedy for conquest, and to maintain its rights and ideals.

God has apparently chosen the German people for a high mission. Among the present civilized States it is Germany where the natural method of healing has originated and is developing powerfully. Would that the German people might soon recognize this holy mission more fully.

Germany's throne to-day is occupied by a Hohenzollern of singular energy, imbued with the rare ambition to work and to labor for the welfare of the people and the Fatherland, and to serve also his Saviour and his God. But, alas! he, too, is but performing the labor of the Danaids. Would that an illumination of the right way might come to our great Emperor, then, perhaps, true salvation could soon be brought to the Fatherland, and, moreover, to the entire present civilization.

IDEALS AND POETRY.

Mankind to-day is without IDEALS; it is ever striving for material benefit. The cause I am here teaching could afford many an opportunity for cherishing the highest, holiest ideals. But we must work for the cause in the right way, through our own example and without any ostentation whatever. It is too great and holy a cause, and must therefore never be obtruded upon any one. I would like to impress the words of the great Master upon all my friends and adherents:

"And whosoever shall not receive you, nor hear you, when ye depart thence, shake off the dust under your feet, for a testimony against them."—Mark 6:11.

I should therefore like to see all passion, all loud and violent championship of my cause avoided from the start. Of the Saviour, too, it has been said in the prophecy that He would not shout upon the market place and upon the street.

Science has also destroyed *poetry,* for science has shot up like a weed and has stunted poetry. In all our artificiality to-day it is but rare that poetry shows itself in the form of a weak talent, and this, too, is then pressed into a scientific form so that it loses still more, and becomes accessible only to a small part of the people.

Goethe in his time had to realize that he would not become popular, and to-day, indeed, the people have no knowledge and derive no benefit from the poetry of Goethe.

But the people must again have poetry; they must not be allowed to degenerate through the greed for gain, to sink into the commonplace and low.

Is it not wonderful poetry that has been preserved to us from early ages, from the childhood of humanity and of nations, when men still lived in and according to nature? Let us only call to mind Homer's "Iliad "and "Odyssy," the Greek and Roman myths, Germanic folk-lore and myths, the myths of "King Arthur and the Round Table," of "The Holy Grail," of "Lohengrin," and "Elsa of Brabant," of "Tristan and Isolde," of "Fritjof and

Ingeborg," of "Siegfried and Krimhilde," of "The Sleeping Beauty in the Woods," and of "Little Snow White," etc. And let me also remind you of the troubadour songs (Minnesingers) and of the works from former flood-tides of German and foreign poetry.

In all of them we find real poetry. But this poetry dates from a time when men (even poets) could not yet read and write; when there was no science as yet, like to-day.

These wonderfully poetic works had partially been preserved to us for hundreds, even thousands of years, before there was any art of writing or of printing.

Our people, too, will again have poetry if men will only return to nature. Every one who will again live a natural life will soon find himself surrounded by a wonderfully poetic charm. Imagination, this sublime gift of God to man, will be gently reawakened, and in many cases, where it was morbidly active, like a stormy sea, it will become serene and quiet. In this way the life of man is no longer barren and insipid, as the occupation with science makes it, but it is as if filled with flowers and perfume and surrounded with beautiful pictures and dreams.

The poetic works mentioned above are by no means the most beautiful and the best that men have had and can have in the way of poetry, for they have in great part originated in times when men no longer lived entirely in accordance with nature, but had fallen from nature in many respects, particularly in respect to food (meat-eating, etc.).

But I must still call attention to the most beautiful, most holy work of folk-lore poetry of all time, namely, the *Bible,* particularly the *New Testament.* In the Bible we have a holy poem of the people, which did not arise from a wild, excited fancy, and therefore does not cause our soul to vibrate in restless undulations and moods, but offers it delightful recreation and holy peace.

But men to-day are wholly misguided and benighted; they can no longer understand and comprehend the Bible, and can no longer refresh their souls with its magnificent, holy poetry.

But, dear reader, follow me still a little further; perhaps I can yet unlock for you the Bible as a magic fountain of holy lore, and perhaps you can then again believe and pray like a child, and then you will surely find again all the health of your body, your whole childhood, your youth, your whole happiness and earthly blessedness.

Many things are spoken of and many ideas advanced in my book which are not found in other books on the care of health. But I believe that I have attained to a wider knowledge in many respects, in the school of my own severe suffering and need.

Many most unnatural practices in the intellectual and spiritual realm are still overlooked to-day, but which are great obstacles in the healing of many diseases, particularly nervous diseases. If we can again lead mind and soul into the right channels, and bring men back to recognize the highest Physician, to whom nothing is impossible, and teach them to love; what disease can then still remain unhealed and what human misery can withstand it?

CONCLUSION.

When I began to revise the fourth edition of my book my chief intention was to enlarge it with respect to spiritual influences, and soul life in general. Now that this edition is printed so far, and a great part of my treatise on soul life is written, I have decided to break off here, and have the work appear in two volumes, each complete in itself.

This first volume contains almost everything that was to be found in former editions of my book, but some things have been more fully elaborated, and much new matter has been added. If man is to be made healthy and good, body and soul must never be separated. The contents of this first volume, however, deal especially with the natural care of the body; spiritual matters have been considered only in so far as they were necessary also for this part, while in the second volume the correct soul life is the chief consideration, which will be supplemented with matter pertaining to the care of the body only in so far as the exigencies of the subject demand.

The part on soul-life will nevertheless become much longer than I had at first expected. In this domain I shall certainly present to the reader much more that is new and significant than I have done with regard to the care of the body. But not what we eat is of benefit to our nutrition, but what we digest. The same can be said of mental food. The first volume ought therefore to be read and understood first, and, better still, what is taught therein ought to be tried and made use of; then, indeed, we can again turn to something new, something still more beautiful and holy.

These are the reasons that prompted me to divide the book into two volumes. Things that have been indicated in several places of this volume will therefore be found discussed in detail in the second volume.

With regard to soul-life, in the second volume, I shall attempt to deduce my proofs as thoroughly and as logically as heretofore, and likewise draw the final conclusions. For this purpose many points brought out in the first volume will be more fully elaborated.

Here too, in the simplest manner and with the help of God, I hope to throw light upon many a dark spot, to teach men to again recognize and understand the "Word of God" correctly, and also to refresh and save many who are to-day sorrowful and burdened, and about to despair. Still many others I hope to lead from scientific delusions, from obscurity and confusion, many from self-deceit and sanctimoniousness, from self-conceit and pietism to true piety and godliness.

The true natural method of healing and living and of caring for the body is the only true beginning of all good and the salvation of man. Likewise all true salvation of the soul, all higher blessedness to which men have hitherto aspired without this foundation, have been nothing but delusion, nothing but sham and deceit, never anything permanent and enduring, never anything thorough and complete.

Also the immediate, direct care of the soul upon earth can be of real use, and carry with it real results and blessings only in union with nature.

It is the safest thing in every case, therefore, to become acquainted with the natural method of living and healing, to open one's mind to it and adopt it. Both nature and God are mild and indulgent, in this respect, and do not demand too much at once. All the old beliefs, all the deep-rooted errors, the great number of unnatural habits to which men are now addicted, come into consideration. It is impossible to break with all of them at once, but a beginning can at least be made.

Let us in the first place drop all unnaturalness in the treatment of disease (medicine, serum, operations, etc.) and direct our attention once more to water, light, air, earth, food and the natural human healing forces. I have shown sufficiently how everyone can adopt the true natural method of healing and living in every respect, either partially or entirely, and think I have also shown how the transition can be graded so that each one can proceed either slowly or rapidly.

Of course the sooner anyone *can and does return to nature the greater will the benefit be both for his present state of health, or in all cases of sickness.*

Only by a return to nature does the soul also find the true, sure way to salvation. On the way to nature man also finds God. But all noble, high aspirations of the soul, the salvation of the soul, that have again been established in this manner, have a particularly great power of reaction on the body.

Yes, trust in God, faith, prayer, hope, and the sum of all that is good, sublime, and noble, for which we can and must strive, *love;* all these, for which the natural mode of life alone gives the true foundation, and everything that they revive and effect in us, reacts upon the sick body with wonderfully healing power. It is particularly on account of his more highly developed soul that man occupies a higher, a privileged position upon earth. Therefore if the true natural foundation is laid, man can once more exert a powerfully healing influence on the body through the soul.

Of course we shall then at the same time enter upon the sphere of eternal, unclouded, perfect blessedness for which we need not wait until we reach heaven, but in which we shall already participate here upon earth, and do so the more fully the more we have completely adjusted ourselves with body and soul to the true, eternal, divine harmony. Yes, it will be the more difficult to attain to blessedness in heaven the less we have already reached it upon earth, and the unnatural mode of life does a great deal of harm even to the salvation of our soul, and obstructs our entrance upon eternal blessedness.

With this first volume as a guide, everyone can build for himself a magnificent edifice, but it cannot be perfectly completed and cannot receive its true dedication and crowning glory without the help of the second volume.

May this first volume of my work prepare many hearts to receive the highest blessing. It will then have gained its best purpose.

May God grant it!

Supplement

THE JUNGBORN.

ITS ARRANGEMENTS AND PURPOSES.

(*Extract from the prospectus of the Jungborn.*)

I shall not, as I had announced on page 9, here describe the Jungborn in detail, but only briefly.

The Jungborn is for my cause what the foundation head is for the river. The practical realization of my teachings, the spirit that is cultivated here, the great successes that are here achieved in curing disease, are constantly to give new life to the cause. All those who at the Jungborn can at once re-enter into full harmony with nature, who can here for a time live a pure nature-life, quite removed from the world of artificiality, civilization and science, and become fitted with the true spirit of the method, can do very much to spread the great and holy cause.

At the Jungborn civilized man has an opportunity to lead a pure nature-life with all its true delights, and its wonderful curative effects, such as never has been the case since the fall of man from nature.

The Jungborn offers opportunities for the most extreme, most complete nature-life possible under present conditions; it is a true model for the cause.

The Jungborn is situated in the most beautiful part of the Hartz, at the entrance to the lovely protected Ecker valley. The most aromatic, delicious *forest air* prevails here—Hartz-air—and the visitor receives a wonderful, charmed impression of a *grandly romantic nature.*

The guests under treatment live in charming little light-and-air cottages (and during the warmest months in Summer in light-and-air halls), surrounded by pines and other trees, and situated in large beautiful parks, which are surrounded by high plank walls so that everyone can at any time go directly from his room (and bed, at night or day, in the rain, etc.,) to take a *light-and-air bath, a sun bath,* etc.

In the light-and-air parks the patients can, moreover, sleep in the open air at night and utilize the *earth power* by lying on the bare ground, taking *earth baths,* going *bare-footed,* etc.

The *bath* is taken *in the open* in the light-and-air parks (in small bathing tanks). The Jungborn has its own waterworks, the pipes of which are laid through all the parks, so that there always is an abundance of water for bathing and sprinkling.

Besides two large parks for men and women respectively, and other small parks, there is an especially beautiful, open, general park (the "Friedrichspark"),* where patients that do not wish to be separated (married couples) can live in light-and-air cottages.

The inhabitants of this park are, of course, at liberty to use the light-and-air parks for all purposes.

In the "Friedrichspark" the other larger, heatable buildings (dining hall, etc.) are situated.

The rooms in the light-and-air cottages are nicely furnished, although display is avoided.

Earth and clay compresses are most extensively employed at the Jungborn. They are probably taken by every patient.

Proper attendants are at the service of the patients for the purpose of rubbing and stroking the body by way of applying and transferring *human curative power and animal heat* in the most natural and effective manner. Sandals, health shirts, and clothes are always kept on hand, and it is left to the option of the patients to wear them or not.

---

*The Jungborn, especially the beautiful "Friedrichspark," was entirely laid out according to the plans of an eminent professional man, the Inspector of Promenades in Brunswick, Friedrich Kreis, after whom the chief park is named. But I wish to state, furthermore, that I am otherwise greatly indebted to the Inspector of Promenades, Fr. Kreis, for the sincere interest he has taken in, and the great services he has rendered to, the Jungborn.

In the large parks of the Jungborn are large *fruit plantations*. Their purpose is to adorn the parks, and also to give the patients an opportunity for physical work (even while taking light-and-air baths), but particularly to arouse the interest of the patients in fruit culture, and to teach them how much joy and pleasure there is in it.

At the Jungborn the *fruit diet* is strictly observed. In the first place *nuts* and all sorts of delicious fruit: tree-fruit, berries, grapes, etc., according to the season, and some tropical fruit are always on the table. Besides this there is *milk* from pasture cows, and butter and bread, also *cottage cheese, vegetables* (with few potatoes), salads, and fruit preserves.

The bill of fare of the Jungborn table is without severe deprivations, even for beginners, and I have convinced myself again and again that it always met with great approval on the part of all patients.

Every patient has the choice to adopt a complete fruit diet or to proceed less strenuously (fruit with milk, butter, bread, vegetables, etc.).

It is considered a matter of great importance that every patient is served and treated with kindness and friendly consideration. Great value is also placed on preserving the *liberty* and *independence* of every patient.

The significance of powerful *spiritual influences* (brotherly love, trust in God, etc.) is greatly taken into consideration, and such influences are promoted.

As for the rest, all the teachings previously described are most carefully observed.

The *curative successes* are, of course, the greatest possible, and probably surpass everything else that has hitherto been achieved in this respect.

I do not usually like to publish cases of cures, but have yielded to necessity to report a few.

Whoever has followed me so far must know of himself what cures must of necessity be achieved at the Jungborn with the purest, most complete and true natural healing method and natural mode of life.

During the *cool seasons* (particularly during the *Spring* and *Autumn,* the greatest and best cures were always achieved.

With a purely natural life, such as is lived at the Jungborn, diseases soon lose all their painful and distressing features. The difference between the sick and the well, therefore, soon disappears at the Jungborn. Thus it comes about that the social atmosphere is generally a very cheerful and happy one.

The patients often claim that they feel as if they had been transplanted into a new world—into fairy land, as it were.

The Jungborn is not only visited by actual invalids; many wish to escape for a time from our present world of hurry and unrest, of envy, ill-well and selfishness, and wish to see and learn here how to forestall and avoid the general ailments and misery of to-day, by natural healing and a natural mode of life. May God's blessing continue to rest on the Jungborn and its good, great cause.

VOLUMES II. AND III. OF MY WORK.

I had intended to include in this edition, with the description of the Jungborn, everything that was involved in the complete practical realization of a purely natural method of healing and living, as well as the enlargements that were necessitated by a more complete effectuation of my views.

But in preparing the work for the press, such an abundance of matter continued to present itself that it seemed advisable, after all, to publish this one volume by itself for the present.

For the present, and simultaneously with this volume, a second volume of my work goes to press. It treats of the Jungborn, and contains further and more explicit practical instructions for a true natural method of healing and living, as well as observations on its final objects and consequences

The soul-life does not now appear in a second volume, as I had stated in the Conclusion, but will appear later in a third volume of my work.

In the second volume I have described the Jungborn and its contrivances (the light-and-air cottages, opportunities for bathing, beds, clothes, etc.) to the smallest detail, in order that they may in this way serve as an example and model to others.

I am in no wise desirous to call forth and promote business enterprises through my cause; my only object is to help everyone to be his own physician and to arrange his life, as much as his circumstances will permit, according to the Jungborn.

But by giving a most explicit description of and full publicity to the Jungborn, I moreover wish to avoid future imitations of it by persons of artifice and cunning, with vulgar business tactics, and a confusion of purposes resulting from sordid actions. In this way institutions often arise after the pattern of the Jungborn, with an attempt to disguise the imitation, which are almost entirely unfit for use, and which consequently remain empty, as objects of ridicule and scorn for envious persons and opponents, and to the greatest injury to the cause.

I have described in detail the course of treatment and the whole life at the Jungborn, as it naturally comes about as a result of close communion with nature, all the phenomena that appear thereby, and everything that must be observed and taken into consideration: the exact size of the bandages for the earth or clay compresses, minute directions for preparing and applying every earth compress, thorough careful instruction with regard to the application of *human healing power,* a description of every form of rubbing, stroking and kneading—so that anybody can at once make any kind of bandage or compress with earth or clay, and that human healing power can also be at once applied and practised without mistake by everybody and everywhere, for purposes of rejuvenation, and for the achievement of the greatest curative results.

The second volume contains furthermore: A complete bill of fare and cookery book for fruit-eaters for every day and every season, with consideration of all fruits and side-dishes, such as milk, butter, bread, cottage cheese, vegetables and salads, which must certainly be very welcome to housewives. It contains, moreover, directions for the treatment of milk, the preparation and cooking of barley coffee, and of the vegetables and salads that always met with great approval at the Jungborn; the preparing at home of barley coffee, of the right kind of bread (not our present black bread, or white bread, or groat bread), of good, fresh butter, for the drying of fruit and vegetables, for the preserving of fruit and vegetables, etc.

I have proved the entire erroneousness of the present gluten theory from clearly discernible processes in nature, and have taken great pleasure in showing a good, correct bread (Jungborn bread), since I know that we cannot yet generally avoid bread, even not among fruit-eaters, and that even vegetables, preserves and salads will disappear sooner than bread.

In the second volume I have also given information to fruit-eaters about: Foods and drinks for social gatherings, for feasts, for excursions and travel, for individual persons (in the army, at the university, etc.), for the plain simple circumstances of laborers, the necessary, most appropriate and best utensils for fruit-eaters (fruit-knife, nut-cracker, grating machine, stew-pans, etc.).

I was particularly anxious to prove how business men and manufacturers to-day, engaged in an intensely nervous struggle for existence, in which there is nothing exalted or holy, no longer regard the health and life of their fellow-men and both consciously and unconsciously contaminate, adulterate, poison, etc., articles of food (butter, bread, cheese, all kinds of food-stuffs and articles of luxury), as well as cooking utensils (enamels, glazings, etc.).

In this way I tried to expose the innumerable abysses that to-day, in spite of all health boards and police, are forever belching forth poisons, and the many dreadful murderers that are constantly and everywhere lurking in the dark to rob and kill mankind.

I have dwelt more fully upon the right, natural mode of procedure in extraordinary cases (sudden accidents and deaths, epilepsy, insanity, etc.), moreover on fractures (of bones, inguinal hernia, etc.). I have also more fully explained my position with regard to our present household remedies, herbs and homœopathy, which many adherents of the natural healing method still retain in good faith, and with regard to operations.

I have thoroughly discussed the rearing of children and school-education, with its present perversities and great dangers, and have given a full solution of this question.

The significance of making one's own clothes (even furniture, houses, etc.), also spinning and weaving and home industry in the future, have received my attention, but I have dwelt more particularly upon fruit-culture, upon its great importance and the new era of civilized mankind, full of health and happiness, that depends upon it.

The question, why men are not healthy and happy, and whether and how salvation and redemption can come to civilized mankind, I have answered concisely, without subterfuges and without fear of the extremest conclusions, and have especially shown how every individual can at once find his complete salvation.

After the preceding explanations, and expositions, many of the subjects considered in the first volume, as well as all the aims of our cause, could be more explicitly and clearly discussed and carried to their final culmination in the second volume.

I therefore believed myself justified in painting the new era that is dawning for mankind truthfully and in the most glowing colors. I could here also allow myself to enter more fully upon the true soul-life, upon the most high, the most holy ends of all our thinking, imagining, doing and striving, The complete practical directions for the true soul-life, the full exposition of this final purpose, will, however, appear in the third volume.

The myth of the fountain of youth still unconsciously cherishes faint hopes in the German heart of a coming salvation of mankind, of true human happiness that is to be.

The Jungborn is the first practical realization of the myth of the fountain of youth. In the conception Jungborn not the least thing is wanting for the first true beginnings of a complete paradise of man sometime to be regained. Here, therefore, we can already see that distant goal—the perfect health and unclouded happiness of man.

For this reason the second volume of my work bears the title, "The Jungborn."

I have divided my book into three volumes, especially out of consideration for those who are obliged to consider the price in obtaining the work. I have therefore so arranged the first volume, that everyone can accomplish a complete cure by following its directions.

I advise anyone who can obtain only the first volume to use whole wheat bread rather than ordinary white bread.

As for the rest the second volume will certainly offer everyone an abundance of the most important and useful material, and much that is interesting and surprising. It is certainly still more adapted to call forth the right perceptions, real confidence, and the greatest hopes.

The third volume will finally crown the whole.

Many a one, no doubt, will welcome the division of the work into three volumes, because it will enable him to acquire them gradually.

The holy fervor that inspires me, and the great pains I am taking in writing and publishing my books, give me the firm conviction that no one will bring a useless sacrifice in buying them, for I know that they will be of the greatest use and bring the richest blessings.

SOURCES OF SUPPLIES.

From the many inquiries that are constantly made of me I infer that it will be a favor to my readers if I state reliable sources, where many things that are necessary for fruit-eaters, who wish to live according to my book, can be bought.

In case anyone cannot get the things in the place where he lives, I will name some business addresses that have served me well in my experiences of getting supplies for the Jungborn.

A. C. Kuthe, Celler street, Brunswick, supplies nuts (hazelnuts and walnuts), oranges, lemons, figs, dates, dried fruit, table oil, dried vegetables, unblued sugar, etc. A price-list will be sent to anyone on request.

Adolf Kotte, Wernigerode, keeps Jungborn beds on stock. He will supply complete Jungborn beds or single parts of the bed, bandages for earth applications, Jungborn shirts, Jungborn suspenders, as well as all kinds of porous cotton and linen cloths for health shirts; also ready-made shirts of choice material are always on hand. Samples of the cloth and price-lists will be sent.

Carl Wenning, Schuh street, 8, Brunswick, supplies all the rest of the things that cannot be had at A. C. Kuthe's and Adolf Kotte's. Jungborn sandals, lemon squeezers, fruit knives, Jungborn nut-crackers, nut grating machines, kitchen and table utensils, bath-tubs, especially *the wooden bath-tub according to my design for the natural bath.*

As I have already stated, the wooden bath-tub is better adapted and more to be recommended for the bath, besides being cheaper than the zinc bath-tub.

The inside size of this bath-tub is 1.10 m long at the top, and 60 cm broad behind, the length and breadth at the bottom being, of course, somewhat smaller. The inside depth is 21 cm in front and 27 cm behind.

The tub is made of pine wood, notched with turned spigot, and zinced hoops and handles.

Price-lists will also be sent on request.

I have always found the parties here mentioned to be reliable and worthy of recommendation.

SUBSTANTIAL IMPROVEMENT AND ENLARGEMENT OF THE JUNGBORN.

The Sanitarium Jungborn is closed from Oct. 15 to April 15.

Substantial improvements have been under way, aiming at the perfection, increased beauty, and enlargement of the Jungborn through the addition of new buildings and parks,

Adjoining the present dining and reception rooms a *larger and more beautiful reception room,* with a large balcony and veranda has been built.

I have also introduced charming log houses in Northern style (likewise only of wood), which are firmly built, capable of being heated, and will keep especially warm. These, in addition to the other comfortable apartments of the Jungborn (dining-room, reception-rooms) may be used in the cooler seasons for sleeping and living purposes by such patients who have but little animal heat, or who are confined to their beds.

These log houses were likewise constructed according to a new plan of my own. The log houses consist of only two rooms, (elegantly appointed) a little larger than the rooms of the light-and-air cottages, and a beautiful balcony. Adjoining each room is a small space (for a nurse in case of need). These log houses are likewise meant to serve as models for the ends in view, and are in every respect more beautiful, more healthful, and altogether better adapted to their ends (brighter, quieter) than the warm rooms in the usual large houses, (such as inside the present sanitariums).

In this way the sojourn is made pleasant to even the most spoiled and effeminate persons in the *cooler seasons, spring and autumn, when the quickest and greatest results are achieved here.*

In the park for women and the Friedrichs Park new light-and-air cottages have been built. A number of pavilions have also been erected (at elevated points, etc.).

All kinds of small improvements (water-closets, etc.), have been introduced. The parks (covering an area of over twenty acres) have been made more beautiful by new soft lawns and sandpaths (for going barefooted) by ponds (also small waterfalls) and new plantations, flower-beds, etc., and one of the light-and-air parks has been considerably enlarged by the addition of some woodland.

By the establishment of new waterworks in the light-and-air parks special provision has been made for the most healthful refreshment during the hot season (also for going barefooted on wet lawns).

Besides the two principal light-and-air parks for men and women respectively, there are now also four smaller separate light-and-air parks to meet special requirements (children and patients who may at first feel embarrassed in taking the light-and-air baths, *i. e.,* going naked).

The magnificent surroundings of the Jungborn, with their rarely romantic scenery and their wonderful wood magic, have also been made more available for the use of the Jungborn guests by placing of benches, seats, etc.

The great fruit plantations belonging to the Jungborn are continually becoming more productive of the most delicious, aromatic berries and tree fruit, so that there is a constantly increasing supply of the most exquisite fruits.

The Jungborn in its perfection may indeed be expected to satisfy the demands of the *finest* and *most fastidious public,* although many of the modern effeminating and enervating luxuries, and nerve-straining means of amusement are still wanting, for, after all, the achievement of the *greatest curative results* is the main thing for the Jungborn.

In the course of time also the most appropriate helpers have grown, so to speak, under my hands, who now, with the enlargement of the Jungborn, are able to support me with their help and advice. An able woman, in particular, who has already proved her efficiency during the last Summer, has been secured for the *management and care* of the greatly enlarged department for women.

The Jungborn has now been in existence for five years. All sorts of disturbances and obstacles to the new cause (also difficulties with the authorities) and other circumstances, which during this time proved to be hindering and paralyzing factors, have now been gloriously conquered.

During all the difficulties that have hitherto beset the Jungborn, I have realized again and again that the Jungborn and its ideas are God's cause, and that I must therefore devote all my strength to it. *But it is especially the wonderful cures through the simple, purely natural healing method of the Jungborn which I myself have again and again observed in the most difficult cases, where all other means, even those of the old nature-cure method, have failed, and which here often called out the greatest admiration,* which induced me to perfect and enlarge the Jungborn.

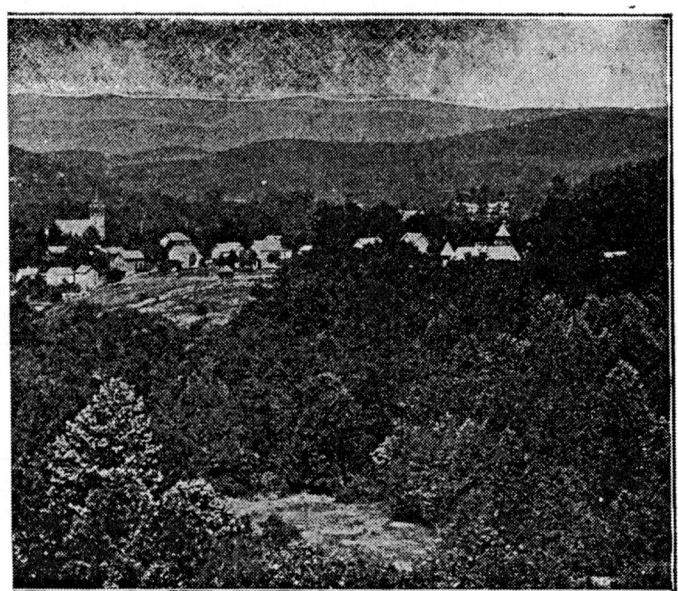

View of Butler from the American Jungborn, Bellevue, Butler, N. J.

I have also always clearly realized how important it is for the patient if he can, at least for a time, be taken out of his ordinary circumstances and live in an institution in the closest purest communion with nature and in the real atmosphere and under the spiritual influence of the cause. Success will in this way come much more quickly and surely.

The many institutions which have in this short time been established after the pattern of the Jungborn are mostly wanting in many respects, often, indeed, in the purity of their methods, and in the true spirit.

So, too, the magnificent idyllic site of the Jungborn, the pure balsamic air of the pine forest, etc., cannot easily be supplied elsewhere.

The great popularity which the Jungborn has enjoyed from the beginning alone makes it possible for me now to continue to make more and even the greatest sacrifices for it and its great cause.

May God's blessing then continue to rest on the Jungborn, for everything depends on God's blessing.

To all readers of my book, "Return to Nature!" To all friends and well-wishers of the new, purely natural method of healing and living, and to *all sufferers, and all manner of sick* I now particularly recommend the Jungborn in its new and perfected form, *as a never-failing source of health.* May it continue to receive their abundant patronage.

ADOLF JUST.

Postscript.—I am, also, willing at any time to give advice by letter in special cases, for a moderate consideration.

"**God's Blessing Gained, All is Obtained.**"

THE
Organization and Establishment of the "American Jungborn."

WHERE IS THE FOUNTAIN OF REGENERATION TO BE FOUND?

In the first half of the last century the Nature-Cure Method of to-day took its rise with Priessnitz, and then it has been gradually developed by Pioneers Schroth, Father Kneipp, Kuhne, Rikli, and others.

In its course of development, slowly casting off all its former defects, the Nature-Cure Method has attained the stage of the uttermost simplicity and perfection in the Jungborn, and has reached there the highest limit.

I founded and established the Jungborn according to views that are fully and particularly described in the book, "Return to Nature," and indeed from the first day of its appearance it met with a most enthusiastic reception.

Man, the image of God, originally lived as every other creature in perfect union with God and was guided in all by God's voices (instinct, the senses and the conscience) in pure Nature without any artificial aid (Paradise). In this state of full happiness man wore no clothing whatever, he principally fed on what mother Earth produced voluntarily and in superabundance, fruits and nuts. His home was the forest. Man did not suffer from sickness nor sin, nor did he enjoy life as animals do; but peace and abundance of heavenly happiness was his enjoyment.

Yet man became disobedient against God. He did not want to submit any more to the stern Laws of Nature (the fall was a forbidden meal). Man did not feed any more on fruit; hunting, agriculture, cookery, etc., began, and he commenced to wear clothing and to live in unhealthy houses, cities, etc. Man no more remained in direct connection with the earth, which constantly bestowed upon him its refreshing and strengthening influence (Antæus-legend). In the same measure as man grew more unnatural and sinful, sickness and all misery arose.

But even in this state man, when sick, for a long time followed his instinct and applied water in a certain form (the Natural Bath) and especially earth.

The men were in a magnetical union. They could exchange their vital force and thus co-operate together. To-day if a man wishes to heal his sickness and become well again, he ought to unconditionally submit to the inflexible and unimpeachable laws of Nature as soon as possible.

Man shall not taste or even touch medicines, poisons, nor undergo operations, etc., which are hallucinations of the restless man thrown into a dreadful labyrinth of culture and science.

But one shall also avoid many remedies of the Natural Healing Method of to-day, as Steam Baths, Electricity, and so many other artificial applications, since delusions and seeming results are obtained by these as well as by all poisons and perversities of nature, but in reality Health only gets injured.

Erring Humanity tries to undermine in vain the immovable Laws of Nature.

Man shall humbly return to Nature in the simplest way. To-day he naturally can enter into close connection with her only temporarily and partially, as the present effemination and fastidiousness of civilized humanity have to be taken into account. No severity nor painful privations must occur during the Cure. If the matter is rightly adjusted, Nature always guides the patient joyfully and happily back to the beautiful land of Health.

On these ideas the "Jungborn" is based; but where is it situated?

The American Jungborn is situated at Bellevue in the suburbs of Butler, N. J., in the most beautiful part of the Ramapo

Mountains, protected from the Northern winds in the delightful Grace Valley. We have here a wonderful grouping of hill and dale, with romantic clusters of rocks and murmuring springs. In the midst of most beautiful bewitching Nature, we are surrounded by rare forest charms. Here blows the purest and most fragrant Mountain-air.

LIGHT-AIR-COTTAGES.

At the Jungborn the patients live in pretty little so-called "Light-Air-Cottages" (see picture cut), built only from wood, and after an entirely new design; they stand in the open country in the midst of magnificent parks and forests, surrounded by pines, fruit-trees and shrubbery. (During the hottest time of Summer, Light-Air-Halls are used.)

Each Light-Air-Cottage contains but two rooms, each left free on three sides. In the Light-Air-Cottages the atmosphere is not rendered unfit for breathing, as is generally the case in large dwellings where many people live and sleep together, or by stone walls, where miasma arises from sewers, cellars, etc.

The Light-Air-Cottages for gentlemen are built in a large park for gentlemen, those for ladies in a separate Ladies' park. Both parks are surrounded and protected by high and solid board fences.

Therefore everybody may live and sleep at the Jungborn in his room "sans-gene," the windows, doors, shutters, etc., always being open, and thus breathe the purest and most invigorating ozone of the forests.

The cosy little Wood Cottages, which are provided with double, hollow board-walls, can be closed entirely and, in a cool, unpleasant temperature, are warmer and more agreeable than stone houses, which are always damp and cold.

LIGHT-AIR, SUN- AND RAIN-BATHS,

From the Light-Air-Cottages one may at any time take a Light-Air-Bath, *i. e.,* go without clothing, or later on dressed with a Light-Air Bathing-Gown or Suit, especially just after arising from bed, which is most beneficial; also take a Sunbath and run naked in the rain.

In nice pleasant nights the patients may sleep entirely under the open sky and enjoy the full charm of silent Nature.

In the Light-Air-Parks one does not feel confined in spite of the high planks, since the parks are very large and beautiful, and the grand romantic view of Grace Valley opens itself to the eye.

"The Light-Air-Cottages at the Jungborn are situated right in the Light-Air-Park, and one may in this manner right from out his room take a Light-Air-Bath at any time, day or night, rain or shine, and is not in the least deprived of any comfort. Thus the best opportunity is offered in the Jungborn to take Light-Air, Sun-Baths, etc. Therefore the Light-Air-Cult is frequently and very diligently practised."

Only he who has tried Light-Air and Sunbaths to such an extent as they are offered in the Jungborn, will experience how he is embodied by light and air, and how soon his whole system feels regenerated as by a new life, by a formerly unknown freshness, and a rare feeling of comfort. The miserable fear of catching cold will soon be overcome.

In a more open, large, very nice and universal park, called, "Regeneration Park," there are also Light-Air-Cottages for families. The Light-Air-Parks are, of course, at a free disposal to the inhabitants of the Light-Air-Cottages.

As the patients live in small Light-Air-Cottages that contain at least two rooms, and are scattered in the large parks, the Jungborn people are not as densely crowded as it is generally the case in Sanitaria.

There are also easily heated rooms (dining-rooms, rooms for entertainments, etc.), at free disposal. All rooms in the Light-Air-Cottages and other Buildings are furnished without luxury, simply, yet elegantly.

FINE BEDDING.

Special attention was given to wholesome, warm and comfortable beds, *i e.*, very fine quilts, made from best curled wool, and porous white covers.

WALKING BAREFOOTED.

Naturally, best opportunity is afforded for walking barefooted in the Light-Air-Parks as well as outside of them.

THE NEW NATURAL BATH.

In the Light-Air-Parks the new Natural Bath, which I introduced (no full- neither half-bath), and which so often showed its most beneficial and comforting influence, may also be taken outdoors amidst the fragrance of the firs.

MASSAGE AND HEALING MAGNETISM.

Most able persons are employed and always ready to properly apply (especially directly after the bath) human healing powers (healing Magnetism and Massage, and transmission of Life- and Nerve-Power) in the most simple, natural and effective form.

THE EARTH-POWER.

The Jungborn patients may make the most of the power of Earth in every respect, *i. e.,* when walking barefooted or naked, and sleeping on the ground at night, they can come again into direct contact with the earth which sends forth such a wonderfully healing power to her creatures (legend of Antæus).

EARTH OR CLAY-PACKS AND BANDAGES.

Earth, respectively Clay, this natural remedy of old, that has been born anew in the Jungborn, is extensively applied in the shape of bandages and packs at various skin diseases and external and internal ailments in order to reduce heat, sooth pain and loosen morbid matter, thus effecting the most startling cures. The Earth and Clay Applications, besides all the other treatments at the Jungborn, have met with great enthusiasm and were most favorably received and imitated, carrying with them the most wonderful results.

FRUIT DIET.

The Jungborn is the first institution where entire fruit diet has been introduced. To the various kinds of nuts, which must be deemed principal ingredients of human food, and to the manifold domestic delicious and aromatic fruit, as berries, apples, etc., some imported foreign fruit is added (Oranges, Figs, Dates, Grapes, etc., are used.)

At the Jungborn the finest fruit is raised and gathered from our own trees.

To those, that are not yet used to a strict fruit diet, the table offers the following:

"The richest milk and butter from the cows and goats in our pastures, a new plain and natural and very palatable bread (Jungborn bread), which is already highly in demand; stewed fruit, vegetables, with some potatoes; salads (from cucumbers, cabbage, beans, celery, asparagus, tomatoes, lettuce), soft pot-cheese, which is much liked with fresh berries and stewed fruit; we also serve pure malt-coffee for breakfast."

This variety in our bill of fare has always met the approval of our patients. No more doubt should exist about the fact that nuts and fruit, on account of their nourishing, easy digestible, and blood purifying qualities are most important in human diet. Nevertheless, it is left to the pleasure of our patients, whether they will eat pure fruit-diet (raw fruit and nuts) or prefer the above variety in vitals (milk, bread, vegetables, etc.).

FRUIT ORCHARDS.

The extensive fruit and berry orchards, especially in the large Light-Air-Parks offer a fine opportunity to the patients for outdoor exercise and farm work, thus teaching them a new, simple natural method of fruit culture (Stringfellow's).

OUR OWN WATER-WORKS.

The Jungborn is lavishly supplied with water from our own works; thus there is sufficient water for bathing, sprinkling, etc.

FREEDOM AND INDEPENDENCE OF THE CURE.

Every patient has full liberty in his treatment and is taught independency in his cure. Thereby many oppressing bonds, which erring humanity imposes upon sick people, vanish. Unworthy slavery ceases.

Here man is freed from so many banes of civilization; here he can study Nature in all its bountiful benevolence and majestic grandeur; here at Nature's bosom he will soon be delivered from all human ailments and suffering, and will find the fountain of new life and vigor.

LECTURES.

From time to time lectures about true, natural Healing and Health Culture are delivered; it is shown how the treatment is to be applied in all cases and professions; also considering the great influence of spiritual life, and true Christianity in regard to sickness. From the beginning these lectures have been in highest favor with the patients and of greatest benefit and blessing everywhere. Thus at the Jungborn each guest is given the opportunity to go through a thorough course of studies and will learn how to escape many dangers and errors for himself and family, and will be led to new joy and happiness, and to the highest blessings in time and eternity. To secure these advantages young men and women have already been recommended to the Jungborn. The living Word tells more than the written one.

It is, of course, at the liberty of the patients to partake of these lectures.

LADIES' DEPARTMENT.

The Ladies' Department is under the Direction and Care of Mrs. B. Lust, who has a staff of thoroughly experienced lady attendants.

PHYSICIAN.

To comply with the regulations of the State Authorities, a regularly licensed physician is in connection with the Jungborn. He holds his office hours at certain times in the Jungborn, and may be consulted by the patients at their convenience.

NEW DRAWING-ROOMS.

Adjoining the dining-room and amusement-hall a larger and more beautiful place for entertainments with a balcony and porch will be erected.

A light and pleasant lecture-room, separated from all other apartments, will also be built; thus the audience will not be disturbed by any outside noise.

NORTHERN LOG-HOUSES.

There are also introduced more solid, charming northern log-houses, which are very warm and can be heated in extreme cold. Such patients who lack natural heat of the body or are confined to their beds, may, besides the other comfortably heated rooms (dining-rooms, entertainment-hall), use such houses for sleeping and dwelling purposes during the cooler season.

A Log-House is also constructed according to my own and new ideas. It contains but two finely furnished rooms, and a pretty balcony; the rooms are somewhat larger than those in the Light-Air-Cottages. Connected with each room is a nice little alcove for a nurse or attendant. The log-houses shall also serve as samples for above mentioned purposes. They are far prettier, healthier, lighter, and more quiet than the heated rooms in our city houses, and the general Sanitaria.

Even the most delicate and fastidious person will enjoy his stay with us, also in the cooler seasons—Spring and Autumn,—when the quickest and most successful cures take place.

New Light-Air-Cottages are constructed. Lately a new system of canalization, including sewers and water closets is added, which has improved the sanitary condition and cleanliness of the institution remarkably. Some more new arrangements and small improvements were made.

The parks are greatly beautified by laying out of soft, blue-grass lawns, fine sand-paths, most inviting for walking barefooted; ponds and cascades vary with beautiful flower-beds, and other plantations, leading into extensive woods.

Besides the main Light-Air-Parks for Gentlemen and Ladies, there are four smaller Light-Air-Parks which serve for certain cases, where patients or children, who are somewhat bashful to run naked in the Light-Air-Bath, may be separated from the others.

In the course of time I have been able to find most suitable help for house- and Sanitarium work; also people who assist in enlarging and developing the Jungborn.

The Jungborn in its perfection can meet the most extended demands.

The Jungborn has existed for seven years and we have gloriously overcome all troubles and hindrances, which could be expected with such a new enterprise, and which often restrained and partly paralyzed our work.

In all difficulties which we have experienced so far, I have again and again recognized the great importance of our work at the Jungborn, and become convinced that I must exert my strength to the utmost to accomplish it. "The wonderful results, which even in severest cases of sickness were effected through the simple Natural Healing Method of the Jungborn, and which often have caused the greatest admiration of so many, have led me to enlarge and complete the Jungborn to such an extent."

The best and most convincing proof for the Jungborn and its work are a great number of institutions which were copied from our style; yet they often lack the purity and simplicity of our method, and especially the right spirit.

Of special value to the Jungborn is its picturesque and favorable situation, the aromatic air of the Ramapo Mountains, etc.

"The great attendance, which the Jungborn enjoyed from its beginning, enables me to sacrifice more and more to the Jungborn and its work."

May God's blessing rest on the Jungborn for evermore. Amen!

WONDERFUL CURES.

Many people cannot imagine the beneficial and wonderful healing effect, a true connection with benign Nature has (without human errors) with the true spirit and the real psychical influence.

"But the wonderful cures, which are daily realized at the Jungborn from all acute and chronic diseases, as, catarrh, diseases of the lungs, stomach, liver, kidneys, throat and heart diseases, diseases of the eye and ear, rheumatism, gout, abdominal and female troubles, skin and sexual diseases, above all nervous diseases, etc.; also many cases, which were proclaimed incurable and where all other natural-healing methods were of no avail, must doubtless convince everybody."

In the *"Kneipp Water-Cure Monthly"* and in the *"Naturopath"* a number of startling cures, which were effected at the Jungborn, are mentioned.

"Therefore I want to call the attention of those who long have moaned and suffered and given up all hope, to the Jungborn. I want to recommend it as a Fountain of Salvation, which never fails, unless an extreme stage of disease is reached or some defect is there."

"*During the cool seasons, especially Spring and Autumn, I have observed the quickest and most remarkable cures.* The treatment is of such a kind, that it will be ever agreeable to the patient. But during the cool seasons the effect is generally a quicker one."

The right connection with nature soon awakens the vital spirits of men and creates a rare joy of life. The humor of the Jungborn patients therefore is most happy and gay, as seldom found in a Sanitarium; this has often been observed.

The duration of a cure varies considerably. Of course, a treatment at the Jungborn can never last too long; here we must say, "the longer, the better." The stay of a patient generally depends on the progressing of the treatment. Some patients remain at the Jungborn some weeks, others a few months, others again six full months; the average time of the cure is from four to six weeks.

ENTERTAINMENTS AND EXCURSIONS.

Diffcrent kinds of entertainments are provided for; also outdoor Bowling Alley, and Golf Links, exercises and plays, Lawn Tennis, Croquet, Ball Games (the latter also during the Light-Air-Baths, etc.).

From the Jungborn, which is situated in the most picturesque parts of the Ramapo Mountains, beautiful excursions can be made to a number of lakes, as Greenwood Lake, Echo Lake, Pompton Lake, and others are within reach for a day's outing, and may be approached either by private conveyance or by railroad. The mountains are from 1,100 to 1,400 feet high.

The view from the celebrated "Keck-Out" Mountain, three miles from Jungborn, is beyond description, and at once reminds the spectator of the Alps in Switzerland. It is only of late that this northern part of New Jersey, with its mountain ranges and its attractive sceneries, has become the favorite spot of the people of New York and neighboring cities as a mountain air resort, being recommended for its pure, bracing and invigorating air by numerous prominent physicians of New York City.

GENERAL RULES AND PRICES.

Patients, convalescents and those in need of recreation are welcome at the Jungborn. Epileptics, mentally deranged, and patients with contagious diseases cannot be admitted. To the latter we count consumptives, too far progressed, and those where a high grade of sexual disease is apparent.

Admission fee and first consultation is $2.00 to $5.00. Board and treatment per day, $1.00, $2.00, $3.00, $5.00, and $10.00. Reduced prices for children according to age. If two persons occupy one room, the rate will be less for each (a few very large rooms excepted). The day of arrival and leaving, counts for one full day. If more than one member of a family is admitted, consultation fee is only charged for one. Visiting patients pay admission fee the first time only. Invalids, who need special care and nursing, have to pay accordingly. For serving meals in private rooms an extra charge of 25 cents per meal or 50 cents per day will be made.

A reduction of prices may be allowed in extraordinary cases.

Lodging in the neighborhood of the Jungborn is offered at Butler and Bloomingdale at the rate of $1.50 to $2.00 per week or by the day in hotels and boarding houses.

For those who dwell outside of the Jungborn, a fee of 25 cents to $1.00 per day is charged for the use of the Light-Air-Park, bathing, advice, etc., and an extra fee for treatments in the Institute.

Dinner or supper for visitors, 50 cents. Breakfast, 35 cents each person. Payment to be made monthly, weekly or daily in advance.

Butler is 38 miles from New York City and 17 miles from Paterson, N. J.

It is to be recommended that everybody brings a common woollen blanket along; nothing else is needed in the line of bedclothing. Jungborn Health-Clothing, shirts, sandals, caps; also woollen blankets, etc., can be bought here.

An invalid chair can be had for free disposal at the Jungborn.

Many ladies like to wear so-called "hangers." made of light

washable goods or porous worsted, coarse woollen stuffs (also Reform Dresses). The ladies can have their clothing made at home or buy it here.

Simplicity in dressing prevails at the Jungborn. Everybody is pleased with the plain style of dressing regardless of fashion. It is well to remember this when getting ready for a trip to the Jungborn.

The Jungborn is open all the year round.

Applications should be made early enough to secure admittance and accommodations.

Butler Station is 15 minutes distant from the Jungborn.

Arriving guests will please mention whether they wish a carriage or the porter to meet them at the depot, for which a small charge is made.

Visitors who wish to inspect the Jungborn, are asked to put 25 cents into the poor-box; this regulation is necessary to avoid a great crowd of visitors. The closed Gentlemen's and Ladies' Parks cannot be seen. Whoever wishes to inspect or visit the Jungborn may stop at the boarding house, which is situated close to the Jungborn.

We kindly ask you to send us the addresses of friends, acquaintances and patients to whom we will gladly forward our Prospectus and a sample copy of our monthly magazine, "The Naturopath" free of any charges.

BENEDICT LUST,
Naturopathic Physician.

Jungborn, Butler, N. J.

POINTERS

FOR TRUTH SEEKERS

PLEASE READ THIS, INSTEAD OF ASKING US.

It's taking people an unconscionable while to understand the first doctrines and principles of Naturopathy. They write us every day for "literature describing our system"—they tell us how they have undergone this or that "Method" of Physical Culture or Diet or Personal Magnetism—they beg us for "testimonials" of cures—they don't seem to grasp the fact that Naturopathy includes every movement for the betterment of humanity, from the grossest Physical Culture to the purest New Thought. After hundreds of requests to recommend the best Books discussing separate branches of Naturopathy, we decided to look the field over, select representative works, and give the public our exact opinion. Some of these Books we advertise elsewhere—some we don't—it makes no difference. We consider them among the very best, and suggest them for what you'll find in them, not for what we'll get out of them.

NATUROPATHIC LITERATURE

KNEIPP SYSTEM

Kneipp's World-Famous Books.

MY WATER-CURE.—Tested for more than fifty years, and published for the cure of diseases and the preservation of health. 1,000,000 copies sold abroad. 100 illustrations, 389 pp. Elegant Edition, $1.65; stiff cover, 75c.; paper cover, 50c. **Special American Edition**, cloth, $1.00; paper, 50c.

THUS SHALT THOU LIVE.—Hints and advice for the well and the ill, suggesting a plain, rational mode of living, and a natural method of curing. 380 pp. Elegant Edition, $1.65; stiff cover, 75c.; paper, 50c.

MY WILL.—A Legacy to the Healthy and the Sick. This book explains best the Kneipp Water-Cure System in all its branches. 29 photographs from life. 388 pp. Elegant Edition, $1.65; stiff cover, 75c.; paper, 50c.

CODICIL TO MY WILL.—The last of Father Kneipp's renowned works, giving lessons on diet and cooking, on the human body, on practical home gymnastics, on various diseases and accidents, with the treatment therefor. 408 pp. Elegant Edition, $1.65; stiff cover, 75c.; paper, 50c.

THE CARE OF CHILDREN in Sickness and Health.—Contains instructions for mothers on their own welfare, the rearing of children, and the curing of ailments incident to childhood. 260 pp.

NOTE.—Kneipp books are published also in French, German, Italian, Spanish, Polish, Bohemian, Portuguese, Hungarian, Dutch, etc. Price list and Kneipp-Brochure free on application.

Elegant Edition, $1.65; stiff, 75c.; paper, 50c. **Special American Edition,** cloth, 75c.; paper 50c.

KNEIPP'S PLANT ATLAS.—Illustrates the curative herbs recommended by Very Rev. Mgr. Kneipp in his works. Published in English, French, German, Bohemian, Polish, Spanish, Hungarian, and Dutch. Edition I (Albertype printing), $2.00; Edition II (natural colors), $3.85; Edition III (plain), 55c.

PRACTICAL GUIDE TO KNEIPP'S METHOD OF CURE.—Published in English, French, German, 10c.

KNEIPP APOTHEKA.—B. Lust. Of manifold usefulness in every household, 10c.

NATUROPATHY.

NATURAL METHOD OF HEALING.—F. E. Bilz.—The compendium, par excellence, of the Naturopathic School. Every rational measure, from Massage to Magnetism, is discussed in detail, both theoretically and practically. The Kneipp Cure, Nursing, Dietetics, Curative Gymnastics, Medicinal Herbs, Hydropathy, Heliotherapy, Hygeiotherapy—every conceivable phase of the Natural Regime; Disease, particularly chronic, sexual, and youthful, with their symptoms, origin, purpose, and specific treatment; Anatomy, as pictured in 9 adjustable colored models; Hygiene and the Art of Keeping Well. These are a few of the themes developed. A Cyclopedia for reference, a Text-book for study, a Manual for daily use. Over one million copies sold abroad. Gold Medal, 1899, German Hygienic Exposition. 2,000 pp. of text. 700 illustrations. 2 Volumes, attractively bound, $7.50, $8.00 express prepaid. Prospectus sent for the asking.

THE NEW CURATIVE TREATMENT OF DISEASE.—M. Platen.—The therapeutic thought of the scientific world translated into the American vernacular. The book is written by a German, but it breathes American spirit; the "atmosphere," to borrow an artist's term, is pellucid, you don't have to grope through mazes of archaic circumlocution and technical terminology to reach the point. To begin with, Anatomy is not presented in the diffusely didactic orthodox style, that instructs a trifle, bewilders much, interests not at all. It is crystallized into eight anatomical plates, separable and dissectible, picturing the organs and systems of the human body in their entirety. With this as a basis, the author goes straight into the vital problems of everyday life—Eating, and Drinking, and the other unrealized potencies that twentieth century thought is investigating.. In a word, Prophylaxis is the key—not the dreading of the beneficent germ-scavenger, but the forbidding and the clearing of the corruption-mass that feeds him. Diseases, particularly those incident to children and to womanhood, are treated in detail and by various methods of Nature Cure. Given the knowledge this book imparts and the spirit that radiates from it, and one should never know what it means to be weary or weak or diseased. About 2,000 pp., many illustrations, 17 colored plates, 8 anatomical models. Two Volumes, handsomely bound, $7.50. Express prepaid, $8.00. Full descriptive matter mailed on application.

RETURN TO NATURE.—Ad. Just.—Beauty, simplicity, directness,

power; a book not written, but evolved, not a treatise, but a life-experience. Years of the severest bodily ills, utter failures on the part of all the Schools of Therapeutics, despair that instinctively turned to Nature herself, the dawning of the Truth, the realizing of its power, and the telling of it out of a full heart—such is the story of this plea for self-hood. You are not ready to read until you have studied the portrait of the man: most Nature Curists are materialists, but you feel, intuitively, that this man is an etherealist, and that the mental motive is back of the purely physical means. The opening pages soothe rather than startle, breathing a peace and a conscious poise that are very essential before the radical truths that follow. Then with kaleidoscopic swiftness the thought becomes revolutionary, iconoclastic-sensational the ultra-purist would call it. For the sex organs are mentioned as plainly and as reverently as the lover tells of the lips of his betrothed. The Just Bath is perhaps the distinguishing feature of the different physical measures. Based on a personal study of animals in their native habit, it is absolutely without analogue in all the previous range of Hydropathy. Unlike any other single water-application, it has a direct effect on Digestion, Sex, Circulation, Secretion, Exertion, and Nerve Power—the elements most needing vivifying. In the opinion of the publishers "Return to Nature" is the simplest and the strongest work ever brought out in any language. Not so much the actual facts and treatments and proofs, though they are unique and invaluable, but the insight into the New Century thought is what makes the book indispensable to the thinker. If you possess, in every particular, pulsating, energizing, empowering Health, you might not be interested—for yourself, and at the present. But not one man in ten thousand does. And whatever stage you may be, simply locate yourself in the pages of a life-history like your own, and follow the book to the close. If you once get in touch with this man who has suffered, his vision will clarify yours, his heart-beats will quicken your own, and you will have the spirit of Mental Healing with the measures of the Physical. Which is the ideal. $2.00 postpaid. A new enlarged Edition is in preparation. Price $3.00.

THE NEW DOCTOR; OR, HEALTH AND HAPPINESS.—L. M. Biddle.—Therapeutic truths in every-day garb; Nature teachings in story-form. Attractive, convincing, inspiring, this book is essentially a help in the home, where the tyro, whether child or adult, needs a bit of a sweet persuasion, along with solid instruction. 255 pp. $1.00.

THE NATURE-CURE CAUSE AND CURE OF ALL DISEASES.—Dr. M. E. Rose C. Conger.—Twelve chapters of terse facts and telling statements. A bold assertion of the bolder beliefs, backed by the proofs of half a life-time in the healing vocation. Wholly antagonistic to Drugs, Druggists, and Druggers. Includes studies of organs, systems, diseases general and special, causes and remedies, baths, gymnastics, dress, recipes, tobacco and alcohol, pregnancy, child-birth and child-culture. Testimony of 100 eminent physicians, etc., etc. Price $2.00.

THE NEW METHOD IN HEALTH AND DISEASE.—Dr. W. E. Forest. —Naturopathy from a physician's viewpoint. But particularly

Hygeiopathy, for the individual and the family. The demand for twelve editions is sufficient comment on the merits of the work. $1.00 ....

THE NEW SCIENCE OF HEALING.—Louis Kuhne.—A convincingly concrete exposition of the oneness of all Disease, and the consequent basal uniformity of treatment traces ailments from the embryo to the corpse, and shows just how impure blood retains its deadly character through infinite multiplicities of external form. The work is a detailed account of Pathological Genealogy, set forth in colloquial phraseology, and appealing to the reason of layman and physician. The author is an acknowledged pioneer in the field of German investigation, his methods have been imitated by innumerable plagiarist Hydropathists, and "The New Science of Healing" is his most representative book. Translated into 26 languages. 420 pp. (3rd Edition.) Price, $2.65.

NATURE VERSUS DRUGS.—A. F. Reinhold.—The classic Drug-Denunciation of modern times. Revolution, Renovation, Reconstruction are the clarion calls from every page. Not a book for the tradition-blinded, mealy-mouthed, convention-bound hibernator in antiquity. Not cold type dissertation, but a live, throbbing, thrilling appeal for knowledge and freedom and health and nature. The author eats microbes, sleeps head down, courts "catching cold," and makes habits of other fatal feats. Moreover, he tells you exactly why and how it is that unthinking, perverse modes of life trisect a man's earthly span. As an animal, man should live to 125; he dies at 35. The why and the how not are most ably discussed. The book goes to the extreme of radicalism, but that it reaches the depths of realism is attested by many statements from the very physicians it so scathingly arraigns. 546 pp., 174 illustrations. $2.50.

MURDEROUS FADS IN THE PRACTICE OF MEDICINE.—Dr. M. J. Rodermund.—Written by the man who dabbled in the most virulent virus and then shook hands with family and friends, to the consternation of press and public. Vaccination is termed the "Prince of Frauds," and $1,000 is offered to the first man who can demonstrate its accord with Nature and its beneficence in a single case. Expensive laboratories, a life-time of research, and unwavering convictions are the background for this bold defiance of professional ostracism. Other fads, fancies and foibles commonly accepted without question are stripped of their antediluvian foggery, their mystic chicanery, their authoritative setting, and the scanty remnants of Truth are a pitiful witness to the world's perversions. 654 pp. Price, $3.00.

HYDROPATHY.

RICHARD METCALFE, HYDROPATHIST, THE MAN AND HIS WORK.—This treats of the life work of one of England's most eminent hydropathists, enumerates and illustrates diseases successfully treated by him, includes treatises on Hydrophobia and its cure, and concludes with a most explicit Hydropathic Materia Medica. A valuable English interpretation of the Water-Cure. 75c.

LIFE OF VINCENT PREISSNITZ.—Richard Metcalfe.—The tribute of a great English Hydropathist to the founder of the system. Describes the early methods in detail, contrasts them with the modern, presents numerous illustrative cases, emphasizes the cardinal principles of the Water-Cure, and closes with a comprehensive chapter of Bibliography. Illustrated. $1.75.

THE ROYAL ROAD TO HEALTH.—Dr. Chas. A. Tyrell.—Advocates the Internal Bath. J. B. L. Cascade Treatment. $1.00.

THE NEW INTERNAL BATH.—Dr. Laura M. Wright.—A strong and practical presentation of a matter commonly misunderstood, misconsidered, and misapplied. Especially helpful to the man whose fetish is a cathartic or liver pills. 25c.

DIETETICS AND COOKERY.

NATURAL WAY IN DIET; OR, PROPER FOOD FOR MAN.—L. H. Anderson.—A typical representative of the modern movement toward perfect nutrition. Mal-assimilation is assumed now as the basis of all disease, and the first therapeutic measure is the regulating of the dietary. This book will prove a valuable adjunct toward this end. $1.25.

A COMPREHENSIVE GUIDE-BOOK TO NATURAL HYGIENIC, HUMANE DIET.—Sidney H. Beard.—Is even more than the name implies. Contains essays on Hygienic Living, Moderation, Woman's Mission, Travelling Hints, Substitutes for Animal Foods, Health Recipes, and other vital topics. The author is a leading exponent of the golden-age tenets; that alone is ample assurance of the book's merits. 50c.; cloth, $1.00.

THE GOLDEN AGE COOK-BOOK.—Henrietta Latham Dwight.—This cleverly written book in elegant binding, was especially written to aid those who, having decided to adopt a bloodless diet, are still asking how they can be nourished without flesh. That flesh-eating is not necessary to the perfect health of man is attested by many eminent scientists. Reduced from $1.50. Now only $1.00.

FRUIT AND NUT DIET.—O. Hashnu Hara.—Practical Hints upon natural forms of diet. 10c.

EATING FOR STRENGTH.—Dr. M. L. Holbrook.—For the invalid, the student, the athlete. Shows the exact effect of various foods and drinks, the relation of eating to health and disease, and makes explicit and emphatic mention of important points omitted in similar works. Distinctly modern and American, and one of the few really popular books on the food question. $1.00.

SCIENCE IN THE KITCHEN.—Mrs. E. E. Kellogg.—The embodiment of ten years' experiment and experience in the Laboratory Kitchen connected with the Battle Creek Sanitarium. A complete culinary manual, treating of the Pocketbook, the Market, the Kitchen, the Dining-Room, the Pantry, and the other departments of model housewifery. Over 800 carefully tested recipes of dishes used at the greatest Sanitarium in America. $1.90.

QUISISANA HYGIENIC COOK-BOOK.—Lina Kuepper.—The basis of cookery at the Quisisana Sanitarium (Naturopathic). Adapted menus for the different seasons of the year, and 300 hygienic recipes. 50c.

WHY I AM A VEGETARIAN.—J. Howard Moore, A. B.—Hygienically,

athletically, aesthetically, ethically, this plea for satisfying food is without a peer in all vegetarian literature. The facts are unanswerable arguments, the thought is chaste and expressive, but, more than all, the manifest motif is a love for all animal creation. 25c.

FRUITS AND HOW TO USE THEM.—Mrs. Hester M. Poole.—Superlatively the best discussion of the perfect food. Fruits have a wider sphere of usefulness than any other single nutritive element. Antiseptic, laxative, depurative, soothing, sustaining, they are being made a daily delight, by people who think. The book is the best guide to their use. $1.00.

FAT OF THE LAND AND HOW TO LIVE ON IT.—Dr. Ellen G. Smith.—The title of the closing chapter, "In a Nutshell," is an epitome of the chapters preceding. The prose of everyday eating is transformed into the poetry of ideal nutrition. Every cognate question is measured by the main point, and such seemingly foreign topics as Cooking Utensils, Social Requirements, Bakeries, Alcoholics in Food, and Farm-Yard Slaughter, each yield their quota of truth. The chapters on Vegetable oils, Fruits, and Nuts are especially apt. $1.50.

FRUITS AND FARINACEA THE PROPER FOOD OF MAN.—J. Smith and Dr. R. T. Trall.—A conclusive corroboration of the New School of Dietetics. Lessened expense, increased vitality, prolonged longevity, and intensified enjoyment, are inevitable results attending the adoption of this system. Illustrated. $1.50.

JUST HOW TO COOK MEALS WITHOUT MEAT.—Elizabeth Towne.—Quaint, picturesque, irresistible The author's experiences in the author's own style. A biography, a letter, a chat, a cook-book, and a sermon—all in one. 25c.

MECHANOTHERAPY.

THE ART OF MASSAGE.—Dr. J. H. Kellogg.—The standard work on the subject. Resume of twenty years' experience at the greatest health establishment in America, and among the most expert masseurs on the continent. $2.25.

MASSAGE AND THE ORIGINAL SWEDISH MOVEMENTS.—Ostrom.—One of the few final authorities. A work purely scientific and practical, and unadulterated by modern mercenarism. 4th edition, 105 illustrations. $1.00.

PHILOSOPHY OF OSTEOPATHY.—A. T. Still.—The conception of the "Founder of Osteopathy" and President Kirkville's school. $2.50.

PHYSICAL CULTURE.

AMERICAN DELSARTE CULTURE.—Emily M. Bishop.—A true interpretation by a true disciple. $1.00.

FASTING, HYDROPATHY, EXERCISE.—B. O. Macfadden and Dr. Felix Oswald.—Everyday knowledge, forgotten facts, strange theories, and fervid appeals, unite to form a most interesting and instructive book. Compiled by the foremost apostle of Physical Culture in America. $1.00.

NEW SCHOOL OF PHYSICAL CULTURE.—Rohde and Haskins.—How to Box to Win, by Terry McGovern; How to Build Muscle, by James J. Corbett; How to Breathe, Stand, Walk, or Run, by J. Gardiner Smith, M. D.; How to Punch the Bag, by Gus E. and Arthur R.Keeley. Every author is at the pinnacle of his profession, and the work may be taken as an ultimatum. The best book written for energizing the over-studious lad. $1.00.

ILLUSTRATED HINTS FOR HEALTH AND STRENGTH.—A. P. Schmidt.—Purposely for Busy People. Not a calisthenic drill, or an athlete's vade mecum, but a very few vitalizing movements, with no appliances but a brain and a bit of muscle. The illustrations are particularly happy, and they illustrate, moreover. This book is a radical departure from the ordinary commonplace chaos sent out by physical culturists. $1.50.

DELSARTE SYSTEM OF EXPRESSION.—Genevieve Stebbins.—A text-book and self-instructor in aesthetic physical training. Sixteen charts, nineteen sets of gymnastics, etc., etc. $2.00.

BREATHING AND VOICE-CULTURE.

POSITIVE PREVENTION AND CURE OF TUBERCULOSIS.—A. F. Reinhold.—Replete with startling facts and pointed advice. A companion book to "Nature vs. Drugs," though less of a philippic, and more of a manual. $3.00.

DIAGNOSIS AND DELINEATION.

MAN AN OPEN BOOK—CRANIOGNOMY.—J. S. Doolittle.—The immanent truths of Phrenology, Temperament, Vocation, Development, and the comprehensive study of the individual. Keen analysis, deft handling, apt illustration, attractive style, and, back of all, versatile intellection and humanity-loving spirit, distinctly differentiate this book from like publications. $1.00.

FACIAL DIAGNOSIS.—Louis Kuhne.—No thermometer, no pulse, no percussion, no speculum, none of the common playthings of the orthodox diagnostician. Instead, a single element—knowledge. The result, not an axiomatic announcement of unexplained disease but a foretelling of it, and a forbidding, and withal a clarifying of the whole matter. A book especially for fleshy people and for the anaemic. $2.00.

AM I WELL OR SICK?—Louis Kuhne. 25c.

THE ART OF BREATHING.—Leo Kofler.—The Basis of Tone-Production. Indispensable to Singers, Elocutionists, Lawyers, Preachers, and Good Health. Price, $1.50.

CARE AND DEVELOPMENT OF THE LUNGS AND MUSCULAR SYSTEM.—P. von Boeckmann.—A 54-page book, containing valuable information in regard to Muscle Building, Chest Expansion, Proper Breathing, etc. Special chapter for women. Illustrated by cuts and diagrams. Author has largest and most powerful lungs in the world.—11½ inches expansion, 410 cubic-inch lung capacity. Book accepted by National Medical Library, Washington, D. C. 12c.

SPECIAL AND ORGANIC DISEASES.

INTESTINAL ILLS.—Dr. Alcinous B. Jamison. A book designed for physicians, medical students, and non-professional readers interested in the causes of disease. Proctitus (chronic inflammation of anus and rectum) is posited as the cause of costiveness, diarrhoea, auto-intoxication, uric acid, anaemia, and the huge host of ills incident to faecal poisoning, and usually misunderstood and mistreated. A unique work, packed with thoughts and thought-incentives. $2.00.

THE STOMACH: ITS DISORDERS AND HOW TO CURE THEM.—Dr. J. H. Kellogg.—Theories not speculative, but materialized and proved at the institution best equipped in America for studying the stomach. $1.50.

MENTAL THERAPEUTICS.

SCIENCE AND HEALTH.—Mrs. Mary Baker Eddy.—The doctrines of the founder of Christian Science. $3.00.

MEN AND GODS.—C. C. Post.—A bold, brilliant affirmation of Man Omnipotent. It batters straight at the bulwarks of dogma, creed, tradition, superstition; and you can fairly feel the narrowing confines of your own childish conceptions crumbling into the nothingness that fabricated them. 50c.

PRACTICAL HYPNOTISM.—O. Hashnu Hara. 50c.

HYPNOTISM EXPLAINED. Rev. L. Schlathoelter. 60c.

THE ROAD TO SUCCESS.—O. Hashnu Hara. $1.00.

JUST HOW TO WAKE THE SOLAR PLEXUS.—Elizabeth Towne.—A practical, analogue adaptation of Heliocentric Philosophy. How to control emotions, banish fear, develop self, breathe for health, and do other things the unfoldment idea carries with it. 25 cents.

CONQUEST OF POVERTY.—Helen Wilmans.—Not how to do it;—how it was done. The record of a vision, a revelation, a transformation, as wonderful as the awakening of Saul of Tarsus. From the possession of a frail body, a life half gone, and twenty-five cents, to the ecstacies of superb health, the dictatorship of an entire town, the apostleship of a world-wide belief, and the reception of tens of thousands every year—that is the history of half a decade. The author is the leader, in so far as they acknowledge any, of the Mental Science advocates of America. 50c, cloth, $1.00.

HOME COURSE IN MENTAL SCIENCE.—Helen Wilmans.—The Criterion Course—Twenty Lessons. $5.00.

CONQEST OF DEATH.—Helen Wilmans.—Sensitized visionaries have at rare intervals hinted timidly at physical immortality. But the material side had atrophied, and evanescence was the outcome of the hypothesis. This dogma destroyer has already translated most of her theories into cold cash and redundant health. There are idioms in the translation, but the spirit and possibility is just as valent for every other human being. If you want to pierce, in a measure, the penetralia of existence, get this book—and go alone to read it. 400 pp., 36 half-tones. $3.00.

THE LIBRARY OF HEALTH.—Charles Brodie Patterson.—By the Editor of "The Arena." Perhaps the most popular of all the New Thought and Practical Psychology expositions. Excellent books for beginners. Three volumes. $2.25.

CONCENTRATION AND THE ACQUIREMENT OF PERSONAL MAGNETISM.—O. Hashnu Hara. $1.00

MEMORY AND MIND.

MEMORY AND INTELLECTUAL IMPROVEMENT.—O. S. Fowler.—Applied to self-instruction and juvenile improvement. No recent work equals this in direct arrival at the root of the matter. $1.00.

POWER OF WILL (KING ON HIS THRONE)—Rev. F. C. Haddock.—For students, teachers, professional workers, and all who desire self-culture and the mastery of life. In five parts: Theory and Life, Physical Regime, Mental Regime, Destruction of Habit, Contact With Other People. One of the few books that both instruct and inspire—deeply metaphysical, broadly practical, intensely vital. $2.50.

MANHOOD.

MANHOOD WRECKED AND RESCUED.—Rev. W. J. Hunter.—How strength and vigor is lost, and how manhood may be restored by self-treatment. In eight chapters: The Wreck; An Ancient Wreck; A Modern Wreck; A Youthful Wreck; A Wreck Escaped; The Rescue Begun; The Rescue Continued; The Rescue Completed. A single book that obviates the humiliation of confession, the cost of consultation, the danger of medical treatment, the deadliness of neglect, and, beyond all, the fear of helpless ignorance. $1.00.

CHASTITY; OR, OUR SECRET SIN.—Dr. Dio Lewis.—This was the author's favorite book. In it he thought he reached the highest altitudes of his life. The salient point in connection with the work is this: that the heartiest commendation and support has come from the Presidents of Colleges and Female Seminaries, where such questions are most relentlessly tabooed. Every delicate phase of the sex-life is discussed, unreservedly and exhaustively. And women as well as men who are striving for purity and perfection, cannot afford to be without such a guide. $2.00.

MACFADDEN, B. A.—Virile Powers of Superb Manhood. $1.00.

SHEPHERD, E. R.—True Manhood. $1.25.

Address all orders to:

B. LUST, 124 EAST 59th STREET, NEW YORK.

Books sent prepaid on receipt of price.

JOHN WERWEIN'S NATURE CURE & FRUIT SANITARIUM
Hammonton, Atlantic County, N. J.

BEAUTIFULLY located on a lake, amongst Pine Woods, Fruit Orchards and Vineyards. Well adapted to the Just Methods. Prices moderate. Write for circular to

JOHN WERWEIN, Hammonton, N. J.

WE HAVE TRANSPLANTED
THE JUST=CURE

to American soil, where it flourishes even more cosily than in its native home at Stapelburg, Germany. The Fruit-Nut Dietary that Mr. Just so wisely prefers is more varied and appetizing here than in Germany, the periods of rain and cold are less frequent and trying, and the climatic conditions as a whole are quite superior to those of the Hartz Mountains.

Seasons for air-sun baths lasts from April 15th to December 1st—almost till the snow-baths begin.

If you can afford the time, money, energy, and anxiety that a European trip always involves, we advise you by all means to take the Ideal Nature-Cure as given in Germany by its founder, Adolph Just.

But the voyage will cost you several hundred dollars, the treatment 8-20 marks daily, and the whole expedition will mean a vast amount of care and wear and worry. If you are a confirmed invalid, you will need an attendant for an ocean voyage; more expense. And if you attempt to be your own courier, you will find more annoyance and irritation going and coming than all the relief and recreation to be had from your stay.

Now we don't believe any more than you do in the "just-as-good" substitution game. And if we did not expect to offer you something far better than even the German-born Just-Cure, we would not risk our reputation in soliciting your support.

Perhaps the thing that differentiates us from typical Nature-Curists is our inveterate habit of teaching patients how to live so ideally that they will never be ill again.

Our patients don't come back—except to bring their sick friends for treatment.

The Institute in the heart of New York City has its attractions no less than the Sanatorium and Nature Camp among the peaks of the Ramapo Mountains. A most unique description of this "American Jungborn" at Butler, N. J., appeared in "Naturopath," June, 1902, pages 251-254.

This special number mailed for four cents postage. Treatment at Sanatorium directed by Mr. Benedict Lust and Mrs. Louisa Lust, Naturopaths. Weekly rates being $16 and upward entire expense. Charge less by the month or season. Consultation free at Institute. Examination $2, treatments weekly or single, hygienic board for patients and transients.

Prospectus and full information on request.

SANATORIUM JUNGBORN, BELLEVUE,
BUTLER, NEW JERSEY.
or
NATUROPATHIC INSTITUTE AND COLLEGE,
124 East 59th Street, NEW YORK CITY.

PERFECT ...

... HEALTH

How to Get it and How to Keep it
By One who Has it

TRUE SCIENTIFIC LIVING

"I have yet to meet a case in the treatment of which it has not proved helpful. I am convinced that its power to heal has no limit."—JOSEPH F. LAND, M. D., 130 West 126th Street, New York.

PUBLISHER'S GUARANTEE.

Any person who purchases this book and adopts its teaching and follows it for one month, and is not entirely satisfied with the improvement in his health, may return the book and the price will be refunded.

References as to Above Guarantee.

F. S. Jerome, V. Pres. 1st Nat. Bank, Norwich, Ct.
N. L. Bishop, Sup't of Schools, Norwich, Ct.

Price in Linen, $1.00. Sent prepaid on receipt of price.

CHARLES C. HASKELL

DEPT. B   NORWICH, CONN., U. S. A.

AGENTS WANTED.   (Mention this Book.)

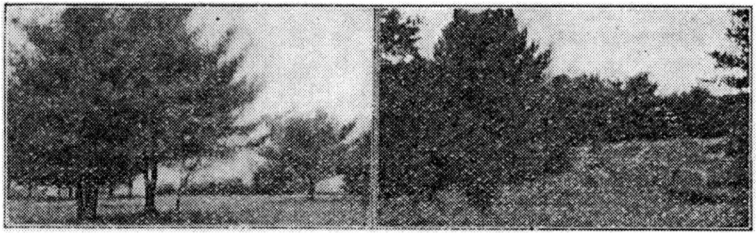

View of Air-Bath Park for Men.   View of Ladies' Air-Bath Park.

SANITARIUM BETHESDA

MILTON, MORRIS COUNTY, NEW JERSEY.

• • •

This Sanitarium is conducted strictly in accordance with the laws of nature and the principles and ideas set forth by Adolph Just. Absolutely pure fruit diet. Milk and sweet butter produced on the spot.

Ideal location. Pine Woods. Beautiful Lake for Boating and Swimming, and Creek for taking the Natural Bath. Without doubt the most lovely and healthiest situation in the State of New Jersey.

The arrangements are most convenient and sanitary. Remarkably successful results have been obtained in cases of hopeless—so-called "incurable" diseases.

Sleeping in the open air or on the bare earth or on grass; or, if necessary in light-and-air huts. Clay applications and air baths. Nervous diseases are most rapidly benefited by this treatment.

For Prospectus apply to

CHAS. LAUTERWASSER,

252 LITTLETON AVENUE, - - - NEWARK, N. J.

OR BETHESDA, MILTON, MORRIS CO., NEW JERSEY.

STOP CHOKING YOUR PORES — TEACH THEM TO BREATHE

If You Live IN the Flannels of your Fathers,
You will Live OUT the Ailments of Your Ancestors.

The Naturopathic Linen Tricot Health Underwear

Manufactured by Lenz & Co., Boblingen, near Stuttgart, Germany.

Is imported from Germany, for people who recognize German genuineness, and want to embody German hardihood.

It is recommended by the Author of this book in his fifth German Edition, Father Kneipp ("Thus Shalt Thou Live," pp. 15—20), Dr. Baumgarten, and other distinguished authorities.

If you are in touch with modern thought, the superiority of coarse Linen as underfabric need not be emphasized; and if you are not, no amount of reason or persuasion could convince you.

Send a postal for a free sample.

**Transmits Perspiration. Stimulates Transpiration. Electrifies by Gentle Friction.
Prevents Colds, Catarrh, Pneumonia and all Congestions.
Improves with Washing. Wears Amazingly. Feels Good—No Scratching.
Keeps you Warm all Winter, Cool all Summer, and Hardy all the Time.
Makes you Want to Return to Nature, to Health and to Happiness**

PRICES FOR WOMEN'S AND MEN'S UNDERWEAR.

Following prices are for sizes 32 to 40, 42 to 52; 50c extra for pair or $1.00 per garment:

Undershirts, natural gray, Quality 50 and 60	2.25
Undershirts, bleached, Quality 30 and 40	2.50
Drawers, natural gray, Quality 50 and 60	2.50
Drawers, bleached, Quality 30 and 40	2.75
Filet Undershirts (neat, extra light and porous for hot weather)	1.75
Extra heavy knitted for extreme cold climates	2.75
Drawers	3.00
Shirts, with or without collar	3.00
Kneipp Linen-tricot socks, natural gray, No. 7, to 11	.55c
11¼ to 12½	.65
Kneipp Linen-tricot socks, black, No. 7 to 11	.70
No. 11¼ to 12½	.80

Linen stockings for ladies, wheelmen, sports, etc:

Gray, No. 6 to 9 ....80c; 9¼ to 12½	.95
Black, No. 6 to 8 ....90c; 8¼ to 12½	1.00
Piece Goods, natural gray, 26 inches wide, per yard	.75
Piece Goods, bleached, 30 inches wide, per yard	.85
Yarn, Thread, for mending stockings and underwear, per skein	.25

Measure for Undervests and Shirts.

1. Total length. 2. Circumference of breast (full measure). 3. Length of sleeve from middle of back to wrist (bend arm when taking measure). For shirts add width of neck wanted.

Measure for Drawers.

1. Circumference of body. 2. Length of leg from step to ankle. 3. Total length of drawers.

Complete Catalogue of Kneipp, Just & Naturopathic Supplies, Free by Mail.

THE KNEIPP AND NATUROPATHIC SUPPLY CO.

General Depot for the United States: 111 East 59th St., New York.

NUTS AND FRUITS

THE DIET ADVOCATED BY THIS BOOK.

What you eat makes you what you are. If you want to be dull, brutish, apathetic and finally sick, eat flesh food. If you want to have full use of all your mental, vital and physical powers, so that life is a delight and not a burden, eat the Diet the Creator meant for you—the natural diet, **nuts and fruits**.

We have made it a specialty to extract all **Nut Meats** from the shells by means of machines ingeniously constructed and patented, so as to deliver the meat pure and appetizing; we deliver all meat fresh extracted, always in first-class condition, and in a better and more perfect shape than anybody else can do.

We recommend mainly for all sanitary purposes, "**PECAN NUT MEAT**," the finest nut meat in the world in taste and flavor, much superior in quality to walnuts, filberts, Brazils and peanuts.

Of our Senior, Mr. R. C. Koerber, the originator of the Pecan Industry, the official reports of the U. S. Dept. of Agriculture of 1896, say, page 60: "An industry was established a few months since at Austin, Texas, by R. C. Koerber, for cleansing, polishing and burnishing pecans, a business which he has since transferred to New York." Page 61: "The industry of preparing the kernels, or meats, of pecans for market, though yet in its infancy, has assumed large proportions. It was begun by Mr. Koerber in 1884, and his books show that in 1887 he prepared 20,000 lbs., and in 1890 more than 100,000 lbs.," etc.

With similar machines which extract the pecan meat, we open hickory nuts, Brazil nuts, filberts, walnuts, etc. We also stuff fruits, dates, figs, raisins and prunes with all kinds of nut meat; we also manufacture Nut Marmalade, Almond, Pecan, Brazil and Peanut Butter, etc.

WE OFFER FOR SALE:

Shelled Almonds, Shelled Walnuts, Shelled Pecans, Shelled Filberts, Brazil Nut Meat, Hickory Nut Meat, Black Walnut Meat, and Pignolias.

Salted Almonds and Salted Pecans,

Arabia Dates, seeded and stuffed with pecans, walnuts, almonds, crystallized ginger, citron or orange.

Turkish Prunes, seeded, stuffed with walnuts and pecans, crystallized. Turkish washed figs in original baskets of 1 or 2 lbs.

Our ladies' ideal food, "**Corona,**" in fancy wooden boxes; a combination of selected fruits filled with nut meats. Raisins stuffed, etc.

NUT BUTTER of different kinds. **DATE BUTTER. NUT MARMALADE.**

All our packages are sealed with the name "Koerber" on it
All goods in large and small quantities.

THE KOERBER NUT MEAT COMPANY.

156 Reade Street,   **NEW YORK.**

Incorporated under the laws of the State of New York.

We send out specimen samples of our delicious preparations, Nut Meats, Nut Butters, Nut and Fruit combinations, jams, Marmalades, etc., with price list, pamphlets and descriptions; postage prepaid upon receipt of 25c in cash, stamps or money order.

THE KNEIPP CURE

◆ ◆ ◆

My Water Cure.

◆ ◆ ◆

A translation from the Reverend Father Kneipp's famous world renowned German book "My Water Cure."

Kneipp's "Water Cure" has been tested for more than 65 years, and is at present known and adopted in every country of the world. The book, called "My Water Cure," has been translated into a great many foreign languages, and is a complete guide to regain one's health —without the use of any drugs or medicines.—Its 200 illustrations aid materially the applications of the various bandages, packages, compresses and other healing components included in Hydrotherapy.

A great variety of diseases are gone through alphabetically.— their cause and development described exhaustively, and then the mode of application of the Water Cure treatment is detailed very minutely in each case.

Kneipp also advocates in many instances the additional use of various herbs in form of teas.—All these herbs are described in his book, and to each description is appended the exact benefits to be derived from their use.—

A part of the book is devoted to the description of several kinds of strengthening foods as Whole-Wheat Bread, Strength-giving Soup, and Honey-Wine.

Part III of the book contains a large number of reported cures— all alphabetically arranged—with the exact mode of application in each instance; giving full particulars of the progress of each malady— manner of treatment and duration of Cure. This part will prove of the very greatest interest to invalids and sufferers from all those diseases, enumerated and described in this work.

In conclusion all the various Kneipp-Gushes are depicted with exact directions how to apply each one.

Especial stress is laid upon the fact that this book covers everything pertaining to a Home-treatment.

Anyone possessing this book will be enabled without the aid of anybody else's help to treat himself, his wife or children **at home,** without having need of having recourse to any other remedies except those Natural ones indicated in this valuable volume.

The low price is another strong point in its favor, and we cannot insist enough on the advisability of sending for this book. Price, paper cover, 50 cents; postpaid, 60 cents. Cloth, $1.00; postpaid, $1.12.

Published by

KNEIPP MAGAZINES PUBLISHING CO.
124 EAST 59th STREET, NEW YORK.

INSURE YOUR CHILD'S HEALTH
FOR 50 CENTS THROUGH

Baby's Kneipp Cure

The American version of the German work that originally brought from German mothers a whole railroad car load of grateful letters. An actual fact—Father Kneipp filled an express car with the loving messages of mothers blessed through this little book.

Of course, you might not want your child to be German all through. But you certainly can't improve on the splendid German sturdiness of the youth born and reared under the Kneipp regime.

Ella Wheeler Wilcox eulogized this system in the New York "Evening Journal," September 5, 1901—and she ought to be good enough company for ordinary folks.

You won't have any conception of what ideal childhood means, till you read this book. It is not enough to prevent absolutely the possibility of all the so-called "Diseases of Children," to rescue your little ones from the frightful mortality that threatens child-life, to save the mammoth doctor-bills that croup and measles and whooping-cough entail.

That would seem to be your money's worth—for 50 cents.

But that's only a fractional part of what this book includes.

A perfectly strong, active, vigorous babe, all sunshine and sweetness and smiles, cooing and crowing, with never a tear or wail till it learns the perpetual laugh that a healthy child can't repress; a beautiful body, glowing with radiant life, the keenest of brains discriminating truth in a way that makes education a delight, and a divine little soul, longing to unfold into the power and peace of ideal manhood—is this a faint picture of your dream for your child?

If you read, understand, and follow the teachings of this "Baby's Kneipp-Cure," and fail to realize your dream, you get your money back, and pay for the time you've wasted.

Send for detailed table of Contents. Roughly it is thus:—Part I, Advice to prospective parents, mother's food, dress, baths, etc., soul-culture; Part II, Care for children in health; all about sleeping, eating, clothing, teething, playing, working, studying, maturing—from hour of birth to period of puberty. Part III, Care of children in sickness; Nature treatment of 100 diseases of Babyhood, Childhood, and Youth, from Toothache to Scarlet Fever. Part IV, Ideal food for children, recipes and rules for natural, nourishing, inexpensive meals. What to Eat and What to Avoid.

```
Paper Edition..........................50c, by mail 60c
Board.................................75c, by mail 85c
Cloth (Elegant).....................$1.65, by mail, $1.75
```

If you're merely curious, perhaps the paper cover will be durable enough. But if you want to use the book, we suggest the stiff binding. The elegant Edition would make a most sumptuous and sensible Betrothal or Wedding Present.

KNEIPP MAGAZINES PUBLISHING CO., 124 East 59th ST., N. Y.

THE JUNGBORN BREAD

IS RECOMMENDED BY ADOPH JUST IN THIS WORK. So far it is only baked at the Hygienic Bakery, 100 E. 105th Street, New York, in this country. It is baked according to original recipe of Adolph Just and keeps for sometime. Can be shipped to any part of the United States. Price, one pound loaf, 5 cents; two pound loaf, 10 cents. (By mail, 25 cents for one pound loaf, and 40 cents for two pounds.) We sell the original recipe for making this bread for 50 cents. With an order for one hundred pounds of the Jungborn Flour, price, $3.00, this recipe is given free.

MINNESOTA WHITE SPRING WHEAT, the best in the world and fresh weekly, is used for

LUST'S JUNGBORN BREAD.

Washed, dried, ground and not separated after grinding, the finer bran, wholesome gluten and rich phosphates provide naturally the muscle-tissue and consequent strength and vigor ingredients for all mankind, weak or athletic.

LUST'S JUNGBORN BREAD

is made without fermentation, is absolutely free from fat and its lasting sweetness is but that which is natural to the wheat. In the baking-moulds only pure olive oil is used and largely due to this unusual practice the bread remains, days after baking, palatable, wholesome and free from distasteful, injurious conditions so common in "health bread" offerings. A single slice of

LUST'S JUNGBORN BREAD

contains more nutriment than an entire loaf of the light, white, spongy kinds usually offered as good food, and is generously beneficial to sufferers from Indigestion, Dyspepsia, Sour Stomach, Diabetes, etc. As a corrective in Constipation it will earn for us everlasting regard.

LUST'S JUNGBORN BREAD

with nuts or Nut Butter and your choice of fruits, will gratify, satisfy and maintain in good health any rational being.

Fresh ground Jungborn Flour sells as follows: 1 pound 5 cents; 10 pounds 40 cents; 100 pounds $3.00; 200 pounds or one barrel, $5.50. The Jungborn zwieback is the same as the Jungborn Bread, but it is prepared as zwieback in order that it may keep longer. It can be kept for any length of time, and can be shipped to any part of the world. Price for one package, 15 cents; one dozen packages, $1.50. We also have a nut fruit loaf, which serves as a substitute for cakes and pastries, etc. In the second volume of his book, Adolph Just speaks of such bread. It is composed of different kinds of nuts, fruits, figs, dates, prunes, raisins and Jungborn Flour. Price 2½ pound loaf, 25 cents; by mail, 65 cents.

Pure Extracted Bee Honey, per pound bottle, 25 cents; per dozen bottles, $2.50.

Wheat Berries, (Grains) same price as the Jungborn Flour.

Nuts, shelled and unshelled, choice Peanuts, best Chaberts Walnuts, Pignolias, Pecans, etc.; write for special catalogue and price list for Nuts and Preparations.

We also have three kinds of ground nuts or nut butter, as recommended by Adolph Just, of which the No. 1 kind is made of peanuts exclusively. It sells as follows:

½ lb. Jar   20 cents..............per doz..........$2.00
1 lb. Jar   30 cents..............per doz.......... 3.00
4 lb. Can   80 cents..............per doz.......... 8.00

For price of Nut Butter made of Pecans, Almonds, Walnuts, etc., and of Pecans exclusively, see price list which will be furnished on request.

We deliver our bread and foods free anywhere in New York City and Brooklyn. Branches are established all over Greater New York. Write for list of branches. Agents wanted all over the country.

Special Prices for Jungborn Sanatoria. For Circulars and Full Particulars Address,

LOUIS LUST & CO.,
S. E. Corner Park Avenue and 105th Street,
or
Depot of Naturopathic Supplies,
124 E. 59th Street, — — — **New York.**

... Free Information Bureau ...
for our Readers, Patrons, Patients, Students and Friends.

Impartial advice as to best choice of Naturopathic specialties.

Revised lists of Sanitaria, Nature Homes, Vegetarian Restaurants, Hygienic Manufactures, New Thought Books and Periodicals, Local Practitioners, Masseurs, Physical Culturists, Magnetic Healers, and all firms, institutions and individuals competent to serve practically the seeker after Health, Truth and Success.

Consultation gratis at office, 10 to 12 a. m., 7 to 8 p. m., every week-day.

Correspondent inquirers should enclose 25 cents for stationery, postage, and clerical expenses.

NATUROPATHIC INFORMATION BUREAU,
124 East 59th Street,   NEW YORK CITY.

I Will Take a Few Private Pupils

for my Preliminary Courses in Naturopathy, including Physiological Anatomy, Kneipp-Cure, Massage, Dietetics, Phototherapy, Just Method, Comparative Therapeutics, History and Biography of Nature-Cure Systems, and Practical Prophylactics.

Being both a medical Graduate and Naturopathic Physician I am in a position to teach from experience the relative merits of Allopathy, Homeopathy, and Naturopathy.

Physical Culturists, Masseurs, Nurses, Magnetic and Mental Healers, Doctors, Teachers, and Prospective Naturopaths are specially welcome in these Private Classes of Personal Instruction.

Theories demonstrated in actual clinical cases at our Institute and Sanatorium. Hours for classes and individual tuition adapted to preference of students.

Synopsis of Courses, with full information, 10 cents, stamps.

BENEDICT LUST, NATUROPATH,
124 East 59th Street,   NEW YORK CITY

Cultivate a Taste for Kneipp Malt=Coffee

One month will demonstrate its wonderful merit as a health producer. It will conquer and cure your nervous and dyspeptic troubles because it does not contain the poison caffeine. It combines the highest degree of nourishment and palatability possible to embody in a hygienic coffee substitute.

No other hygienic coffee substitute in the world is so scientifically, so carefully, so excellently prepared, at so great an expense, and with such scrupulous regard for purity as Kneipp Malt-Coffee. Its great popularity is due to uniform high quality.

Kneipp Malt-Coffee is put up in the whole grain which precludes the possibility of adulteration. Avoid coffee substitutes put on the market in the ground form. You know not what they contain. **There is no coffee substitute as good as Kneipp Malt-Coffee.**

The surest way to secure the genuine Kneipp Malt-Coffee is to look for the portrait and signature of Father Sebastian Kneipp and the signature of the Kneipp Malt Food Co. on every package.

Kneipp Malt-Coffee is never sold in bulk.

If on inquiry your grocer does not handle Kneipp Malt-Coffee, send us his name and address. For your trouble we will send you **free sample prepaid;** also our treatise on Coffee, Its Use and Abuse.
Address

KNEIPP MALT FOOD CO.,

Department D. Manitowoc, Wis.

HENRY MILLER'S MALTED BARLEY COFFEE

FOR TWENTY YEARS HENRY MILLER'S MALT-COFFEE has been known for its purity and superior quality. This coffee is put up in the whole grain—the malted barley—from the best Montana Barley. It has no other ingredients, nothing else is put in inthe process of malting and roasting; it is simply malted and roasted barley. The writer of this book, Adolph Just, recommends especially the use of this coffee. It is just what Just, Sebastian Kneipp and Vincent Priessnitz recommend as the very best substitute for narcotic drinks. It is used by the followers of Naturopathic principles, and by Sanatoria all over the world. It is warranted pure and genuine. The United States Health Reports, Volume 14, No. 20, Nov. 29th, 1895, says: "Common justice impels us to say that the result of careful investigations stamps Henry Miller's Malt-Coffee as being of the highest value."

The price of Henry Miller's Barley-Coffee is, five pounds 50 cents; 10 pounds $1.00. A sample package will be sent postpaid to any part of the world for 25 cents. On receipt of a postal, we will send, C. O. D., express prepaid, orders to anywhere within one hundred miles of New York City. Agents wanted in all parts of the United States, Canada, and Mexico. We also sell German Jungborn Flour and whole wheat flour.

There is no other Malt-Coffee in the market that comes up exactly to the requirements of Adolph Just.

Address orders, or write for circulars, etc., to

HENRY MILLER, 176 Fulton Street, New York, N. Y.
—Mention this book.

Healthy, Durable, Cheap, Practical.

MAHR'S POROUS UNDERCLOTHING.

Recommended by ADOLPH JUST and Physicians.

Gold Medal Diploma of Honor at all Expositions.

MAHR & HAAKE, Pinneberg, Germany, Inventors and Sole Manufacturers.

Mahr's Porous Underwear and Garments
  are a grand novelty of the very highest importance for the health of mankind.

MAHR'S UNDERWEAR, made of best Egyptian Maco on the Corell weaving process, is in every respect the most perfect make ever known in the line of sanitary clothing, which is unhesitatingly acknowledged by prominent medical authorities.

MAHR'S UNDERWEAR will keep its porosity in the use even after several times' washing, as the Corell-made twisting of the threads absolutely excludes any their getting tight, whereas almost all other systems, offering knit-work, fail to accomplish that chief requirement of a natural underwear.

MAHR'S UNDERWEAR acts very favorably on the system and the state of health in general, as by the almost imperceptible **rubbing** brought about by the **Corell weft**, the blood is made to **circulate much better.**

MAHR'S UNDERWEAR excels by its **soft, agreeable and cleanly** wear as well as its great durability, protects the body from **effemination**, keeps its warmth in a cool temperature and may, therefore, fairly be said to be the most **perfect clothing system of the day.**

MAHR'S UNDERWEAR is airy in hot weather and absorbs the **sweat by-and-by**, and to a slight extent only, without **feeling cold.**

MAHR'S UNDERWEAR is an **excellent outfit for the tropics and is**, indeed, already worn there by many customers **to their greatest satisfaction.**

MAHR'S UNDERWEAR, on account of its great advantages, meets the requirements of all countries.

MAHR'S UNDERWEAR is to be had in the following kinds:

For gentlemen and boys: Shirts, day-shirts, jackets, sweaters, drawers, shirt-drawers, bathing- and air-robes, socks, cyclists' stockings, sporting caps, bathing breeches; also pants, coats, overcoats, etc.

For ladies and girls: Shirts, jackets, shirt-drawers, night-gowns, breeches, under-coats, bathing-dresses, stockings, corsets, night-caps, waists, Reform costumes, etc.

FOR CYCLISTS AND TOURISTS the sporting shirts, stockings and caps are a wear that meets a real want.

MAHR'S CORELL WEFT is also manufactured for garments in modern colours, thus offering an excellent stuff for ladies' dresses, sporting dresses, etc.

MAHR'S GARMENTS are very well-fitting and elegant.

OF MAHR'S POROUS CORELL WEFT there are furthermore made beddings, bathing sheets and robes, towels, etc., etc.

Material also sold by the yard.

Write for samples and price list to American Depot:

BENEDICT LUST, 124 East 59th Street, New York.

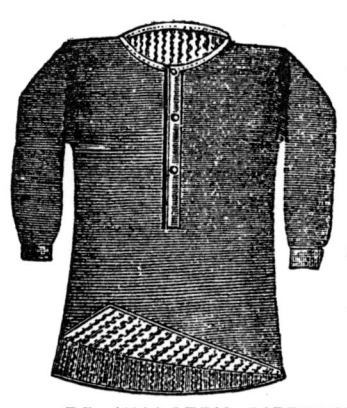

DR. WALSER'S
Chinagrass Rippenkrepp Health Underwear

Mesh Garments with two Layers.

Manufactured exclusively by
CARL MEZ & SOHNE IN FREIBURG, BADEN, GERMANY.

Patented in Germany and America.

Several Medals awarded at Hygienic Expositions.

DR. WALSER'S RIPPENKREPP HEALTH UNDERWEAR made of the best Maco with Chinagrass ribs is the cheapest and most practical for adherents of the Just, Kneipp and other Natural Healing Methods. The Rippenkrepp Health-Underwear holds a great deal of air, offers the best protection for colds, does not lose its porosity, does not shrink in the wash, only the linen-threads come in contact with the skin, at the same time being much more durable than the real linen.

Prices for Dr. Walser's Rippenkrepp Health Underwear.

Following prices are Gentlemen and Ladies (Sizes 32 to 40; 42 to 52 cost 50 cents extra each piece or $1.00 per suit):

Undershirts, unbleached, with Chinagrass ribs..................$2.50
Undershirts, bleached, with Chinagrass ribs................... 2.75
Drawers, unbleached, with Chinagrass ribs..................... 2.75
Drawers, bleached, with Chinagrass ribs....................... 3.00
Shirts, with or without collar (can be worn without underwear).. 3.25
Sporting and Night-shirts....................................... 3.50
Rippenkrepp-texture, bleached or unbleached, with Chinagrass
    ribs, width 22 inches............................per yard .65

Above prices for sizes 32 to 40, 41 to 52 50 cents extra each piece or $1.00 per suit.

Suits or Combination Suits to order $1.50 extra to above prices.

HOW TO SEND MEASURE FOR UNDERWEAR:

1) Total length; 2) Circumference of chest (give it as large as possible); 3) Length of the sleeves from the centre of the back to the wrist (bending your arm); For shirts the exact measure of the neck should also be indicated besides the above measures.

DRAWERS:

1) Circumference of the body; 2) Length of leg from crotch to ankle; 3) Total length of drawers.

General Depot for the United States:

Kneipp Health Store, 111 E. 59th St., N.Y.

WHOLESALE AND RETAIL.

A complete catalogue and samples will be furnished on application.

KAUF- UND VERSANDHAUS "JUNGBORN"
GUSTAV JUST, Ilsenburg a/Harz, Germany.

AMERICAN DEPOT—NATUROPATHIC HEALTH STORE
for Jungborn Articles and Supplies.

To meet the manifold wants and numerous desires of the public, I opened a "NATUROPATHIC HEALTH STORE" for "Jungborn Articles and Supplies.

I shall endeavor to attend promptly to the wishes of my customers, and ask for confidence and support at such enterprise.

My principle is to sell only **HIGH GRADE ARTICLES** of finest quality and at **reasonable terms**. These articles are especially recommended for the new, true and natural method of living by **ADOLF JUST, Ilsenburg at the Hartz Mts., Germany.**

"JUST'S POROUS UNDERWEAR AND GARMENTS:" Shirts for gentlemen, ladies and children; also porous material, bleached and unbleached, for Jungborn shirts.

POROUS MATERIAL FOR OUTER GARMENTS (suits, capes, light coats, etc.); ready made capes for men and boys. I do highly recommend very durable, porous material for suits in all colors.

"HEALTH FOOT WEAR: Sandals, sandal shoes, air shoes, very fine but not striking so they are suitable to be worn in cities and on any occasion; porous **Socks in fancy colors.**

"JUNGBORN REFORM BEDDING:" Fine porous woollen quilts, mattresses and pillows, porous white sheets and slips, etc.

ARTICLES OF FOOD: Nuts and Fruit (Filberts, walnuts, pine nuts, brazil nuts, pecans; dates, figs, oranges and bananas), Nut butter and Jungborn Wheat Bread, Fruit and Nut Bread (Fruitloaves). Malt-Coffee, Preserves, Fruit Juices, Dried Vegetables, and Fruit of the highest grade.

LIGHT HATS AND POROUS CAPS.

We endeavor to promptly fill all orders. Our extended sale enables us to furnish the **best quality of goods at Standard Prices.** To all friends and believers in Vegetarianism and Natural Healing Methods, I do highly recommend my Naturopathic Health Store and Supplies.

We keep also in stock all other articles which are needed by friends of Natural Living and Healing.

Bath Tubs for the Natural Bath; Mills for Grinding Nuts and Whole Wheat, Bake Ovens, Churns, Nut-Crackers, Fruit-Knives, Lemon-Squeezers, Clay, Literature. All Bandages for Clay Packs, etc., etc.

Naturopathic Books and Pamphlets of every description, etc., etc. **A COMPLETE CATALOGUE** will be sent on request **free of charge.** We kindly ask you to favor us with an order.

In Europe write to: **GUSTAVE JUST, ILSENBURG A HARZ,** Germany.

In America to:

BENEDICT LUST,
124 EAST 59th STREET,   -   -   NEW YORK
or, **AMERICAN JUNGBORN**, Bellevue, Butler, N. J.

POROUS REFORM CLOTHING

We Have Had from Our Many German Friends, who have already procured the first and second volumes of the German edition of "Return to Nature" so many inquiries for the porous underwear and outer garments as are now almost universally used in Germany, that we have decided to import such goods for the benefit of the American adherents to the Just method. These porous reform-clothes are made strictly according to the Just system. They are strong, durable and allow the air to penetrate to the skin, allow the excretions of the skin to pass off unobstructed, increase the circulation of the blood to the surface of the skin, whereby congestion of the inner, vital organs is avoided. The production of warmth and the giving off of warmth is normally regulated, and through the hardening process of the skin, the whole system is vitalized in conformity to the giving off of watery and fatty secretions. Anyone can take the Just Cure to the full extent at home in the city or country by wearing such clothes; they are also a great help in the treatment and cure of the different nervous diseases which prevail among the people. They are of great value especially to horsemen, hunters, gymnasts, bicycle-riders, physical culturists and other sportsmen. They are invaluable for every man or woman of sedentary habits, who are as a consequence of faulty clothing sickly, suffering from nervous diseases, Anaemia, Jaundice, Gout, and Rheumatism, invaluable to all those who are habitual sufferers from Catarrh or Colds, and especially to all those whose daily vocations oblige them to sit much or who are apt to perspire too freely.

This Reform Outer Clothing is made from the very finest and best, clean healthy wool from the live sheep under guarantee of the inventor. Wool which comes from the living and healthy sheep possesses strong "para-magnetic" electrical properties, (vital electricity) or, in other words, healing power. Wool of sheep that have died a natural death or have been killed lack those beneficial, healing properties.

Everyone interested is invited to write for samples, price list, etc., remembering that one cannot be a Justianer in the full sense of the word without wearing such clothing.

HAVE YOU HEARD OF THE COMMON SENSE

NATUROPATHIC AIR SHOE?

A real boon and a blessing to all those suffering from hot and sweaty feet. May be had in Gray, Brown, or Black, made of strong knitted linen, have the best leather soles—and let the feet exhale freely, allowing the air free access to the pores. **They are a Great Comfort** to any one especially in hot weather and keep the feet warm in cold and cool weather. **Look Neat and Stylish.** Ladies' sizes **$3.50.** Gentlemen's **$4.00.**

Sandals made of leather for Gentlemen.................$2.50
Sandals made of leather for Ladies................... 2.25
Sandals made of leather for Children................. 1.75

To take measure put your feet firmly on a sheet of paper (with stockings on) and mark the outlines with a pencil; then with a tape measure around the foot where it is broadest, right behind the toes, and send these measurements with your order. Send for our free catalogue of Health Supplies, etc.

NOTICE.

Already Now, at the moment we are going to press with this volume of "Return to Nature" we have several hundred inquiries for the second volume of Adolph Just's great work. This book has been published in Germany and is called "The Jungborn." Besides this several parties have asked for the third volume, announced by Ad. Just in the first and second volumes and called "The Life of the Soul." Now, to all those inquirers, we desire to say that we have decided not to publish the second volume, at the present time, since Adolph Just in Germany has come out by this time with a fifth edition of his book, very materially enlarged and perfected. This covers the first and second volume in one book, giving their respective contents in one. We have therefore decided to soon commence the translation of this new book. The price of same will be $3.50 bound, or $3.00, paper cover. All of those who have already ordered the second volume will receive this book. (The book, "Life of the Soul," is in preparation by A. Just in German.)

The contents of this Fifth Edition are not essentially the same, since it is the revision and perfection of four previous German editions. It is entirely re-written, revised and improved, and all the latest experiences and experiments of Ad. Just, which he has made in the last few years, are contained therein. It contains alphabetically every disease and its treatment, gives also a critic of the latest inventions and discoveries along the technical medical lines of the world. It contains everything that the second volume, published in the German language gives to the public there, regarding "The Jungborn," Cooking, Table Utensils, The Preparation and Keeping of Food, The New Simple Vegetarian Cook-book; it speaks about poisons in the different colors of wall-paper, clothing, etc., Science and Art; Clothing and Bedding; Clothing and Bedding for Laborers; Furniture; Agriculture; The True Natural Veterinary Healing Method; Feeding of Cattle; Vivisection; A New Voice Culture; Walking; Physical Culture; Soul Life and True Christianity in Regard to Disease; Influence of the Body on the Soul and Spirit; Influence of the Soul and Spirit on the Body; The Bible and the Christian Faith; The Bible versus Diseases. The Bible and Natural Healing Methods; The New Paradise; Medical Science; Operations; Fear of Death; The Responsibility in Diseases; Homeopathic and House Remedies; Patent Medicines and Quackery; Sea-shore, Mineral and Air-Cure Resorts; The Old Nature-Cure; Everybody His Own Physician; The Diagnosis of Diseases; Immorality; Marriage; The Natural Method in Training and Caring for Children; School Education; Vacations; Vaccination; The False Return to Nature; The Table for Single Persons; Eating and Drinking when Travelling; How to Live Cheap and According to Nature, etc., etc.

Besides this, the book contains, alphabetically arranged, a systematic index, which covers thousands of questions, and in view of all this it will prove still more than the present volume, the book of books on Naturopathy. Everyone who owns a copy of this book (first

CPSIA information can be obtained at www.ICGtesting.com
Printed in the USA
LVOW121531030212

266962LV00001B/251/A